Managing and Preventing Obesity

Related titles

Dietary supplements
(ISBN 978-1-78242-076-7)

Satiation, satiety and the control of food intake
(ISBN 978-0-85709-543-5)

Reducing saturated fats in foods
(ISBN 978-1-84569-740-2)

Woodhead Publishing Series in Food Science, Technology and Nutrition: Number 270

Managing and Preventing Obesity

Behavioural Factors and Dietary Interventions

Edited by

Timothy Gill

ELSEVIER

AMSTERDAM • BOSTON • CAMBRIDGE • HEIDELBERG
LONDON • NEW YORK • OXFORD • PARIS • SAN DIEGO
SAN FRANCISCO • SINGAPORE • SYDNEY • TOKYO
Woodhead Publishing is an imprint of Elsevier

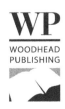

WP
WOODHEAD
PUBLISHING

Woodhead Publishing is an imprint of Elsevier
80 High Street, Sawston, Cambridge, CB22 3HJ, UK
225 Wyman Street, Waltham, MA 02451, USA
Langford Lane, Kidlington, OX5 1GB, UK

Notice
No responsibility is assumed by the publisher for any injury and/or damage to persons or
property as a matter of products liability, negligence or otherwise, or from any use or
operation of any methods, products, instructions or ideas contained in the material herein.
Because of rapid advances in the medical sciences, in particular, independent verification of
diagnoses and drug dosages should be made.

British Library Cataloguing in Publication Data
A catalogue record for this book is available from the British Library.

Library of Congress Control Number: 2014944414

ISBN 978-1-78242-091-0 (print)
ISBN 978-1-78242-099-6 (online)

For information on all Woodhead Publishing publications
visit our website at http://store.elsevier.com/

Typeset by RefineCatch Limited, Bungay, Suffolk
Printed and bound in the United Kingdom

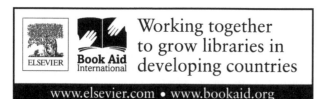

Contents

List of contributors

J. L. Baker Institute of Preventive Medicine and University of Copenhagen, Copenhagen, Denmark

J. Baranowski Baylor College of Medicine, Houston, TX, USA

T. Baranowski Baylor College of Medicine, Houston, TX, USA

M. Bes-Rastrollo University of Navarra, Navarra, Spain

S. Boylan University of Sydney, Sydney, NSW, Australia

G. A. Bray Pennington Biomedical Research Center, Baton Rouge, LA, USA

P. Clifton University of South Australia, Adelaide, SA, Australia

C. S. Diep Baylor College of Medicine, Houston, TX, USA

C. D. Economos Tufts University, Medford, MA, USA

M. Fogelholm University of Helsinki, Helsinki, Finland

M. Fong University of Sydney, Sydney, NSW, Australia

N. R. Fuller University of Sydney, Sydney, NSW, Australia

T. P. Gill University of Sydney, Sydney, NSW, Australia

C. Grace King's College Hospital, London, UK

D.P. Hatfield Tufts University, Medford, MA, USA

C. P. Herman University of Toronto, Toronto, ON, Canada

F. Hu Harvard School of Public Health, Boston, MA, USA

M. Hunsberger University of Gothenburg, Gothenburg, Sweden

R. Jackson-Leach London School of Hygiene and Tropical Medicine, London, UK

W. P. T. James London School of Hygiene and Tropical Medicine, London, UK

K. Keller The Pennsylvania State University, PA, USA

B. Kelly University of Wollongong, Wollongong, NSW, Australia

L. King University of Sydney, Sydney, NSW, Australia

N. S. Lau University of Sydney, Sydney, NSW, Australia,

L. Lissner University of Gothenburg, Gothenburg, Sweden

N. D. Luscombe-Marsh CSIRO Animal, Food and Health Sciences, Clayton South, VIC, Australia

M. A. Martinez-Gonzalez University of Navarra, Navarra, Spain

M. P. Poelman VU University, Amsterdam, The Netherlands

J. Polivy University of Toronto, Toronto, ON, Canada

L. Pomeranz Temple University, Philadelphia, PA, USA

B. M. Popkin University of North Carolina, Wilmington, MC, USA

J. Proietto University of Melbourne, Melbourne, VIC, Australia

M. Rayner University of Oxford, Oxford, UK

C. A. Roberto   Harvard School
of Public Health, Boston,
MA, USA

B. J. Rolls   The Pennsylvania State
University, PA, USA

J. Soo   Harvard School of Public
Health, Boston, MA, USA

R. Stanton   2866 Moss Vale Road,
Barrengarry, NSW, Australia

I. H. M. Steenhuis   VU
University, Amsterdam,
The Netherlands

R. J. Stubbs   University of Derby,
Derby, UK

P. Sumithran   University of Melbourne,
Melbourne, VIC, Australia

A. M. Thow   University of Sydney,
Sydney, NSW, Australia

G. Tognon   University of Gothenburg,
Gothenburg, Sweden

W. M. Vermeer   Leiden University
Medical Center, The Netherlands

R. Williams   The Pennsylvania State
University, PA, USA

Woodhead Publishing Series in Food Science, Technology and Nutrition

Preface

The changing diet of humans through our history is subject to a great deal of contention. However, what is not in dispute is that our diet has changed significantly in both a qualitative and quantitative sense as we have moved through periods as hunter-gatherers or subsistence farmers to a situation today where we are now consumers of highly processed and ready-prepared foods. At the same time our patterns of physical activity have also changed from the demands of high activity necessary for survival and strenuous occupations to those of limited physical burdens and sedentary occupations or leisure pursuits. For most of history, humans have experienced food shortages, hunger and under-nutrition as they struggled each day to secure sufficient food to meet their needs. However, with improved agricultural processes, mechanisation, improved storage and processing of foods we are now in a situation where a significant proportion of the world's population now has more food energy than is necessary to meet their reduced requirements. As a consequence conditions associated with over-nutrition and excess weight gain are now dominating human health and well-being.

Obesity has become a major public health and economic problem of global significance. According to World Health Organization (WHO) estimates, more than 1.4 billion adults aged 20 and older (or 35% of the world's population),were overweight in 2008. Of these over 200 million men and nearly 300 million women were obese. Prevalence rates continue to rise rapidly in all areas of the world, including low-income countries, and obesity associated illness is now so common that it has replaced the more established public health concerns, such as under-nutrition and infectious disease, as the most significant contributor to global ill health.

Obesity impacts on both quality and length of life and is associated with a wide range of chronic conditions such as diabetes, hypertension, cardiovascular disease and many cancers, as well as non-life-threatening but debilitating conditions such as arthritis, back pain and breathlessness. Obesity also places enormous financial burdens on governments and individuals and accounts for a significant proportion of total health care expenditure in developed countries. Obesity is now the sixth most important contributor to premature death in the world.

In recent years, our knowledge of the epidemiology and causation of obesity has improved dramatically but we still have an incomplete understanding of the drivers of obesity. We know that obesity results from a prolonged period of energy imbalance where the energy intake from food and drink exceeds energy expenditure for metabolic processes and physical activity. However, there are many aspects of our current diet and lifestyle that have potential to contribute to this energy imbalance that leads to weight gain and the development of obesity. Overconsumption of food energy may potentially be facilitated by the composition of the diet, by serving sizes, by where, when or how we eat, as a response to external cues or driven by the appeal of price, marketing or nutrition guidance. Understanding these issues is important in formulating appropriate dietary strategies to assist with weight loss or the prevention of weight gain in the community.

Whilst there has been much written about the aetiology of obesity in recent years, most books that examine the problem of obesity provide only limited coverage of dietary aspects, because they need to address the wide-ranging aspects of the issue. Therefore, in planning this book it was decided that there would be great merit in examining in more detail the broad range of dietary issues that may receive only cursory attention in more general texts. Authors were requested to prepare short chapters which focused on a single aspect of the relationship between diet and the prevention and management of obesity.

This is not a textbook or encyclopaedia, but rather an edited collection of short, relevant (and sometimes personal) review chapters by experts on the most important developments and topics in obesity management. These chapters are arranged in five sections that deal with different aspects of the relationship between diet and obesity:

> Part One deals with general issues and background to the problem of obesity, its development and strategies for its management.
> Part Two examines the role of different dietary components in obesity management and weight control.
> Part Three explores the role of eating patterns and other behavioural factors in obesity management.
> Part Four addresses structured dietary interventions in the treatment of obesity
> Part Five tackles the difficult issues around government and industry interventions in the prevention of obesity.

The focus of each chapter means that authors cannot explore all the interrelated aspects of their topic. To ensure each chapter is complete, there may be some overlap between chapters. In addition, given the scale and complexity of the subject, there are many potential issues which are not addressed in depth. However, we hope that the breadth and scope of the contents help ensure that most of the important topics relating to dietary aspects of obesity are covered. It is likely that as research evidence builds in this area over time, that some of the insights and conclusions presented within these chapters may be challenged and replaced. However, the concepts and principles are likely to stand the test of time.

Timothy P Gill
Boden Institute, University of Sydney, NSW, Australia

Introduction: an overview of the key drivers of obesity and their influence on diet

T. P. Gill
University of Sydney, NSW, Australia

1 Introduction

Obesity results from a prolonged period of energy imbalance where the energy intake from food and drink exceeds energy expenditure for metabolic processes and physical activity. Excess energy is stored as fat within the body and is associated with a wide range of health, social and psychological problems.

Energy balance within the body is usually well regulated by a range of physiological responses which monitor food intake, metabolism and storage and send signals to influence appetite and to a lesser extent energy expenditure. Physiological energy regulation mechanisms operate within each person to keep weight and body fat stores stable in the long term (Schutz 1995). However, powerful societal and environmental forces influence energy intake and expenditure through effects on dietary and physical activity patterns, and may overwhelm the physiological control of body weight. The susceptibility of individuals to these forces is influenced by genetic and other biological factors such as gender, age and hormonal activities, over which they have little or no control.

The breadth of these 'drivers of weight gain' is addressed in this chapter but discussed in more detail in later chapters.

1.1 Key influences on energy balance and weight gain

A number of analyses have attempted to define the key determinants of obesity and there remains a degree of controversy over which factors have made the greatest contribution to the recent rise in the rates of obesity throughout the world. Comprehensive assessment of the situation has been undertaken by the World Health Organization in the *Expert Report on Diet, Nutrition and the Prevention of Chronic Disease* (WHO 2003) and the World Cancer Research Fund report *Food, Nutrition, Physical Activity, and the Prevention of Cancer: a Global Perspective* (WCRF 2007).

These reports examined the current literature and identified a range of key factors which either increase or decrease the risk of weight gain and the development of obesity. The results of both assessments are summarised in Table I.1.

Managing and Preventing Obesity. http://dx.doi.org/10.1533/9781782420996.1

Table 1 Summary of the strengths of evidence on behaviours that might promote or protect against weight gain and obesity – agreement from WHO 2003 and WCRF 2007 reports

Evidence	Decreases risk	Increases risk
Rated convincing or likely in both reports.	Regular physical activity. High intake of low energy-dense foods.*	Sedentary lifestyles. High intake of energy-dense foods.*
Rated probable or possible in both reports.	High dietary fibre intake. Promoting linear growth. Breastfeeding.	Sugar-sweetened soft drinks and juices. High proportion of food prepared outside of homes. High exposure to television (marketing).
Rated possible in one report only.	Low glycaemic index foods.	Adverse social and economic conditions in developed countries (especially for women). Large portion sizes. Rigid restraint/periodic disinhibition eating patterns.
Rated insufficient.	Increased eating frequency.	Alcohol.

* Energy-dense foods are high in fat/sugar, and energy-dilute foods are high in fibre and water such as vegetables, fruits, legumes and whole grain cereals.
Source: Developed from WHO 2003 and WCRF 2007.

1.2 The complex web of influences on the aetiology of obesity

Although the WHO and WCRF reviews touched upon the array of behavioural and environmental influences in the aetiology of obesity at an individual and population level, they did not capture the interplay of these factors and how they operate at a societal level. One of the first attempts to represent the nature of the prevailing, multi-layered environmental factors that influence energy balance in the modern world was the International Obesity Task Force 'causal web' (Kumanyika *et al.*, 2002). The causal web illustrated that although food intake and energy expenditure ultimately influence energy balance, there are an array of forces operating at different layers of society that impact directly or indirectly upon these behaviours. The implications of this representation are apparent. Addressing obesity prevention will require action at many levels and must include a focus on many of the distal factors that influence our food and activity environment.

Although the causal web suggests that the genesis of and thus, the solution to obesity is complicated, its linear format does not clearly illustrate the complexity of the interactions between the various layers. The Foresight Programme of the UK Government Office for Science expanded on the causal web approach by using a systems approach to produce a complex conceptual model with 108 variables known as the 'obesity systems map' (Vandenbroek *et al.*, 2007). The relationships between the variables are illustrated with more than 300 solid or dashed lines to indicate positive and negative influences. All the variables are interconnected and these connections give rise to feedback loops. At the core (or engine) of the map is energy balance, surrounded by variables that directly or indirectly influence this key process. The relationships between each factor and their influence on the energy balance core is represented by a complex array of multi-directional arrows that illustrate the complex interaction between environment, behaviour and physiology. The original spaghetti-like, causal loop map has been simplified by dividing the factors represented into seven cross-cutting, principal themes (Figure 1):

- Biology: an individuals starting point – the influence of genetics and physiology.
- Food consumption patterns and behaviours: the quality, quantity and frequency of an individual's food intake.
- Food environment: the influence of the food environment on an individual's food choices.
- Physical activity behaviours: the type, frequency and intensity of an individual's physical activities.
- Activity environment: the influence of the environment on an individual's activity behaviour.
- Individual psychology: psychological influences food intake and consumption patterns, or physical activity patterns or preferences.
- Societal norms and influences: the impact of how society views and responds to the issue of obesity.

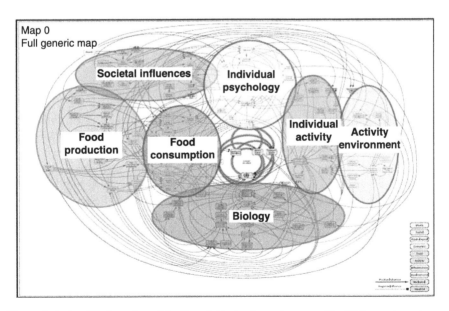

Figure 1 A simplified version of the Foresight obesity system map identifying main sectors of influence

Source: Vandenbroeck *et al.* 2007.

A complete version of the Foresight Obesity System Map can be found at https://
www.gov.uk/government/uploads/system/uploads/attachment_data/file/296290/
obesity-map-full-hi-res.pdf

The Foresight map approach to defining the broad-ranging drivers of obesity
and the inter-relationships between these factors has not met with universal approval.
It has been criticised for being overly complex to the extent that it creates a sense
of confusion and despair, when clarity is what is needed to effectively address this
problem (Finegood *et al.*, 2010). Others have also questioned how comprehensive
such a map could be, in that it implies that all potential drivers of obesity are captured
within the map. It is probably true that very few people completely understand all
the intricacies of the system it describes and that the map is not truly complete,
as it reflects only the perceptions of the stakeholders engaged in its development.
However, it has served some useful objectives in improving our perception of the
nature of the obesity problem and the approach that will be required to successfully
address it. Some of the principles that the Foresight map and process have reinforced
are:

- the wide range of political, social, environmental, behavioural and physiological factors
  that influence individuals' and society's capacity to achieve energy balance, and the
  complex, multifactorial nature of the systems that give rise to obesity;
- the breadth of action that will be required to restore energy balance;
- the futility of attempting to address obesity by focusing attention solely on individual behaviour change or within one domain of action;
- the need to consider the interaction between factors that either enable or amplify, or
  conversely, inhibit the behaviour change process required to achieve energy balance;
- the interaction between factors within the system, which is currently driving energy accretion
  and disrupting individual efforts to achieve energy balance.

2   Behavioural factors

Food intake and physical activity behaviours are the two key factors that have
potential to directly influence energy balance and weight status. Historically
they have been considered a product of free will under the direct cognitive control
of the individual. However, as previous sections have indicated, there are a range
of biological as well as social and environmental forces that constrain these
behaviours in individuals. However, an appreciation of the dietary and activity
behaviours that have been linked to weight gain and the development of obesity is
important if we are to usefully define these problems and decide how best to address
them.

Both energy expenditure and energy intake contribute to weight gain and the
development of obesity, and it is not possible to clearly apportion the contribution
that each makes to the problem. There has been a lot of unnecessary debate over
which factor is more important in the genesis of obesity. Attempts to selectively
promote one factor over the other as the major cause are counterproductive, as both
will need to be addressed in tackling the problem.

2.1 The formation of habits

When a behaviour relating to food intake or activity is repeated often for a long period of time, it becomes a habit, meaning that it becomes almost an automatic response to certain cues or situations. Habits often remain well after the original reason for adoption of the behaviour has passed, making them difficult to change. Often, people passively adopt or continue a behaviour rather than making an active decision to do so. Once habits are formed, individuals show little inclination to change them. In addition, attitudes and intentions have less of an impact when a habit has been established, making changes to inappropriate food and activity behaviours less likely even when the need for such a change is accepted (Vandenbroeck *et al.*, 2007).

Food and activity habits are often associated with an increased energy intake, and as environments become more 'obesogenic' (obesity-promoting), the behaviours that lead to obesity are increasingly the default or automatic ones.

2.2 Dietary behaviours

A number of dietary factors have been identified as potential contributors to weight gain and obesity by undermining the innate regulatory control of body weight. There are multiple mechanisms by which this can occur, including satiety, palatability, food availability or low energy needs as a consequence of physical inactivity. Despite great interest in this area, evidence linking specific dietary behaviours to weight gain is limited and is largely restricted to observational and intervention studies.

Although surplus energy intake is an obvious cause of weight gain, there is little evidence to link high kilojoule intake directly to obesity. This may be the result of large individual variability in energy requirements, with higher requirements often being associated with higher levels of activity. In addition, total kilojoule intake is not reported accurately or consistently in most dietary surveys (Willett and Stampfer 1986). This has led to the exploration of the role of a range of dietary behaviours associated with weight gain and obesity. The key elements of these behaviours are addressed in separate chapters within this book including:

- Energy density of the diet
- Fat composition of the diet
- Protein intake
- Carbohydrate intake and glycaemic index of the diet
- Fibre
- Alcohol
- Fruit and vegetable consumption
- Consumption of sugar-sweetened beverages
- Portion size
- Increased consumption of takeaway foods and foods prepared away from home
- Eating frequency.

2.3 Physical activity behaviours

Although it may appear obvious that inactive people will gain more weight over time than active people, the true impact of reduced activity on weight gain is not easy to clarify for a number of reasons (WHO Euro 2007, Wareham 2007, Fox and Hilsdon 2007).

Unfortunately, we do not have high quality data on the amount of physical activity undertaken over time and most of the data we do have is self-reported, with little objective validation. In addition, the relationship between physical inactivity/ sedentary behaviour and obesity is complex and is subject to a wide array of confounding factors which are difficult to exclude.

Although data is now available from large prospective studies, it is difficult to exclude the possible influence of reverse causality; that is, a high BMI at the start of the study may be a cause of decreasing physical activity and may also be independently associated with an increased risk of weight gain. In addition, most studies have examined only leisure time physical activity and have ignored the impact of occupational and incidental activity.

Despite these limitations, most reviews of research consistently show the expected inverse relationship between leisure time physical activity and obesity in all but the youngest children (Fogelholm and Kukkonen-Harjula 2000, Summerbell *et al.*, 2009).

2.4 Sedentary behaviours

Sedentary behaviours are not merely the inverse of being physically active. They are different but interlinked behaviours and there is a growing body of evidence that sedentary behaviour may be a distinct risk factor, independent of physical inactivity, for multiple adverse health outcomes including obesity in adults (Thorp *et al.*, 2011). The most commonly utilised indicator of sedentary behaviour is television viewing time and many (but not all) studies have found a positive association between hours of TV watched and increased body weight. A study by Hardy *et al.* (2009) indicated that more than two hours a day of screen time was associated with reduced fitness, increased weight and a greater risk of ill health in schoolchildren. A number of studies have examined the level of sitting time among workers and have found that sitting for more than six hours a day doubles a person's risk of being overweight compared to those who spend less than one hour a day sitting (Brown *et al.*, 2003, Mummery *et al.*, 2005).

3 Environmental and structural factors

The external social, political and economic environment in which people live has a profound effect on the way people behave. Each day, people interact with a wide range of services, systems and pressures in settings such as schools, the workplace, home, restaurants and takeaway food outlets. In addition, these settings are influenced by laws, policies, economic imperatives and attitudes of governments, industry and society as a whole. Each of the features of this complex system, which shapes the environment we live in, has the capacity to inhibit or encourage appropriate dietary and physical activity patterns. This has led some researchers to term the environment in most developed countries today as 'obesogenic' or 'toxic' because it inhibits appropriate dietary and physical activity patterns and encourages energy imbalance (Egger and Swinburn 1997).

3.1   Changing physical activity environment

The availability of open space and access to public transport, the design of suburbs, access to buildings, perceived levels of safety, provision of lighting and many other factors influence our capacity and desire to be more physically active in our daily lives (Ding and Gebel 2012). In recent years, changes in the occupational structure, urban and building design and technology have contributed to a situation where opportunities to be more physically active are now more limited.

The built environment encompasses a range of physical and social elements that make up the structure of a community and may influence obesity-related behaviours. Several characteristics of the urban form (natural and built environment) tend to be associated with increased physical activity, and possibly with nutrition behaviours. These include:

- mixed land use and density;
- footpaths, cycleways and other facilities for physical activity;
- street connectivity and design;
- transport infrastructure and systems linking residential, commercial and business areas.

A number of studies have found that access to proximate and large public open space with attractive attributes such as trees, water features and bird life is associated with higher levels of walking (Gebel et al., 2005). The characteristics of the neighbourhood also have an impact on physical activity. For instance, street layout and the level of connectivity of streets (suburban or more traditional layout) determine route choices and distances, thereby making walking or cycling more or less practicable. Urban design features such as the location of residential, business and commercial areas, in combination with transport services, influence people's access to food.

Recent research has found that people who drove to work were more likely to be overweight or obese than those who walked, cycled or used public transport, regardless of their income level. Additionally, the further people had to drive each day, the greater their weight increase (Wen et al., 2006, Basset et al., 2008).

3.2   Changing food environment

Access to appropriate food outlets, advertising pressures, school food policies, nutrition information and labelling all potentially influence food selection. In past years, the usual environment throughout much of the world allowed only a limited food choice, while today, we have access to a wide variety of cheap, high fat/energy-dense foods that are aggressively marketed.

There is widespread acceptance that the current food supply is not conducive to the maintenance of energy balance. The widely available processed foods have levels of trans fats, saturated fats, salt and sugar well above those recommended for good health and weight control, and provide excess kilojoules. Short-term experimental studies have shown that larger portions of energy-dense food are associated with increased energy intake (Rolls *et al.*, 2007). Specifically, they have shown that both children and adults consume more at a single eating episode when offered larger portions of energy-dense food. Studies from Denmark (Matthiessen 2003) and the USA (Neilsen and Popkin 2003) indicate that:

- the portion sizes of many (but not all) commercial energy-dense foods and beverages and fast food meals seem to have increased over time, particularly in the last 10 years;
- the number of super-sized food items available in grocery stores and supermarkets seems to have increased substantially;
- conventional and fast food restaurants serve larger so-called value meals and offer all-you-can-eat buffets in the competition for customers.

Consumers now spend a significant proportion of their household food expenditure on food consumed away from the home and many people underestimate the number of kilojoules in fast food meals and they tend to consume more kilojoules and fat, and fewer vegetables, fruits and fibre when eating out (Rudd Center 2008).

Access to the right foods at the right price also appears to influence the quality of our diet. The majority of studies that have examined the relationship between store access and dietary intake find that better access to a supermarket or large grocery store is associated with healthier food intakes (Larson *et al.*, 2009). Economic theory suggests that food prices affect food intake. Therefore, manipulating the price of food is likely to have both short- and long-term consequences for body weight (Goldman *et al.*, 2009). Some researchers suggest that the relative cheapness of high energy-dense foods is a major driver of their consumption by less affluent consumers (Drewnowski 2004). Conversely, the high relative cost of low energy-dense foods, such as fruit and vegetables, is seen as a barrier to their increased consumption.

Numerous systematic reviews have concluded that the marketing of unhealthy (or energy-dense, nutrient-poor) foods and beverages to children negatively influences children's eating behaviour, dietary intake and beliefs, and purchase requests to their parents (Cairns *et al.*, 2009, IOM 2006). Much of this literature has focused on the effects of marketing energy-dense, nutrient-poor (EDNP) foods on television, given that this is the main media outlet to which children are exposed. However, marketing has now spread to multiple media platforms including print, the Internet, sports (via sponsorship) and outdoors (IOM 2006).

3.3 Changed living and working environment

Some of the most profound changes to our way of life in recent decades have occurred around the living and working environment. Not only have occupational structures changed but so have working hours and the gender balance within the workforce. Longer working hours, living further from work and the involvement of both partners or parents in the workforce have led to a situation where individuals and families have less time to devote to planned nutrition and physical activity behaviours. As a consequence, certain changes have occurred, which research has identified as having had a negative impact on weight control, and which may have contributed to the rise in obesity (Vandenbroeck *et al.*, 2007, NPHT 2009, Keith *et al.*, 2006). These changes include:

- reduced time for personal physical activity and unavailability to supervise the play and active pursuits of children;
- a greater reliance on sedentary leisure time pursuits;
- the loss of regular meal patterns and family meals, which has been shown to result in greater snacking and a higher kilojoule intake;
- disrupted sleep patterns (short sleep duration has been shown to create metabolic disturbance that interferes with the body's systems for appetite control and has been associated with weight gain, especially in children).

4 Biological factors

Most of the existing scientific information suggests that the increasing rate of obesity within populations is a result of changes in our food intake and physical activity behaviours driven by social, political and economic environments which promote overconsumption of food and limit opportunities for physical activity. However, it is also clear that heritable biological factors explain why some individuals or groups are more at risk of developing obesity compared to others within the community. In particular, our genes and the nutrition and physical activity environment we are exposed to *in utero* and early in life have profound effects on our regulation of energy balance and how and where we store fat generated by excess kilojoules.

4.1 Genetic influences

One of the strongest predictors of a child's weight status is the weight status of their parents. Overweight parents are more likely to have overweight children. This could be a result of the shared family environment, but the fact that adopted children have a weight status closer to their biological rather than adoptive parents suggests a strong role of genetics in weight status. This relationship has been confirmed by examining the closeness in body weight of monozygotic (identical) twins, who have exactly the same genes and very similar weight status, versus dizygotic (non-identical) twins, who share only 50% of their genes on average and have much greater variability in weight status (Bouchard 2007). This does not imply that a certain genetic makeup inevitably leads to obesity but rather, that the propensity to gain weight and become obese is increased. Estimates of how much of the difference in weight status between individuals can be explained by their genes vary depending on what group is being studied and what aspect of weight is being measured – it can be as low as 5% and as high as 70% (Yang and Kelly 2007).

Unlike other inherited conditions, it is extremely rare for a single gene difference to result in obesity. Rather, the inheritance of obesity is thought to be the result of a wide number of genetic variations which result in a series of small but important disruptions to our energy balance regulatory systems (Farooqi and O'Rahilly 2007). So far, around 30,000 genes have been identified in the human genome, and a large number of these have the potential to influence factors associated with energy balance regulation. However, research does not support the commonly held view that genetics endows some people with slow metabolisms, meaning that they can eat hardly anything without gaining weight, and delivers others with a super metabolism, allowing them to expend significantly more energy than others just by existing. Most of the common gene defects that have thus far been associated with obesity influence appetite and satiety regulation or the way the body handles food and stores fat. Some of these genes may have been associated with positive outcomes in past times when food was scarce and work was hard but now, with our changed environment, they contribute to a negative outcome of weight gain.

4.2   Epigenetic influences on weight gain

It is now understood that inheriting a particular gene does not mean that it will always result in the same outcome in different individuals. Part of the reason for this is that it is possible to alter the way the gene is expressed, or translated into action within the body, by subtle changes to that gene. This process is called epigenetics and is a result of small chemical modifications to the DNA material which can result from a range of factors, such as poor nutrition, a lack of physical activity, smoking, exposure to certain toxins and ageing (Bird 2007). It is thought that these epigenetic changes can predispose individuals to obesity by influencing the way food is handled or energy balance is regulated (Campion *et al.*, 2009). It is unclear whether these epigenetic modifications can be reversed but they are clearly heritable and are passed on to the next generation, leading to poor health outcomes. Epigenetic changes in response to poor nutrition and physical activity environments may explain why rates of obesity have increased so rapidly in recent generations, who have inherited physiological traits that exacerbate weight gain as a result of their own exposure to the obesogenic environment (Campion *et al.*, 2010).

4.3   In utero *and early life influences*

It has long been known that good nutrition during pregnancy is important for the growth and development of the foetus, and the health and wellbeing of the mother as well as the ease of delivery. However, recent evidence has revealed that *in utero* exposures, together with early life experiences, have profound effects on the weight status and health of the infant that last well into adulthood. Some of the key perinatal nutrition factors that influence later development of obesity include the following.

4.4   Low birth weight and smoking during pregnancy

Low birth weight infants experience a range of health problems usually associated with under-nutrition and failure to thrive, but it is also clear now that low birth weight infants are at higher risk of a range of chronic conditions later in life (Barker 2004). Such children are more prone to develop abdominal obesity and early metabolic disease, especially if exposed to over-nutrition in childhood. Low birth weight is common among babies born to women who smoke during pregnancy, but smoking is also associated with a 50% increase in the risk of childhood obesity (Oken *et al.*, 2008).

4.5   Excessive weight gain during pregnancy

Women who gain more than the recommended levels of weight during pregnancy are at greater risk of gestational diabetes and having a high birth weight child. Such children have a greater rate of obesity later in childhood (Gillman *et al.*, 2003). Women who enter pregnancy with an existing weight problem and have excessive weight gain during pregnancy further increase their risk of gestational diabetes and the obstetric complications associated with high birth weight children (Whittaker 2004).

Accelerated weight gain during the first weeks or months of life is associated with higher BMI or obesity later in life. A systematic review by Baird *et al.* (2005) found that infants with more rapid early growth had a higher risk of later obesity than infants with normal growth.

4.6   Breastfeeding

A number of reviews have concluded that exclusive breastfeeding for a period of at least six months is associated with a reduced level of obesity later in child-hood. A meta-analysis of 17 studies of breastfeeding duration found that each additional month infants were breastfed was associated with a 4% lower risk of later-life obesity (Harder *et al.*, 2005). However, there remains some controversy around the role of breastfeeding as results of studies have been inconsistent and it is hard to separate associated factors socio-economic status and cultural factors in any analysis.

4.7   Short sleep duration in infancy

There is some indication from a small number of studies of an association between short sleep duration in infants and higher levels of overweight in later childhood (Taveras *et al.*, 2008). However, separating the effect of sleep from the wide range of potential confounders in this relationship is difficult.

Other research shows that short sleep times appear to have no relationship with obesity in teenagers aged 10–16 years, and it is unclear whether longer sleep times are beneficial for obese teenagers (Sung *et al.*, 2011).

5 Summary and conclusions

Although there has been substantial effort invested in identifying the determinants of obesity we still have an incomplete understanding all the drivers of obesity. It is clear that diet and physical activity behaviours are the central elements of the energy balance equation. However, in contrast to popular belief, obesity is not solely caused by a lack of cognitive control over personal dietary and physical activity behaviours. It is now understood that physiology and genetics have a critical role in driving or attenuating these behaviours and the physical, social and political environment in which we live greatly influences out ability to maintain behaviours appropriate to weight control.

A number of analyses have attempted to define the key determinants of obesity and there remains a degree of controversy over which factors have made the greatest contribution to the recent rise in the rates of obesity. What is accepted is that there is no simple single cause of obesity and that complex array of interacting factors is driving changes in weight status at a societal level.

References

Baird J, Fisher D, Lucas P, Kleijnen J, Roberts H and Law C (2005). Being big or growing fast: systematic review of size and growth in infancy and later obesity. *BMJ* 331: 929.

Barker DJ (2004). The developmental origins of adult disease. *J Am Coll Nutr* 23: S588–95.

Bassett DR, Pucher J, Buehler R, Thompson DL and Crouter SE (2003). Walking, cycling, and obesity rates in Europe, North America and Australia. *J Phys Act Health* 5(6): 795–814.

Bird A (2007). Perceptions of epigenetics. *Nature* 447: 396–8.

Bouchard C (2007). The biological predisposition to obesity: beyond the thrifty genotype scenario. *Int J Obes* 31: 1337–9.

Brown WJ, Miller YD and Miller R (2003). Sitting time and work patterns as indicators of overweight and obesity in Australian adults. *Int J Obes* 27(11): 1340–6.

Cairns G, Angus K and Hastings G (2009). *The Extent, Nature and Effects of Food Promotion to Children: A Review of the Evidence to December 2008*. United Kingdom: Institute of Social Marketing, University of Stirling and Open University.

Campión J, Milagro FI and Martínez JA (2009). Individuality and epigenetics in obesity. *Obesity Reviews* 10: 383–92.

Campion J, Milagro F and Martínez JA (2010). Epigenetics and obesity. *Prog Mol Biol Transl Sci* 94: 291–347.

Ding D and Gebel K (2012). Built environment, physical activity, and obesity: what have we learned from reviewing the literature? *Health and Place* 18(1): 100–6.

Drewnowski A (2004). Obesity and the food environment: dietary energy density and diet costs. *Am J Prev Med.* 27(3, Suppl 1): 154–62.

Egger, G and Swinburn, B (1997). An 'ecological' approach to the obesity pandemic. *BMJ* 315: 477–480.

Farooqi IS and O'Rahilly S (2007). Genetic factors in human obesity. *Obesity Reviews* 8 (Suppl 1): 37–40.

Finegood DT, Merth TDN and Rutter H (2010). Implications of the Foresight Obesity System map for solutions to childhood obesity. *Obesity* 18: S13–16.

Fogelholm M and Kukkonen-Harjula K. (2000). Does physical activity prevent weight gain – a systematic review. *Obes Rev Off J Int Assoc Study Obes* 1: 95–111.

Fox KR and Hilsdon M (2007). Physical activity and obesity. *Obesity Reviews* 8 (Suppl 1): 115–21.

Gebel K, King L, Bauman A, Vita P, Gill T, *et al.* (2005). *Creating Healthy Environments: A Review of Links Between the Physical Environment, Physical Activity and Obesity.* Sydney: NSW Health Department and NSW Centre for Overweight and Obesity.

Gillman MW, Rifas-Shiman S, Berkey CS, Field AE and Colditz GA (2003). Maternal gestational diabetes, birth weight, and adolescent obesity. *Pediatrics* 111: e221–6.

Goldman D, Lakdawalla D and Zheng Y (2009). *Food Prices and the Dynamics of Body Weight.* Cambridge, MA: National Bureau of Economic Research.

Harder T, Bergmann R, Kallischnigg G and Plagemann A (2005). Duration of breastfeeding and risk of overweight: a meta-analysis. *Am J Epidemiol* 162: 397–403.

Hardy L, Dobbins T, Denney-Wilson E, Okely A and Booth M (2009). Sedentariness, small-screen recreation, and fitness in youth. *Am J Prev Med* 36(2): 120–5.

Institute of Medicine of the National Academies (IOM) (2006). *Food Marketing to Children and Youth: Threat or Opportunity?* Washington DC: Food and Nutrition Board, Board on Children, Youth and Families, Institute of Medicine of the National Academies.

Kumanyika S, Jeffrey RW, Morabia A, Ritenbaugh C and Antipastis V (2002). Public Health Approaches to the Prevention of Obesity (PHAPO) Working Group of the International Obesity Task Force (IOTF). Obesity prevention: the case for action. *Int J Obes* 26: 425–36.

Larson, NI, Story, MT and Nelson, MC (2009). Neighborhood environments: disparities in access to healthy foods in the U.S. *American Journal of Preventive Medicine* 36(1): 74–81.

Matthiessen J, Fagt S, Biltoft-Jensen A, Beck A and Ovesen L (2003). Size makes a difference. *Public Health Nutrition* 6: 65–72.

Mummery WK, Schofield GM, Steele R, Eakin EG and Brown WJ (2005). Occupational sitting time and overweight and obesity in Australian workers. *Am J Prev Med* 29(2): 91–7.

Neilsen SJ and Popkin BM (2003). Patterns and trends in food portion sizes, 1977–1998. *JAMA* 289: 450–3.

NPHT (National Preventative Health Taskforce) (2009): 'Australia: the healthiest country by 2020. Technical Report No 1. Obesity in Australia: a need for urgent action.' Canberra, Commonwealth of Australia.

Oken E, Levitan EB and Gillman MW (2008). Maternal smoking during pregnancy and child overweight: systematic review and meta-analysis. *Int J Obes* 32: 201–10.

Rolls BJ, Roe LS and Meengs JS (2007). The effect of large portion sizes on energy intake is sustained for 11 days. *Obesity* 15: 1535–43.

Rudd Center for Food Policy and Obesity (2008). *Menu Labelling in Chain Restaurants: Opportunities for Public Policy.* USA: Yale University.

Schutz Y (1995). Macronutrients and energy balance in obesity. *Metabolism* 64 (Suppl 30): 7–11.

Summerbell CD, Douthwaite W, Whittaker V, Ells LJ, Hillier F, *et al.* (2009). The association between diet and physical activity and subsequent excess weight gain and obesity assessed at 5 years of age or older: a systematic review of the epidemiological evidence. *Int. J. Obes* 33 (Suppl 3): S1–92.

Sung V, Beebe DW, Vandyke R, Fenchel MC, Crimmins NA, *et al.* (2011). Does sleep duration predict metabolic risk in obese adolescents attending tertiary services? A cross-sectional study. *Sleep* 34(7): 891–8.

Taveras EM, Rifas-Shiman SL, Oken E, Gunderson EP and Gillman MW (2008). Short sleep duration in infancy and risk of childhood overweight. *Arch Pediatr Adolesc Med* 162: 305–11.

Thorp AA, Owen N, Neuhaus M and Dunstan DW (2011). Sedentary behaviors and subsequent health outcomes in adults a systematic review of longitudinal studies, 1996–2011. *Am J Prev Med* 41(2): 207–15.

Vandenbroeck IP, Goossens J and Clemens M (2007). *Foresight Tackling Obesities: Future Choices—Building the Obesity System Map.* Government Office for Science, UK Government's Foresight Programme http://www.foresight.gov.uk/Obesity/12.pdf

Wareham N (2007). Physical activity and obesity prevention. *Obesity Reviews* 8 (Suppl. 1): 109–14.

Wen LM, Orr N, Millett C and Rissel C (2006). Driving to work and 18. Overweight and obesity: finding from the 2003 New South Wales Health Survey, Australia. *In J Obes* 30(5): 782–6.

Whittaker RC (2004). Predicting preschooler obesity at birth: the role of maternal obesity in early pregnancy. *Pediatrics* 114: e29–36.

WHO Europe (2007). *The Challenge of Obesity in the WHO European Region and the Strategies for Response* (eds Francesco Branca, Haik Nikogosian and Tim Lobstein). Copenhagen WHO.

Willett W and Stampfer MJ (1986). Total energy intake: implications for epidemiologic analyses. *Am J Epidemiol* 124(1): 17–27.

World Cancer Research Fund / American Institute for Cancer Research (2007). *Food, Nutrition, Physical Activity, and the Prevention of Cancer: A Global Perspective.* Washington DC: AICR.

World Health Organization (2003). *Joint WHO/FAO Expert Report on Diet, Nutrition and the Prevention of Chronic Disease.* WHO Technical Report Series No. 916, Geneva.

Yang W, Kelly T and He J (2007). Genetic epidemiology of obesity. *Epidemiol Rev* 29: 49–61.

Part One

General issues

Trends in understanding patterns of obesity and health outcomes

W. P. T. James[1], R. Jackson-Leach[2]
[1]London School of Hygiene and Tropical Medicine and World Obesity Federation, London, UK; [2]World Obesity Federation, London, UK

1.1   Introduction

Although obesity has been described in literature and depicted in paintings for many centuries it is very clear that excessive weight gain in adulthood on a population level is of recent origin and really became of medical and public health concern only in the late 1970s. At that stage the crude definitions of overweight and obesity set out as the body mass index (BMI) were derived from mortality data taken from the pre-Second World War U.S.A.-based Metropolitan Life insurance statistics. BMIs of 25 and 30 are still taken for the clinical and epidemiological classification cut-offs of overweight and obesity in adults despite suggestions to the contrary from Flegal (Flegal *et al.*, 2007, 2013). Her analyses are based, however, on relatively short term US studies which were known since the 1970s as not being a suitable basis for demonstrating the incremental effect of modest increases in BMI; they also fail to take account adequately of several other major issues including the effect of smoking and unintentional weight loss associated with pre-existing disease. A series of integrated cohort studies involving well over a million subjects with long follow up periods from across the globe has confirmed the value of BMI 25 as a reasonable limit in terms of all-cause mortality and ischaemic heart disease mortality rates (Batty *et al.*, 2006; Prospective Studies Collaboration 2009; Adams *et al.*, 2006) with only death rates from haemorrhagic strokes suggesting that a higher BMI, e.g. of 30, might be more reasonable (Asia Pacific Cohort Studies Collaboration, 2004). Indeed the 57 prospective studies analyses with nearly a million subjects found that in both sexes mortality was lowest at about 22.5–25 kg/m and each 5 kg/m^2 higher BMI was associated with about a 30% higher overall mortality. As usual the first three years of follow up had to be discarded because those who were already ill had lower BMIs and early deaths so without this adjustment the curves were J shaped. These data have recently been amplified with data from 97 cohort studies demonstrating clearly that overweight (BMI 25–29.9) as well as obesity is a predictor of both coronary artery disease and stroke in Caucasians and Asians, with only 50% of the excess risk being

Managing and Preventing Obesity. http://dx.doi.org/10.1533/9781782420996.1.17

attributable to changes in the classic risk factors of blood pressure, cholesterol and glucose (Lu *et al.*, 2014).

It is clear that BMI is only a crude predictor because the presence of co-morbidities such as hypertension and diabetes are far more powerfully predictive of an early death than BMI alone, probably because they reflect ongoing processes of cellular and organ damage (Padwal *et al.*, 2011). The Asian criteria of a lower BMI of 23 were not based on mortality data at all but on the accepted greater morbidity of many Asian groups as weight increases, albeit that in Caucasians it has also been known for decades that the co-morbidities of diabetes, hypertension, coronary heart disease and some cancers increase progressively from a BMI of about 20. Nevertheless, internationally adult overweight and obesity continue to be considered in terms of the World Health Organization (WHO) accepted BMIs of 25 and 30.

1.2   The importance of abdominal obesity

It has been known for decades that the distribution of body fat is associated with different levels of co-morbidity and a specific emphasis on fat accumulation in the abdomen was made by Vague in the early post second world war years (Vague 1956). Since then global studies have confirmed the greater sensitivity of measures of waist circumference or waist/ hip ratios in predicting cardiovascular events (Yusuf *et al.*, 2005). Waist/height ratios (W/HtR) have also been advocated (Ashwell *et al.*, 2012) and found to be applicable in children as well as adults with some suggestion that it might be superior to waist or waist/hip ratios alone. Other systematic analyses emphasise the value of adding waist measures to BMI in evaluating the risk of disease or mortality (Carmienke *et al.*, 2013) and in Asian subjects the use of both waist and W/HtR has been proposed for predicting risk (Wakabayashi 2013). There seems general agreement that waist measurement is a better measure than BMI and the simplicity of the waist measure is easy for both the public and professionals to understand and certainly overcomes the need to measure the hip circumference, which in some societies is a culturally problematic measure to make except with female physicians taking considerable care. The original Scottish SIGN guideline and the subsequent WHO choices of waist circumference measurements (WHO 2000) were made simply on the basis that the waist measures chosen would correspond with the BMI cut-offs for overweight and obesity, i.e. 25 and 30. Then the International Diabetes Federation proposed other levels of waist measurement for different ethnic groups but based on very different and non-standardized criteria (Zimmet *et al.*, 2005).

Waist values do not automatically increase in line with BMI increases: strong genetic factors influence fat distribution but smoking and alcohol consumption also amplify the propensity to abdominal obesity. Early nutritional and other handicaps, often inferred from evidence of low birth weights, are also associated with later abdominal obesity when even modest weight is gained in adulthood. Thus, Japanese, Chinese, Indian, and Hispanic populations with a marked history of early childhood malnutrition are particularly prone to abdominal obesity with a high waist circumference even when the BMIs are in the 'normal' range. Then the increased waist values still signify increased risks. Nevertheless, despite all the attention given to waist measurements the BMI is still the measure used for international comparisons.

1.3   Global trends in obesity

We are witnessing a complex evolution in the prevalence of adult overweight and perhaps it is conceptually easier to consider a country such as China or Japan where from the point of view of limiting mortality from either underweight or overweight the mean BMI was 20–21 and the distribution of BMI was Gaussian in the 1970s – 1980s with negligible numbers of either obese or severely underweight (BMI < 17.0) subjects. However as the average BMI increases the Gaussian distribution changes to a markedly skewed one where there is a very big increase in those with very high BMIs for only modest further increases in the median value (Figure 1.1). This feature is reproduced in representative US and UK data and signifies an alarming increase

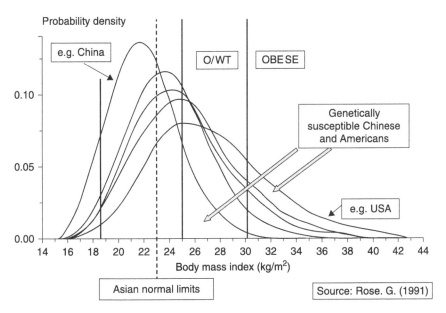

Figure 1.1 The skewed distribution of BMI with increases in the average population BMI. Cross-sectional data taken from the INTERSALT study to illustrate the progressive marked increase in obesity rates for modest increases in mean BMI. Those in the upper BMI range for each population distribution represent the genetically susceptible individuals to weight gain. The usual Caucasian cut-offs for overweight and obesity are shown together with the Asian upper limit of 'normal' BMI. Adapted from Rose (1991).

in the prevalence of morbid obesity with its huge health risks and costs. The reasons are explicable in energetic terms because as excess body energy is stored then there is a maximum to which the expansion of energy consuming lean tissues (normally 25% of initial weight increases) can contribute to the weight gain, i.e. there is a limit to skeletal and visceral metabolic tissue expansion. So if excess intake continues then all the energy has to be stored as fat and little further increase in energy output can be achieved to counterbalance this excess intake. The excess energy slowly but progressively accumulates as fat and the subject then becomes enormously obese as seen so frequently now in the US.

The Chinese data can be amplified by reference to the magnificent China/Oxford/ Cornell study (Chen et al., 1990) where a range of BMIs in different communities (average 20.5 in 1983) within China were observed in association with different diets and activities and particularly where the average fat and sugar intakes were 14.8% and about 3% respectively. The Japanese fat intakes studied by Keys and colleagues (Keys 1970) were similar but in China there has been a deliberate policy of importing fat despite advice to the contrary. As fat intakes increased by a quarter to 18.3% within six years the average BMI rose by 0.8 units to 21.3. Fat intakes have subsequently reached >30% in cities such as Beijing with sugar intakes also rising markedly and obesity, diabetes and hypertension rates escalating rapidly.

1.4   Economic development and obesity

The economic development of countries and particularly the urbanisation of populations is associated with major increases in obesity prevalences (Popkin 2006). Stark changes are seen when relatively isolated rural populations migrate into towns as seen originally with army recruits in Kenya transferring to Nairobi – within 10 weeks their body weights were increasing as their diets changed from an African cereal and root based diet to a more Western British Army diet. More recently relatives studied in both Bangalore India and villages 100–150 km away showed in 2003 BMIs of 19.9 in the villages of Karnataka but BMIs of 25.6 in Bangalore with threefold intake increases in dietary fat, a 6 fold increase in sugar intake and a quadrupling of salt intakes. Little wonder therefore that the corresponding diabetes rates were 9-fold higher (Vas 2003). The isolation of rural communities determines the contrast as the nutrition transition proceeds, so where the rural communities have been blessed by good infrastructure and medical facilities as in the Communist run state of Kerala in Southern India (one of the poorest states in India) the obesity rates were so high in middle-aged adults that their type 2 diabetes rates were already 30–40% in those 50–70 years old (Soman 2007).

The prevalence of obesity and overweight has been increasing rapidly in all regions of the world as very clearly shown by global analyses undertaken by Ezzati and colleagues (Finucaine et al., 2011) prior to the new global burden analyses by the IHME group (Lim et al., 2012) These analyses showed that there have been progressive increases in obesity rates in all regions of the world but we need to remember that in affluent countries there are marked contrasts between the countries, as illustrated

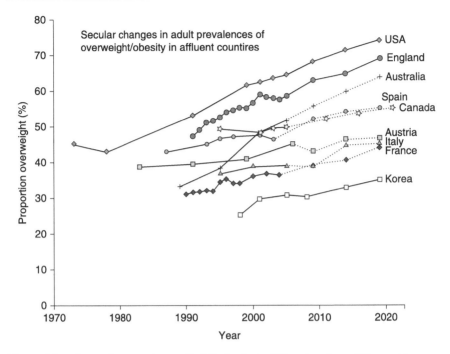

Figure 1.2 Increasing prevalence of adult obesity in different regions of the world.
Source: Wang *et al.* 2011.

by Figure 1.2, which presents an amplification of Wang *et al.*,'s (2011) analyses
There seems to have been an unremitting increase in overweight and obesity rates for
the last 30 years, albeit at different rates. Table 1.1 summarises the regional prevalences of adult overweight and obesity. These prevalences highlight the progressive
increase in weight in the first two decades of adult life and also that men tend to have
higher prevalences of overweight but lower prevalences of obesity than women. This
again probably reflects the greater lean body mass of men and that women reach
the biological limits of lean body mass expansion as they gain weight before men
and therefore they have to store far more energy as fat before they achieve energy
balance.

1.5   Social class differences in obesity

The evolution of overweight in Latin America, and indeed in many countries, first
affects relatively affluent middle-aged women. Then middle-aged men start to become
heavier and this is often seen as clear evidence of economic success and substantial
achievements within many African societies. In due course the whole population is
affected, including children. However as affluence evolves, the more affluent women
(as in Brazil) start to become thinner presumably in part as they became more aware

Table 1.1 The male and female prevalence (%) in the different WHO classified regions of the world at each age group

		18–29 yrs		30–44 yrs		45–59 yrs		60–69 yrs		70+ yrs	
		O/W	Ob	O/W	Ob	O/W	Ob	O/W	Ob	O/W	Ob
Africa	Males	18.1	4.4	23.6	7.8	29.5	11.1	27.8	10.7	18.3	6.5
	Females	13.6	5.1	18.7	10.7	20.5	14.5	30.0	24.3	19.0	16.0
Americas	Males	31.7	18.8	39.2	23.8	41.4	27.8	40.1	27.5	38.5	24.7
	Females	23.4	18.6	28.4	26.1	31.2	31.7	34.8	30.3	34.3	26.9
EMRO	Males	16.3	5.2	27.4	10.2	28.7	12.7	20.6	6.5	21.8	6.6
	Females	19.0	9.7	25.5	24.3	25.2	31.5	21.9	15.9	23.0	12.3
Europe	Males	25.1	6.0	42.0	14.9	45.6	22.3	47.2	26.2	47.6	21.7
	Females	16.6	7.2	28.0	18.1	35.2	30.3	38.8	35.8	37.8	29.8
SEARO	Males	5.1	0.7	11.8	1.9	13.6	2.4	1.7	0.3	3.4	0.6
	Females	7.0	1.5	18.9	4.9	18.2	6.0	5.0	0.9	10.3	1.5
WPRO	Males	16.4	1.7	24.4	4.8	27.1	6.4	27.3	7.1	12.7	1.3
	Females	11.7	2.3	18.3	6.4	22.5	4.9	23.2	9.5	26.0	3.8

O/W signifies BMIs of 25–29.9 and O/b BMIs ≥30.
EMRO – Eastern Mediterranean Region.
SEARO – South East Asia Region.
WPRO – Western Pacific Region.

of external cultural pressures. So they seem to become determined to be slimmer for cosmetic as well as health reasons.

Early studies of middle-aged men (assessed in the famous Seven Countries studies of 16 communities) showed on re-analysis of both their diets and an index of physical activity based on the differences in the average occupational activities, that differences in physical activity and the dietary fibre intake proved to be more powerful predictors of weight gain than their fat intakes (Kromhout *et al.*, 2001). This is in accordance with WHO's first appraisal in 2000 of the global obesity problem (WHO 2000): substantial physical activity as well as dietary fibre were both seen as protective. The weight-promoting effect of dietary fat (Hooper *et al.*, 2012) was incorporated as a determinant of the energy density of the diet with the water-retaining fibre-rich carbohydrate nature of foods contributing to offset substantially the energy density of the fat as well as sugar. Sugar has now been shown to be independently responsible for weight gain (Morenga *et al.*, 2012).

If one takes a global approach to the emergence of obesity, then in poorer communities the average BMI of the population was about 21 but by 1980 was increasing progressively as national incomes rose until a slowing of the increase was seen when GDPs reached about $5,000 with a final peak in women at $15,000 whereas men showed a later peak at $17,000 (Ezzati *et al.*, 2005). Then as societies' economies improved there appeared to be a modest reduction in average BMIs. A new reanalysis, however, now shows that in 2008 the epidemic of overweight/obesity had increased so much in lower income countries that the relationship resembled an inverted U for women, peaking at middle-income levels. BMI increased as the percentage of the population living in urban communities increased and this was evident in both 1980 and 2008. These urbanising effects reflect the impact of the dramatic changes in both physical activity and diet (Danaei *et al.*, 2013).

1.6 Obesity in women and its implications for maternal and infant health

Traditionally the main concern about weight gain has related to the development of physical handicaps such as arthritis and respiratory insufficiency and the metabolic co-morbidities of diabetes and hypertension which typically occur in middle age. However, although it has been recognised for decades that overweight and then obesity begins to increase particularly in the 20–40 year old age range, now a major concern is emerging relating to the risk of increasing infertility as excess weight develops. However, the handicaps of maternal overweight and obesity are much greater than those of infertility as set out by Oteng-Ntim and Doyle (2012) from a collation of systematic reviews and major observational studies. Pre-eclampsia and many other complications of pregnancy are increased with greater risks of maternal deaths, as well as difficulties in delivery. There are also increased rates of birth defect and the likelihood of macrosomia (i.e. birth weights $\geq 4.5\,\text{kg}$).

The development of glucose intolerance and gestational diabetes is of major concern with gestational diabetes now affecting up to 20% of pregnancies in some countries, e.g. Singapore. This condition now affects about 10% of pregnancies in Western Europe and an average of 15% of pregnancies in Eastern Europe, the Middle East and Asia on the basis of WHO criteria (Jenum *et al.*, 2012). On the basis of the modified International Diabetes Federation criteria, however, nearly 40% of South Asian, Middle East, African and South American women are classified as having gestational diabetes with long term consequences not only for the mothers themselves – who are far more likely to develop diabetes a decade or more later – but also the risk for their children becoming obese is ten times greater than normal. The Institute of Medicine (Rassmussen and Yaktine 2009), in their focus on pregnancy outcomes, highlighted the importance of the mother's pre-pregnancy weight in predicting the baby's subsequent birth weight and now cohort studies from Southampton (Gale *et al.*, 2007) show that increases in BMIs within the normal BMI range predict marked increased risks of adiposity in their 9-year-old offspring, particularly in girls. At present there are no internationally collated data which would specify the optimum levels of BMI in pregnancy and the prevalence of pregnancy overweight and obesity, but Table 1.1 clearly shows that women under the age of 44 years have already extraordinarily high prevalences of overweight and obesity.

Current findings re-emphasis that there is a U-shaped curve in the benefits of having babies born within the middle weight range – babies born too small, i.e. <2.5 kg, have a much greater risk of developing the metabolic syndrome as they gain weight later in life but macrosomia (birth weights ≥4.5 kg) is also a powerful predictor of early childhood obesity and the early incidence of diabetes. On this basis we should be regarding the nutritional well-being of young women before and during pregnancy as one of the highest public health priorities. So without early societal interventions we may well see an intergenerational amplification of the problems of obesity and an escalating incidence of much earlier diabetes, hypertension and cardiovascular disease which will then become much more difficult to prevent as well as treat.

1.7   Childhood obesity

Childhood obesity was recognised to be a problem when the WHO Expert Technical group on obesity met in 1997 and indeed WHO had already published in 1995 an analysis specifying, on a standard statistical basis relating to decades long studies on childhood malnutrition, that a child was not really a problem in public health terms until (s)he was outside the two standard deviation unit limits. These limits had been set on the basis of data from a reference population which in practice had been derived from a US population of bottle fed babies (WHO 1995). At that stage there was no real focus by WHO on the obesity problem in children because there was still pandemic malnutrition affecting many regions, if not the whole of the lower income world. The International Obesity Task Force (IOTF) group therefore, aware that this problem had not been considered sufficiently, developed an international classification system for overweight and obesity in children based again on the BMI index with cut-offs derived by taking the adult cut-offs of 25 and 30 and finding the percentiles of growth of collated representative data from six countries in the Americas, Europe and Asia (Cole *et al.*, 2000). It was then assumed that these percentile could be used from aged 2 upwards on the basis that children usually grow according to their percentile position in a population unless they are ill or becoming overweight on a weight for height basis. Recently a simpler, more robust analysis of these IOTF criteria of overweight and obesity have been published (Cole and Lobstein 2012) but now there are also new WHO criteria based in part on a remarkable study of healthy singleton babies from California, Norway, India, Oman, Ghana and Brazil. Carefully chosen mothers had babies who were born at full term and exclusively breast fed with appropriate complementary feeding, immunisations, etc. and studied for three years with similar babies monitored until they were 6 years old. A truly 'standard' growth curve for 0–5-year-olds could then be obtained. To the experts' surprise the children's growth in each country was almost identical and the variability in growth was exceptionally small and not influenced at all by their ethnic background. These growth patterns are very different from those which apply on a national basis in most countries and indicates the remarkable challenge in public health terms to achieve these presumed optimum levels of growth. However, to these standard data WHO then added adjusted data from the original US growth curves to produce their 'reference' values (WHO 2007) which roughly correspond to the IOTF BMI percentile vales of 25 and 30 when aged 18. These WHO reference curves for children from 5 to 20 years of age have now been accepted by governments (de Onis 2013) even though paediatricians find them in practice unrealistic and confusing (Cole and Lobstein 2012). Children with BMIs >1SD for their age show a greater propensity to develop hypertension, higher insulin and uric acid levels and other indices of insulin resistance (de Onis *et al.*, 2013) so this is clearly an unacceptable level of risk of what corresponds approximately to the BMI overweight criteria.

When considering overweight and obesity in children one issue is whether they grow out of their problem so that a finding of overweight can be considered temporary. For children over five years of age, being overweight incurs at least a 40% risk of this overweight/obesity persisting into adult life, but by the mid-teenage years the risk is increased to 60–75% (Power *et al.*, 1997). Table 1.2 summarises an up-to-date collation of both the prevalences and the huge numbers of both overweight and obese children in different regions of the world using the latest IOTF classification system. The different age groups chosen allow one to see how in the poorer regions of the world, e.g. Africa and the Middle East/North African region where data are often limited, overweight and obesity clearly becomes prominent in late adolescence whereas in the Americas, Europe and even the Asian and Pacific regions the primary school children are already showing marked prevalences of overweight. Furthermore, when the absolute numbers are calculated it becomes clear that we are dealing with hundreds of millions of affected children with no evidence of a lower prevalence in later youth so there is also little evidence that children on a population level will grow out of their problem. Indeed these adolescent children will soon amplify the prevalences of overweight and obese young adults. Boys are particularly affected

Table 1.2 The prevalence and numbers of overweight and obesity in children in the preschool years aged 5–9yrs and secondary school 10–17yrs globally

Region based on WHO classification	Overweight %		Obese %		Total O/W+Ob %		O/W number (thousands)		Obese (thousands)		Total: O/W+Ob numbers (thousands)	
	M	F	M	F	M	F	M	F	M	F	M	F
Africa												
5–9yrs	7.9.	8.0.	2.6	1.0	10.5	9.0	4,630	4,519	1,508	580	6,138	5,099
10–13yrs	7.9	8.0	2.6	1.0	10.5	9.0	3,253	3,190	1,062	415	4,315	3,606
14–17yrs	9.3	15.5	4.1	4.5	13.4.	20.0	3,515	5,693	1,550	1,653	5,065	7,346
Americas												
5–9yrs	15.9	13.9	7.5	9.3	23.4.	23.2	6,272	5,274	2,976	3,533	9,249	8,807
10–13yrs	21.3	20.8	11.4	13.3	32.7	34.2	6,732	6,339	3,602	4,054	10,334	10,393
14–17yrs	18.7	18.7	13.7	13.1	32.4	31.8	5,907	5,716	4,346	4,020	10,253	9,736
Eastern Mediterranean												
5–9yrs	3.3	4.1	4.3	5.1	7.6	9.2	1,153	1,365	1,502	1,698	2,655	3,063
10–13yrs	3.3	4.1	4.3	5.1	7.6	9.2	860	1,019	1,120	1,267	1,980	2,286
14–17yrs	20.0	21.1	8.5	6.7	28.5	27.8	5,106	5,142	2,170	1,633	7,276	6,774
Europe												
5–9yrs	13.3	16.8	5.3	6.0	18.6	22.8	3,493	4,178	1,392	1,492	4,885	5,670
10–13yrs	19.7	18.1	5.2	5.5	24.9	23.6	4,168	3,648	1,096	1,111	5,264	4,759
14–17yrs	17.7	15.5	5.6	6.1	23.3	21.5	4,067	3,402	1,296	1,333	5,364	4,736
South East Asia												
5–9yrs	12.6	12.6	5.3	3.9	17.9	16.5	11,707	10,936	4,940	3,385	16,647	14,320
10–13yrs	19.1	18.0	5.7	3.7	24.8	21.7	14,045	12,318	4,191	2,532	18,236	14,850
14–17yrs	17.0	14.7	5.7	4.7	22.7	19.4	12,401	9,969	4,158	3,187	16,559	13,157
Western Pacific/Oceania												
5–9yrs	11.0	6.7	10.6	8.6	21.6	15.4	7,179	3,748	6,931	4,812	14,110	8,560
10–13yrs	10.2	9.1	5.3	3.5	15.5	12.5	5,695	4,377	2,965	1,668	8,660	6,045
14–17yrs	10.5	3.5	3.0	1.9	13.4	5.5	6,224	1,853	1,755	1,014	7,979	2,867

Data based on the use of the IOTF cut-off points with obesity numbers not included in the overweight group.

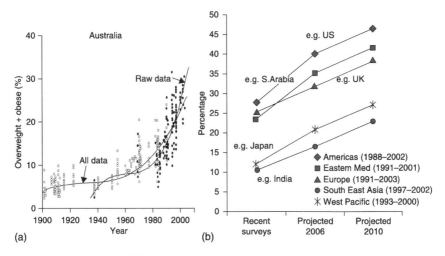

Figure 1.3 Changes in childhood obesity prevalence over time.
Source: (a) Norton *et al.* 2006; (b) Wang and Lobstein 2006.

in the Asian/Pacific region whereas boys and girls elsewhere have roughly the same prevalences; only in Africa is there a suggestion that the dominant problem is in girls.

Traditionally the focus has been on children over 3 years of age but there is now evidence of a worrying prevalence of overweight and obesity in the under 5 age group with increases in the prevalence of both high birth weight babies and obesity in 1–5-year-olds. The majority of 1–5-year-old children with BMIs >1SD of the new WHO limits are in lower income countries with marked increases in these prevalences having occurred since 1990 (de Onis *et al.*, 2010). The era when overweight and obesity in children emerged as a substantial issue is beautifully illustrated by the re-analyses of the growth patterns of Australian children monitored in multiple surveys throughout the twentieth century (see Figure 1.3). Numerous studies have demonstrated that childhood obesity emerged as a major public health problem in the early 1980s in affluent societies and then affected lower income countries about five years later. This is roughly in parallel with the surge in adult overweight and obesity prevalences so this must signify some major changes in the environmental factors.

1.8   Conclusions

Now the epidemic of obesity is predicted to be unsustainable in cost terms for any society, however affluent. Not only will there be the obvious escalating health costs but also the little-recognised indirect costs of work absenteeism. The major effect of reduced productivity when at work as well as the need for early retirement will also add immensely to the societal burden. It is therefore an exceptionally important economic priority to identify the environmental factors responsible and then control or counter these factors on a society-wide systematic basis. It is to these issues that the rest of this book is devoted

References

Adams KF, Schatzkin A, Harris TB, Kipnis V, Mouw T, *et al.* (2006). Overweight, obesity, and mortality in a large prospective cohort of persons 50 to 71 years old. *N Engl J Med* 355: 763–78.

Asia Pacific Cohort Studies Collaboration (2004). Body mass index and cardiovascular disease in the Asia-Pacific Region: an overview of 33 cohorts involving 310 000 participants. *International Journal of Epidemiology* 33: 751–8.

Ashwell M, Gunn P and Gibson S (2012). Waist-to-height ratio is a better screening tool than waist circumference and BMI for adult cardiometabolic risk factors:systematic review and meta-analysis. *Obes Rev* 13: 275–86.

Batty GD, Shipley MJ, Jarrett RJ, Breeze E, Marmot MG and Davey Smith G (2006). Obesity and overweight in relation to disease-specific mortality in men with and without existing coronary heart disease in London: the original Whitehall study. *Heart* 92: 886–92.

Carmienke S, Freitag MH, Pischon T, Schlattmann P, Fankhaenel T, *et al.* (2013). General and abdominal obesity parameters and their combination in relation to mortality: a systematic review and meta-regression analysis. *Eur J Clin Nutr* 67: 573–85.

Chen J, Campbell TC, Li J and Peto R (1990). Diet, lifestyle and mortality in China. Oxford University Press, Oxford, Cornell University Press, Ithaca, and People's Publishing House, Beijing. *See http://www.ctsu.ox.ac.uk/research/research-archive/chinese-ecological-studies/ china-monograph.*

Cole TJ, Bellizzi MC, Flegal KM and Dietz WH (2000). Establishing a standard definition for child overweight and obesity worldwide: international survey. *British Medical Journal* 320: 1240–3

Cole TJ and Lobstein T (2012). Extended international (IOTF) body mass index cut-offs for thinness, overweight and obesity. *Pediatr Obes* 7: 284–94.

Danaei G, Singh GM, Paciorek CJ, Lin JK, Cowan MJ, *et al.* (Global Burden of Metabolic Risk Factors of Chronic Diseases Collaborating Group) (2013). The global cardiovascular risk transition: associations of four metabolic risk factors with national income, urbanization, and Western diet in 1980 and 2008. *Circulation* 127: 1493–1502.

de Onis M (2013). Update on the implementation of the WHO child growth standards. *World Rev Nutr Diet* 106: 75–82.

de Onis M, Blössner M and Borghi E (2010). Global prevalence and trends of overweight and obesity among preschool children. *Am J Clin Nutr* 92: 1257–64.

de Onis M, Martínez-Costa C, Núñez F, Nguefack-Tsague G, Montal A and Brines J (2013). Association between WHO cut-offs for childhood overweight and obesity and cardiometabolic risk. *Public Health Nutr* 16: 625–30.

Ezzati M, Vander Hoorn S, Lawes CM, Leach R, James WP, *et al.* (2005). Rethinking the 'diseases of affluence' paradigm: economic development and global patterns of nutritional risks obesity and other cardiovascular risk factors 2005 in relation to economic development. *PLoS Medicine* 2: 404–12.

Finucane MM, Stevens GA, Cowan MJ, Danaei G, Lin JK, *et al.* (2011). Global Burden of Metabolic Risk Factors of Chronic Diseases Collaborating Group (Body Mass Index). National, regional, and global trends in body-mass index since 1980: systematic analysis of health examination surveys and epidemiological studies with 960 country-years and 9·1 million participants. *Lancet* 377: 557–67.

Flegal KM, Graubard BI, Williamson DF and Gail MH (2007). Cause-specific excess deaths associated with underweight, overweight, and obesity *JAMA* 298: 2028–37.

Flegal KM, Kit BK, Orpana H and Graubard BI (2013). Association of all-cause mortality with overweight and obesity using standard body mass index categories: a systematic review and meta-analysis. *JAMA* 309: 71–82.

Gale CR, Javaid MK, Robinson SM, Law CM, Godfrey KM and Cooper C (2007). Maternal size in pregnancy and body composition in children. *J Clin Endocrinol Metab* 92: 3904–11.

Hooper L, Abdelhamid A, Moore HJ, Douthwaite W, Skeaff CM and Summerbell CD (2012). Effect of reducing total fat intake on body weight: systematic review and meta-analysis of randomised controlled trials and cohort studies. *BMJ* 345: e7666.

Jenum AK, Mørkrid K, Sletner L, Vange S, Torper JL, *et al.* (2012). Impact of ethnicity on gestational diabetes identified with the WHO and the modified International Association of Diabetes and Pregnancy Study Groups criteria: a population-based cohort study. *Eur J Endo* 166: 317–24.

Key A (1970). Coronary heart disease in seven countries. *Circulation* 41(Suppl 1).

Kromhout D, Bloemberg B, Seidell JC, Nissinen A and Menotti A (2001). Physical activity and dietary fiber determine population body fat levels: the Seven Countries Study. *Int J Obes Relat Metab Disord* 25: 301–6.

Lim S, Vos T, Flaxman A, *et al.* (2012). A comparative risk assessment of burden of disease and injury attributable to 67 risk factors and risk factor clusters in 21 regions, 1990–2010: a systematic analysis for the Global Burden of Disease Study 2010. *Lancet* 380: 2224–60. Erratum in: *Lancet* (2013) 381: 628,1276.

Lu Y, Hajifathalian K, Ezzati M, Woodward M, Rimm EB and Danaei G (2014). Metabolic mediators of the effects of body-mass index, overweight, and obesity on coronary heart disease and stroke: a pooled analysis of 97 prospective cohorts with 1·8 million participants. *Lancet* 383: 970–83.

Morenga TL, Mallard S and Mann J (2012). Dietary sugars and body weight: systematic review and meta-analyses of randomised controlled trials and cohort studies. *BMJ* 346: e749.

Norton K, Dollman J, Martin M and Harten N (2006). Descriptive epidemiology of childhood overweight and obesity in Australia: 1901–2003. *Int J Pediatr Obes* 1: 232–8.

Oteng-Ntim E and Doyle P (2012). 'Maternal outcomes in pregnancy'. In *Maternal Obesity* (eds Gillman MW and Poston L), Cambridge University Press, Cambridge, pages 35–44.

Padwal RS, Pajewski NM, Allison DB and Sharma A (2011). Using the Edmonton obesity staging system to predict mortality in a population-representative cohort of people with overweight and obesity. *CMAJ* 183: E1059–66.

Popkin BM (2006). Global nutrition dynamics: the world is shifting rapidly toward a diet linked with non-communicable diseases. *Am J Clin Nut* 84: 289–98.

Power C, Lake JK and Cole TJ (1997). Body mass index and height from childhood to adulthood in the 1958 British born cohort. *Am J Clin Nutr* 66: 1094–1101.

Prospective Studies Collaboration (2009). Body-mass index and cause-specific mortality in 900 000 adults: collaborative analyses of 57 prospective studies. *Lancet* 373: 1083–96.

Rasmussen K M and Yaktin AL (eds) (2009). Weight gain during pregnancy: reexamining the guidelines. Committee to Reexamine IOM Pregnancy Weight Guidelines, Food and Nutrition Board and Board on Children, Youth, and Families. Washington.

Rose G (1991). Population distributions of risk and disease. *Nutr Metab Cardiovasc Dis* 1: 37–40.

Soman CR (2007). Fifty years of primary health care: the Kerala experience. *Nutrition Foundation of India Bulletin* 28: 1–5.

Vague J (1956). The degree of masculine differentiation of obesities: a factor determining predisposition to diabetes, atherosclerosis, gout, and uric calculous disease. *Am J Clin Nutr* 4: 20–34.

Vas M (2003). Personal communication.

Wakabayashi I (2013). Necessity of both waist circumference and waist-to-height ratio for better evaluation of central obesity. *Metab Syndr Relat Disord* 11: 189–94.

Wang Y and Lobstein T (2006). Worldwide trends in childhood overweight and obesity. *Int J Pediatr Obes* 1: 11–25.

Wang YC, McPherson K, Marsh T, Gortmaker SL and Brown M (2011). Health and economic burden of the projected obesity trends in the USA and the UK. *Lancet* 378: 815–25.

World Health Organization (WHO) (1995). *Physical Status: The Use and Interpretation of Anthropometry*. WHO Technical. Report. Series No. 854, Geneva.

World Health Organization (WHO) (2000). Obesity: preventing and managing the global epidemic. WHO Technical Report Series No. 894, Geneva.

World Health Organization WHO (2007). *Child Growth Standards*, WHO, Geneva.

Yusuf S, Hawken S, Ôunpuu S, Bautista L, Franzosi MG, *et al.*, on behalf of the INTERHEARTStudy Investigators (2005). Obesity and the risk of myocardial infarction in 27 000 participants from 52 countries: a case-control study. *Lancet* 366: 1640–49.

Zimmet P, Magliano D, Matsuzawa Y, Alberti G and Shaw J (2005). The metabolic syndrome: a global public health problem and a new definition. *J Atheroscler Thromb* 12(6): 295–300.

Overview of the key current population-level strategies used to prevent obesity

2

C. D. Economos, D. P. Hatfield
Tufts University, Medford, MA, USA

2.1 Introduction

Obesity remains a global public health challenge with unquestionable impacts at all levels of society (Swinburn *et al.*, 2011). Although excess weight accumulation affects people of all ages, races, ethnicities, and income levels, available data from countries worldwide generally reflect disparities in obesity prevalence. These disparities may in part be a function of environmental determinants of obesity, which influence population subgroups differently. In the United States (US), for example, some evidence suggests that low-income and racial/ethnic minority populations are disproportionately exposed to environments that promote excess energy intakes or limit physical activity. Such factors may partially explain disproportionate rates of obesity in these populations (Sallis and Glanz, 2009). A growing understanding of the environmental determinants of obesity has led to an increased focus on environmental and policy-oriented obesity-prevention efforts, which may reduce overall obesity prevalence and help close disparities.

The US Institute of Medicine's 2012 report *Accelerating Progress in Obesity Prevention* (APOP) (IOM, 2012) synthesized the best available evidence and issued recommendations for environmental and policy-oriented obesity-prevention efforts. The report identified strategies that had demonstrated potential, to varying degrees, for rapidly stemming the epidemic. Figure 2.1 provides a visual summary of the areas on which the report focused.

Using the APOP report's findings as a guiding structure, this chapter stresses evidence-based approaches for preventing obesity through community-, social-, and policy-level strategies, which offer particular promise for broad-scale population impact. It also touches upon emerging approaches still being tested. While primary and secondary prevention of obesity is the main focus of this chapter, many of these strategies may also benefit those who are already obese. Individual-level efforts, including more intensive approaches to treatment of obese individuals, are deferred to later chapters.

Managing and Preventing Obesity. http://dx.doi.org/10.1533/9781782420996.1.31

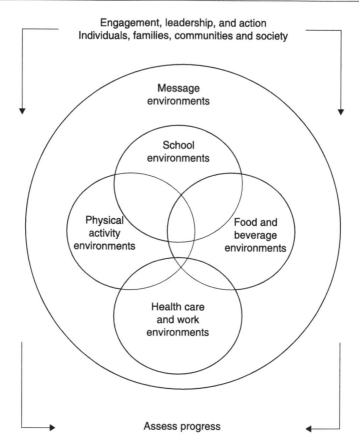

Figure 2.1 Five interacting environments for obesity prevention. Reprinted with permission from *Accelerating Progress in Obesity Prevention: Solving the Weight of the Nation*, 2012, by the National Academy of Sciences, courtesy of the National Academies Press, Washington, D.C.

2.2   Physical activity strategies

Decreasing physical activity (PA) is one factor underlying the increase in obesity prevalence worldwide. While the concept of 'physical activity' commonly conjures recreational exercise and sport, the majority of activity energy expenditure (AEE) is in fact attributable to routine activities like work, transportation, and household chores. As countries develop economically, shifts in these daily activities represent the primary decreases in PA; for example, employment tends to shift from physical to sedentary work, and active transit decreases as people gain access to automobiles (Ng and Popkin, 2012). Comprehensive strategies to increase AEE incorporate efforts to increase PA in these routine activities of daily living in addition to addressing recreation and exercise (Sallis and Glanz, 2009).

The built environment – that is, the physical structures in which people perform their daily activities – is a key determinant of PA. For example, structures like sidewalks and bike lanes, or traffic-calming mechanisms that make those structures safer to use, increase the likelihood that people will bike or walk to work or school rather than commuting in automobiles (Boarnet et al., 2005). Enhancements to public transit, to which commuters must typically walk or bike, can also lead to increases in PA; in fact, public transit users take on average 30% more steps per day than those who principally use cars (Edwards, 2008). Zoning laws and urban planning practices may also help promote PA. For example, mixed commercial and residential designs increase the likelihood that residents will actively commute to do shopping or other tasks (Ding et al., 2011). Recognizing such potential, the US's 2010 National Physical Activity Plan recommended that new building projects include Health Impact Assessments, which help ensure that new developments facilitate rather than impede PA (NPAPCC, 2010).

Increasing access to safe recreational spaces may also increase leisure-time PA, particularly among children in low-income communities where such spaces tend to be limited (Gordon-Larsen et al., 2006). Governments may promote development of recreational facilities by offering economic incentives (IOM, 2009). Other strategies facilitate utilization of existing spaces. Shared-use agreements, for example, can increase PA by allowing children and community organizations to access schools or other public facilities during off-peak hours (Lafleur et al., 2013). Potential levers for encouraging shared-use practices include mandating partnerships between schools and recreational groups and reforming liability laws for school districts that participate in shared-use agreements; however, the effectiveness of such approaches requires further research (IOM, 2012).

Expanding access to recreational facilities may require complementary efforts to make using those facilities safe and easy to use. For example, increasing lighting or police presence can make spaces safer and, in turn, drive utilization (Heath, et al., 2006). Sport and recreation programs may also increase PA, particularly when they are tailored to the needs and preferences of the target population (Ransdell, et al., 2009).

2.3 Food and beverage strategies

Individuals' dietary behaviors – controlling portion sizes, for example, or choosing nutrient-dense foods like fruits and vegetables over foods high in added fats and sugars – play an important role in determining their weight status (USDA and DHHS, 2010). However, shifting dietary behaviors at the population level requires attention not only to individuals, but also to the food and beverage environments they occupy. Efforts to improve food and beverage environments may include strategies to increase access to nutrient-dense products or to reduce access to energy-dense foods and beverages.

Government entities can have a direct and powerful influence on the food environment by setting strong nutrition standards for foods and beverages available in schools and other public facilities. Efforts to restrict access to sugar-sweetened beverages (SSBs) in such facilities hold particular promise for obesity-prevention, given the strong evidence base linking SSBs with obesity (Woodward-Lopez *et al.*, 2011). For example, school-based policies that reduce access to SSBs have been shown to decrease the percentage of children consuming sugary drinks as well as the total calories children consume (Levy *et al.*, 2011). Evidence also supports the effectiveness of expanding access to healthier options. For example, increasing the number of water fountains in schools has been shown to reduce the incidence and prevalence of obesity (Muckelbauer *et al.*, 2009).

The types of foods and beverages available to consumers in the broader retail space are also important predictors of dietary behavior. Consumers who live in areas with greater access to healthy foods, like fruits and vegetables, tend to have higher-quality diets than consumers with comparatively lower access (Larson *et al.*, 2009), while those with high access to convenience stores and fast-food restaurants, where healthy options are often not available, tend to have lower-quality diets (Boone-Heinonen *et al.*, 2011). In the US, insufficient access to healthy foods, and abundant access to less healthy options, tends to be particularly common in low-income and minority communities and may therefore perpetuate disparities in obesity prevalence (Larson *et al.*, 2009).

Zoning or tax policies may encourage expansion of food retailers, like grocery stores, into such environments, or, conversely, prevent expansion of fast-food outlets or other retailers deemed less healthy. However, the impact of such efforts on obesity prevalence is unclear. Some evidence suggests that increasing physical access to healthier foods will only impact consumption if combined with efforts to promote and ensure the affordability of those options (IOM, 2012).

Other strategies may impact consumption by increasing prices of unhealthy foods or reducing prices of healthy items. For example, some research estimates that taxes on SSBs would substantially decrease consumption of these beverages (Wang *et al.*, 2012a), though the extent to which such policies would reduce overall caloric intakes and obesity requires further research. The impact of government agricultural policies on food production patterns and food prices have likewise been scrutinized; some experts have argued, for example, that government subsidies for commodity crops like corn and soybeans contribute to obesity by depressing prices of energy-dense processed foods (Wallinga *et al.*, 2009). However, others note that government subsidies represent a small proportion of the retail food dollar and that their impact on consumer behavior is therefore limited (Alston *et al.*, 2008).

2.4 School strategies

Public-health recommendations in the United States and worldwide place priority on obesity-prevention efforts targeting children. Since childhood weight status tends to track into adulthood (Serdula *et al.*, 1993) and prevention is favored over treatment, aggressive efforts are needed to reverse the population-level energy imbalance underlying the childhood obesity epidemic (Wang *et al.*, 2012b). Schools are a particularly important focal point for obesity-prevention efforts; in the US, children spend up to half of their time in school and consume on average about 35% of their daily calories there (Briefel *et al.*, 2009). Given that children's attendance in school is mandated by law in the US and most other developed countries, the potential reach of school-based efforts, particularly state- or national-level policy changes, is considerable.

2.4.1 School foods

Nutrition standards for the National School Breakfast and National School Lunch Programs have been developed in the US. One study found that individual states with more stringent school nutrition requirements demonstrated less disparity in the prevalence of obesity among school-lunch participants versus nonparticipants (Taber *et al.*, 2013). In many schools, competitive foods – that is, school foods that are not part of the federal nutrition programs – are available through vending machines, school stores, a la carte lines, and other outlets. Comprehensive policies that restrict sales of unhealthy options in all environments, including competitive foods, have been linked with reduced intakes of energy-dense foods and beverages among schoolchildren (Mendoza *et al.*, 2010).

Food- and beverage-related messaging and advertising in schools have also come under scrutiny, given their potential to influence purchase and consumption patterns in children (IOM, 2005). Despite some evidence of a decreased presence of food/beverage commercial messages in schools, a majority of students in the US remain exposed to at least some messages (Terry-McElrath *et al.*, 2014).

2.4.2 School physical activity

While US public-health recommendations suggest that children should accrue at least 30 minutes of daily PA in school (IOM, 2013), children generally fall far short of that goal. Efforts are underway to increase opportunities for quality PA through a variety of creative strategies. One review study found that recess provided up to 40% of children's total daily PA time, though the amount of active recess time varied considerably by the population studied (Ridgers *et al.*, 2006). Some research has suggested that levels of PA during recess can be increased through provision of PA equipment, activity zones, or trained recess staff (Verstraete *et al.*, 2006). Short activity breaks built into class time may further increase opportunities for in-school PA without reducing classroom time (Mahar *et al.*, 2006).

2.4.3 Nutrition/health education

The current level of nutrition education provided in schools is limited, on average reaching just five hours per year in the US (Kann, 2007). By comparison, nutrition experts recommend more intensive and comprehensive approaches, given evidence that at least 50 hours per year of nutrition education are required to facilitate behavior change (Briggs, 2010). It is recommended that state and local education agencies ensure the implementation and monitoring of sequential food literacy and nutrition science education, spanning grades K-12, based on authoritative food and nutrition recommendations (IOM, 2012).

2.5   Healthcare and workplace strategies

The healthcare community, including individual clinicians and health institutions, play an important role in preventing and treating obesity. For example, a US survey showed that overweight adults were more likely to be aware of their weight status and also to have attempted weight loss if their physicians had discussed their weight status with them (Post *et al.*, 2011). However, this same study found that fewer than half of overweight patients and one-third of obese patients had been told by their physicians about their weight status. Other research in pediatric settings has found that only 50% of pediatricians and 22% of general practitioners used BMI-for-age to screen for obesity at every well-child visit (Wethington *et al.*, 2011).

Training physicians and other health professionals to properly diagnose overweight and obesity, and to effectively counsel both overweight/obese and healthy-weight patients on healthy eating and PA, may enable such practitioners to promote healthy weight in their patients (DHHS, 2010). Effective counseling of pregnant women and new mothers also has the potential to impact childhood obesity; healthy pregnancy weight gain (Rasmussen *et al.*, 2009) and breastfeeding practices (Monasta *et al.*, 2010), for example, have both been associated with decreased likelihood of later childhood obesity (DHHS, 2011). At the institutional level, hospitals and other healthcare providers can also develop strong nutrition standards for the foods made available in their facilities. These policies may influence not just immediate but also longer-term dietary behaviors, since consumers tend to perceive items served in healthcare environments as being healthy (Sahud *et al.*, 2006).

Insurance providers also play an important role in enabling and motivating patients to achieve or maintain a healthy weight. For example, providers may make no- or low-cost obesity-prevention programs available to all subscribers or ensure obesity-prevention and obesity-treatment programs are covered under patients' policies. Since obese individuals in the US generate greater healthcare costs per year than do healthy-weight individuals, such efforts may ultimately be win-win propositions that both serve patients' health interests and reduce longer-term costs of care (Dietz *et al.*, 2007).

Worksite-based obesity-prevention efforts offer the potential to reach a large proportion of the adult population and, like insurer-based policies, may benefit both employers and employees. Programs that increase access to healthy foods at worksites, for example, have been shown to favorably impact employees' dietary intakes (Backman *et al.*, 2011), and worksite-based nutrition and PA programs appear to promote improvements in employee weight status (Anderson *et al.*, 2009). Such programs have the potential to yield positive returns on investment for employers, since healthy-weight employees tend to have not only lower healthcare costs but also lower absenteeism and higher productivity than do overweight and obese employees (Goetzel *et al.*, 2010).

2.6   Messaging strategies

Evidence suggests that high volumes of advertising exposure among children (Harris *et al.*, 2009) may impact their health behaviors and weight status. For example, a

2005 Institute of Medicine report found strong evidence of a longitudinal association between exposure to food advertising and adiposity in children and adolescents (IOM, 2005). Given commercial rights to free speech, most efforts to address food advertising to date have entailed industry self-regulation programs, such as the Children's Food and Beverage Advertising Initiative (CFBAI) in the US. Results have been somewhat successful for companies that have signed on to participate. However, enforceable standards that restrict marketing to children may be required for widespread impact (Terry-McElrath *et al.*, 2014).

Conversely, promoting healthful behaviors is an important strategy to counteract and displace unhealthy messages and marketing. Social marketing campaigns, which apply commercial marketing techniques to achieve socially desirable outcomes, have been shown to have a moderate effect on nutrition and PA behaviors (Wakefield *et al.*, 2010). The VERB campaign is an example of a social marketing effort that positively influenced PA outcomes in children, with results that persisted into the adolescent years (Huhman *et al.*, 2010).

There is some evidence from controlled studies that labeling menus with calorie information may reduce the number of calories purchased and consumed, but evidence in real-world settings is more mixed and requires further investigation (Swartz *et al.*, 2011).

2.7 Conclusion: integrating approaches

Interventions focused on the above-noted domains individually appear to have an impact. Multilevel strategies may have further synergistic effects. Recognition of interrelatedness between factors influencing obesity has motivated a shift toward community-level obesity-prevention interventions, through which multiple stakeholders and systems can be brought into play with relatively high levels of control (Economos and Tovar, 2012). Such interventions serve as models for what can be accomplished at the state, region, province, and country levels with sufficient leadership and engagement. A 2013 systematic review synthesizing emerging findings from multi-level, community-based childhood obesity-prevention studies assessed the current strength of evidence supporting such efforts as 'moderate' (Bleich *et al.*, 2013). One successful example is Shape Up Somerville (SUS), a community-engaged intervention that aimed to reduce undesirable weight gain among children by implementing multilevel changes to promote healthy eating and physical activity. Evaluation of SUS found decreases in BMI z-scores over two years among children in the intervention community compared to control communities, as well as decreases in the prevalence, and increases in remission, of overweight/obesity among both boys and girls (Economos *et al.*, 2013). Further findings include reduced consumption of SSBs, increased participation in organized sports and physical activities, and reduced screen time in intervention children compared with controls (Folta *et al.*, 2013). Future work should not only take into account the effectiveness of single environmental or policy strategies, but also use systems methodologies to address how the most promising strategies fit together and reinforce each other's effectiveness (IOM, 2012). Implementation of multi-level, multi-sector strategies will require engagement at all levels of society, including individuals, households, communities, the public sector, the business community and private sector, healthcare, worksites and employers, and citizens and civic organizations. These interrelated and mutually-influencing groups must all be engaged to achieve collective action and maximize impact.

2.8   Sources of further information and advice

The following resources provide additional information on evidence-based strategies for obesity prevention, with a particular emphasis on environmental and policy approaches:

www.activelivingresearch.org

www.healthyeatingresearch.org

www.gov.uk/government/publications/reducing-obesity-future-choices

www.iom.edu/Reports/2012/Accelerating-Progress-in-Obesity-Prevention.aspx

www.nccor.org/

References

Alston, J.M., Sumner, D.A. and Vosti, S.A. (2008) 'Farm subsidies and obesity in the United States: National evidence and international comparisons', *Food Policy*, 33, 470–79.

Anderson, L.M., Quinn, T.A., Glanz, K., Ramirez, G., Kahwati, L.C., *et al.* (2009) 'The effectiveness of worksite nutrition and physical activity interventions for controlling employee overweight and obesity: a systematic review', *Am J Prev Med*, 37, 340–57.

Backman, D., Gonzaga, G., Sugerman, S., Francis, D. and Cook, S. (2011) 'Effect of fresh fruit availability at worksites on the fruit and vegetable consumption of low-wage employees', *J Nutr Educ Behav*, 43, S113–21.

Bleich, S.N., Segal, J., Wu, Y., Wilson, R. and Wang, Y. (2013) 'Systematic review of community-based childhood obesity prevention studies', *Pediatrics*, 132, e201–10.

Boarnet, M., Day, K., Anderson C., *et al.* (2005) 'California's Safe Routes to School Program – impacts on walking, bicycling, and pedestrian safety', *J Am Plann Assoc*, 71, 301–17.

Boone-Heinonen, J., Gordon-Larsen, P., Kiefe, C.I., Shikany, J. M., Lewis, C.E. and Popkin, B.M. (2011) 'Fast food restaurants and food stores: longitudinal associations with diet in young to middle-aged adults: the CARDIA study', *Arch Intern Med*, 171, 1162–70.

Briefel, R.R., Wilson, A. and Gleason, P.M. (2009) 'Consumption of low-nutrient, energy-dense foods and beverages at school, home, and other locations among school lunch participants and nonparticipants', *J Am Diet Assoc*, 109, S79–90.

Briggs, M. (2010) 'Position of the American Dietetic Association, School Nutrition Association, and Society for Nutrition Education: comprehensive school nutrition services', *J Nutr Educ Behav*, 42, 360–71.

DHHS (United States Department of Health and Human Services) (2010) *The Surgeon General's Vision for a Healthy and Fit Nation*. Rockville, MD, Office of the Surgeon General.

DHHS (United States Department of Health and Human Services) (2011), *The Surgeon General's Call to Action to Support Breastfeeding*. Rockville, MD, Office of the Surgeon General.

Dietz, W., Lee, J., Wechsler, H., Malepati, S. and Sherry, B. (2007) 'Health plans' role in preventing overweight in children and adolescents', *Health Aff (Millwood)*, 26, 430–40.

Ding, D., Sallis, J.F., Kerr, J., Lee, S. and Rosenberg, D.E. (2011) 'Neighborhood environment and physical activity among youth a review', *Am J Prev Med*, 41, 442–55.

Economos, C.D. and Tovar, A. (2012) 'Promoting health at the community level: thinking globally, acting locally', *Childhood Obesity*, 8, 19–22.

Economos, C.D., Hyatt, R.R., Must, A., Goldberg, J.P., Kuder, J., *et al.* (2013) 'Shape Up Somerville two-year results: a community-based environmental change intervention sustains weight reduction in children', *Prev Med*, 57, 322–7.

Edwards, R.D. (2008) 'Public transit, obesity, and medical costs: assessing the magnitudes', *Prev Med*, 46, 14–21.

Folta, S.C., Kuder, J.F., Goldberg, J.P., Hyatt, R.R., Must, A., *et al.* (2013) 'Changes in diet and physical activity resulting from the Shape Up Somerville community intervention', *BMC Pediatrics*, 13, 157.

Goetzel, R.Z., Gibson, T.B., Short, M.E., Chu, B.C., Waddell, J., *et al.* (2010) 'A multi-work-site analysis of the relationships among body mass index, medical utilization, and worker productivity', *J Occup Environ Med*, 52 Suppl 1, S52–8.

Gordon-Larsen, P., Nelson, M.C., Page, P. and Popkin, B.M. (2006) 'Inequality in the built environment underlies key health disparities in physical activity and obesity', *Pediatrics*, 117, 417–24.

Harris, J.L., Pomeranz, J.L., Lobstein, T. and Brownell, K.D. (2009) 'A crisis in the market-place: how food marketing contributes to childhood obesity and what can be done', *Ann Rev Public Health*, 30, 211–25.

Heath, G.W., Brownson, R.C., Kruger, J., Miles, R., Powell, K.E. and Ramsey, L.T. (2006) 'The effectiveness of urban design and land use and transport policies and practices to increase physical activity: a systematic review', *J Phys Act Health*, 3, S55.

Huhman, M.E., Potter, L.D., Nolin, M.J., Piesse, A., Judkins, D.R., *et al.* (2010) 'The Influence of the VERB campaign on children's physical activity in 2002 to 2006', *Am J Public Health*, 100, 638–45.

IOM (Institute of Medicine) (2005), *Food Marketing to Children and Youth: Threat or Opportunity?* Washington, DC, National Academies Press.

IOM (Institute of Medicine) (2009), *Local Government Actions to Prevent Childhood Obesity*. Washington, DC, National Academies Press.

IOM (Institute of Medicine) (2012), *Accelerating Progress in Obesity Prevention: Solving the Weight of the Nation*. Washington, DC, National Academies Press.

IOM (Institute of Medicine) (2013), *Educating the Student Body: Taking Physical Activity and Physical Education to School*. Washington, DC, National Academies Press.

Kann, L. (2007) 'Health education: results from the School Health Policies and Programs Study 2006', *J Sch Health*, 77, 408–34.

Lafleur, M., Gonzalez, E., Schwarte, L., Banthia, R., Kuo, T., *et al.* (2013), 'Increasing physical activity in under-resourced communities through school-based, joint-use agreements, Los Angeles County, 2010–2012', *Prev Chronic Dis*, 10, E89.

Larson, N.I., Story, M.T. and Nelson, M.C. (2009) 'Neighborhood environments: disparities in access to healthy foods in the U.S.', *Am J Prev Med*, 36, 74–81.

Levy, D.T., Friend, K.B. and Wang, Y.C. (2011) 'A review of the literature on policies directed at the youth consumption of sugar sweetened beverages', *Adv Nutr*, 2, S182–S200.

Mahar, M.T., Murphy, S.K., Rowe, D.A., Golden, J., Shields, A.T. and Raedeke T.D. (2006) 'Effects of a classroom-based program on physical activity and on-task behavior', *Med Sci Sports Exerc*, 38, 2086–94.

Mendoza, J.A., Watson, K. and Cullen, K.W. (2010) 'Change in dietary energy density after implementation of the Texas Public School Nutrition Policy', *J Am Diet Assoc*, 110, 434–40.

Monasta, L., Batty, G.D., Cattaneo, A., Lutje, V., Ronfani, L., *et al.* (2010) 'Early-life determinants of overweight and obesity: a review of systematic reviews', *Obes Rev*, 11, 695–708.

Muckelbauer, R., Libuda, L., Clausen, K., Toschke, A.M., Reinehr, T. and Kersting, M. (2009) 'Promotion and provision of drinking water in schools for overweight prevention: randomized, controlled cluster trial', *Pediatrics*, 123, e661–7.

Ng, S.W. and Popkin, B.M. (2012) 'Time use and physical activity: a shift away from movement across the globe', *Obes Rev*, 13, 659–80.

NPAPCC (United States National Physical Activity Plan Coordinating Committee) (2010), *National Physical Activity Plan for the United States*.

Post, R.E., Mainous, A.G., Gregorie, S. H., Knoll, M. E., Diaz, V.A. and Saxena, S.K. (2011) 'The influence of physician acknowledgment of patients' weight status on patient perceptions of overweight and obesity in the United States', *Arch Intern Med*, 171, 316–21.

Ransdell, L.B., Dinger, M.K., Huberty, J. and Miller, K.H. (2009) *Developing Effective Physical Activity Programs*. Champaign, IL, Human Kinetics.

Rasmussen, K.M., Catalano, P.M. and Yaktine, A.L. (2009) 'New guidelines for weight gain during pregnancy: what obstetrician/gynecologists should know', *Curr Opin Obstet Gynecol*, 21, 521–6.

Ridgers, N.D., Stratton, G. and Fairclough, S.J. (2006) 'Physical activity levels of children during school playtime', *Sports Med*, 36, 359–71.

Sahud, H.B., Binns, H.J., Meadow, W.L. and Tanz, R.R. (2006) 'Marketing fast food: impact of fast food restaurants in children's hospitals', *Pediatrics*, 118, 2290–7.

Sallis, J.F. and Glanz, K. (2009) 'Physical activity and food environments: solutions to the obesity epidemic', *Milbank Q*, 87, 123–54.

Serdula, M.K., Ivery, D., Coates, R.J., Freedman, D.S., Williamson, D.F. and Byers, T. (1993) 'Do obese children become obese adults? A review of the literature', *Prev Med*, 22, 167–77.

Swartz, J.J., Braxton, D. and Viera, A.J. (2011) 'Calorie menu labeling on quick-service restaurant menus: an updated systematic review of the literature', *Int J Behav Nutr Phys Act*, 8, 135.

Swinburn, B.A., Sacks, G., Hall, K.D., McPherson, K., Finegood, D.T., *et al.* (2011) 'The global obesity pandemic: shaped by global drivers and local environments', *Lancet*, 378, 804–14.

Taber, D.R., Chriqui, J.F., Powell, L. and Chaloupka, F.J. (2013) 'Association between state laws governing school meal nutrition content and student weight status: implications for new USDA school meal standards', *JAMA Pediatr*, 167, 513–19.

Terry-McElrath, Y.M., Turner, L., Sandoval, A., Johnston, L.D. and Chaloupka, F.J. (2014) 'Commercialism in US elementary and secondary school nutrition environments: trends from 2007 to 2012', *JAMA Pediatr*, 168, 234–42.

USDA and DHHS (United States Department of Agriculture and Department of Health and Human Services) (2010), *Dietary Guidelines for Americans*. Washington, DC, Government Printing Office.

Verstraete, S.J., Cardon, G.M., De Clercq, D.L. and De Bourdeaudhuij, I.M. (2006) 'Increasing children's physical activity levels during recess periods in elementary schools: the effects of providing game equipment', *Eur J Public Health*, 16, 415–19.

Wakefield, M.A., Loken, B. and Hornik, R.C. (2010) 'Use of mass media campaigns to change health behaviour', *Lancet*, 376, 1261–71.

Wallinga D., Schoonover, H. and Muller, M. (2009), 'Considering the contribution of US agricultural policy to the obesity epidemic: overview and opportunities', *J Hunger Environ Nutr*, 4, 3–19.

Wang, Y.C., Coxson, P., Shen, Y.M., Goldman, L. and Bibbins-Domingo, K. (2012a) 'A penny-per-ounce tax on sugar-sweetened beverages would cut health and cost burdens of diabetes', *Health Aff* (*Millwood*), 31, 199–207.

Wang, Y.C., Orleans, C.T. and Gortmaker, S.L. (2012b) 'Reaching the healthy people goals for reducing childhood obesity: closing the energy gap', *Am J Prev Med*, 42, 437–44.

Wethington, H.R., Sherry, B. and Polhamus, B. (2011) 'Physician practices related to use of BMI-for-age and counseling for childhood obesity prevention: a cross-sectional study', *BMC Fam Pract*, 12, 80.

Woodward-Lopez, G., Kao, J. and Ritchie, L. (2011) 'To what extent have sweetened beverages contributed to the obesity epidemic?', *Public Health Nutr*, 14, 499–509.

Part Two

The role of different dietary components in obesity management

The role of high sugar foods and sugar-sweetened beverages in weight gain and obesity

B. M. Popkin[1], G. A. Bray[2], F. Hu[3]
[1]University of North Carolina, Wilmington, MC, USA; [2]Pennington Biomedical Research Center, Baton Rouge, LA, USA; [3]Harvard School of Public Health, Boston, MA, USA

3.1 Introduction

A confluence of factors based on scientific findings over the past two decades have led to a growing greater concern about the role of sugar in our diet, particularly in beverages. At the same time, there appears to be an increasing push to promote sugar in both foods and beverages globally and certainly there are large increases in consumption of sugar-sweetened beverages (SSB) across the world.

The role of sugar in our history and in our diet certainly is not new. Scholars such as Yudkin discussed its role decades ago and warned of its potential health effects (Yudkin, 1964, 1972). Similarly, sugar has had a long complex role in global history (Mintz 1979, 1986). However, it is more recent developments that have led to much greater attention to sugar as it has affected the risk of obesity.

The path breaking work of Mattes and Rolls have been particularly important in highlighting a major issue – we do not adequately compensate by reducing food calories when we consume beverage calories (Mattes, 1996, 2006; DiMeglio and Mattes, 2000; DellaValle *et al.*, 2005, Flood *et al.*, 2006). This led to dozens of clinical and epidemiological studies and finally to a series of randomized, controlled clinical trials in adults and adolescents.

At the same time Bray *et al.* (2004) and Havel (Elliott *et al.*, 2002) first raised concerns that dietary fructose was metabolized primarily in the liver and in contrast with glucose might have important detrimental effects of lipogenesis in this organ (Bray *et al.*, 2004; Bray, 2007, 2010). This early work showed that the rise in the consumption of high fructose corn syrup paralleled the increase in obesity and provided a significant amount of free fructose in the diet. It speculated that the consumption of high-fructose corn syrup (HFCS) in beverages may play a role in the epidemic of obesity. HFCS in sugar-sweetened beverages might also play a role in the risk for diabetes and other cardio metabolic problems. Subsequent research has shown that fructose coming from any sugar has the same effects and that it is the

Managing and Preventing Obesity. http://dx.doi.org/10.1533/9781782420996.2.45

fructose *per se* and not its form of a caloric sweetener that poses the serious cardio metabolic threat.

In the following sections of this paper, we review the current patterns of use and consumption of sugar in food and particularly SSBs, the biological effects of fructose and sugar, and knowledge about the health effects of sugar-sweetened beverages.

3.2   Sugar in our food supply

3.2.1   Sugar in foods

First we provide a picture of the general use of added sugars in the food supply using data from the one country for which we have the details on ingredients and can figure out the food items that contain caloric sweeteners. Then we proceed to present data for a few countries on trends in consumption of sugar-sweetened beverages (SSBs).

The only country for which we have data on the extent of added sugar in the food supply is the United States, where scanned data on food purchases can be linked with nutrition facts panels and full ingredient lists to identify all foods and the calories from these foods and beverages with and without caloric sweeteners (Ng *et al.*, 2012). Of the 85,451 uniquely formulated foods purchased during 2005–2009 (sold in many different package sizes), 74% contain caloric sweeteners (68% with caloric sweeteners, 6% with both caloric and non-caloric sweeteners). Caloric sweeteners are in >95% of cakes/cookies/pies, granola/protein/energy bars, ready-to-eat cereals, sweet snacks, and sugar-sweetened beverages. Across unique products, corn syrup is the most commonly listed sweetener, followed by sorghum, cane sugar, high fructose corn syrup and fruit juice concentrate. Also, 77% of all calories purchased in the US in 2005–2009 contained caloric sweeteners. Figure 3.1 provides the trends over this period in proportion of calories from beverages with caloric sweeteners.

Generally speaking, there are no data on added sugar in the food supply of most countries. The United States estimates this using a complex estimation procedure but does this based on recipes rather than using ingredients (Westrich *et al.*, 1994, 1998; U.S. Department of Agriculture, 2012). Furthermore, in the US, fruit juice concentrate, is recognized and used as a caloric sweetener; however, fruit juice concentrate used as a sweetener is not measured as one in neither the USDA calculations of added sugars [termed the MPED (My Pyramid Equivant Database)] nor national aggregates of consumption of sweeteners (U.S. Department of Agriculture, 2012). Yet this study shows that fruit juice concentrate is used as a sweetener in 7% of the 85,451 unique consumer packaged goods (CPG) products, and is used frequently in juices, sugar-sweetened beverages, diet sweetened beverages, salad dressings, yogurt, granola/energy bars, ready-to-eat cereals and baby food. It is also the fifth most commonly listed sweetener. We included fruit juice concentrate in our analysis

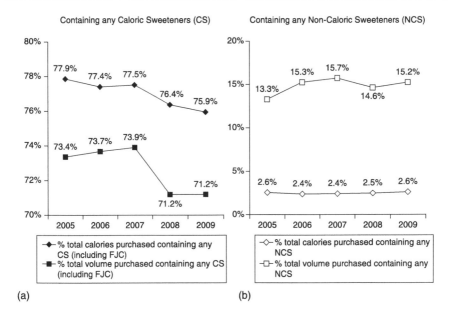

Figure 3.1 Total calories and volume of consumer packaged food and beverages purchased in the United States containing caloric sweeteners (CS) and non-caloric sweeteners (NCS), 2005–2009 (%).

Sources: Nielsen Homescan 2005–2009, Gladson Nutrition Database 2007 and 2010

Ng *et al.* (2012). Copyright © 2012, with permission from Elsevier

3.2.2 The sweeteners provided by beverages

Globally there looks like a marked shift toward marketing sugar-sweetened beverages mainly in low and middle income countries and promoting noncaloric or diet beverages in higher income countries (Kleiman *et al.*, 2011). We explored patterns and trends of carbonated soft drinks and other beverages. In one case study using the two largest and most influential producers of sweetened beverages, the Coca-Cola Company and PepsiCo, who together control 34% of the global soft drink market, we examined their product portfolios globally in three critical markets (the US, Brazil, and China) from 2000 to 2010 (see Figure 3.2). On a global basis, total revenues and energy per capita sold increased, yet the average energy density (kilojoules per 100 milliliters) sold declined slightly, suggesting a shift to lower-calorie products. In the US, both total energy per capita and average energy density of beverages sold decreased significantly, while the opposite was true in the developing markets of Brazil and China, with total per capita energy increasing greatly in China and, to a lesser extent, in Brazil (see Figure 3.2).

What is most striking in looking at countries across the globe (unreported results) is that in the US and selected European countries diet and low caloric sweetener beverages increased as a proportion of sales. Among high income countries UK and US data stand out as showing the largest shift toward increased use of low calorie or

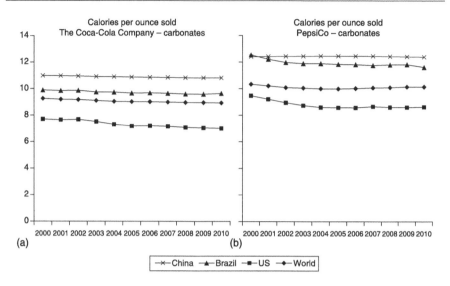

Figure 3.2 Trends 2000–2010 in calories per ounce sold: global, the US, Brazil, and China. *Sources:* Kleiman *et al.* (2011) *Obesity Reviews.* (© 2011 The Authors. *Obesity Reviews* © 2011 International Association for the Study of Obesity.)

diet beverages with mainly non-nutritive sweeteners, although there is a new category of beverages emerging that combine caloric and diet sweeteners (Piernas C, 2013). In both the UK and the US we have seen marked increases in consumption of diet beverages (Ng *et al.*, 2011; Piernas C, 2013) and in the US we showed a marked decline in kcal/ml of all these diet and sugar-sweetened beverages (Kleiman *et al.*, 2011). For example US adults averaged 176 ml/day of diet beverages in 2007–8 while US children averaged 43 ml/day in the same year. Among higher income countries, only South Korea seems to have emerged from the last three decades with a very low intake of sugar-sweetened beverages (Lee, 2012). In contrast in both Europe among adolescents 13–16.9 years (e.g., 227 kcal/d) and in the US and UK, we have found very high levels of intake (Duffey *et al.*, 2011; Ng *et al.*, 2011).

The most striking change is the huge increase in sugar-sweetened beverages across low income countries. We only have trends data for limited countries such as Mexico at the individual level and China and Brazil at the aggregate level. In Figure 3.3 we show for China and Brazil the shift upwards in sales of these beverages by the two major global SSB companies – PepsiCo and Coca Cola – in the past decade. These increases are also seen in studies on individual intake in Brazil.

Elsewhere we have presented data which have explored in depth trends in caloric beverage intake for Mexico (Barquera *et al.*, 2008, 2010). In these studies we found Mexicans consumed over 21% of daily calories from beverages. For children, whole milk dominated along with sugar-sweetened beverages and juices with added sugars while the latter two dominated with adults. These results showed a doubling of calories from 1999–2006. More recently we have examined trends in sales of SSBs in

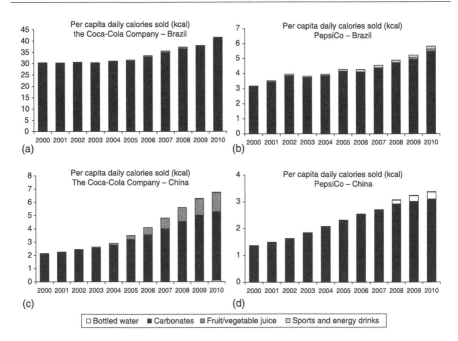

Figure 3.3 Brazilian and Chinese trends 2000–2010 in daily calories.
Sources: Kleiman *et al.*, *Obesity Reviews* (10 Nov 2011). (© 2011 The Authors. *Obesity Reviews* © 2011 International Association for the Study of Obesity.)

Mexico from 1999 to 2011–12 and find intake has increased over time. Commercial data show sales of sugar-sweetened beverages of $66/capita/yr in 1998 that almost quadrupled to $240/capita/yr in 2011. The increase actually accelerated in the 2005–11 period over the earlier period.

3.3 Biological mechanisms for some effects of sugar in beverages

Water is an essential component of the human body, and the thirst mechanism is designed to provide information about bodily needs for water. Human preferences for sweet tastes has led to a profusion of beverages in which sugar and related sweeteners were added to make them more palatable. For a long time, the sugar in beverages was viewed as similar to sugar added to solid foods. A revolution in our thinking has occurred in the past several decades as we learned that beverage calories were not completely compensated for by reducing the intake of solid foods (Mattes, 1996, 2006; DiMeglio and Mattes, 2000; DellaValle *et al.*,005; Flood *et al.*, 2006; Rolls *et al.*, 1990). Whether the calories in beverages are in the form of a fat, protein or carbohydrate, we now know that caloric compensation is incomplete (Mourao *et al.*,

2007). Over the past 50 years there has been a marked shift in our consumption of added sugar from foods toward beverages. Added sugar in solid food was relatively constant from 1977–78 until 2003–4 while sugar added in beverages increased remarkably (Duffey and Popkin, 2008). Furthermore, as noted earlier, much of this was represented by an increase in sugar sweetened beverages, fruit drinks and fruit juices. This resulted in an extensive literature that has explored both the mechanisms and effects of consuming these beverages.

The mechanisms by which added sugar and hence energy in a liquid form may affect energy intake and weight gain are complex and part of a larger impact of beverages with extensive sugar on our entire metabolism and ultimately our health. Figure 3.4 lays out some of the mechanisms. One recent animal study provides in an animal model one potential pathway – namely that fructose produces a smaller increase in satiety than glucose; however this hypothalamic brain signal pathway would need to be followed with human studies to understand the implications of this research for humans (Page *et al.*, 2013).

In addition to the effect of passive overconsumption of calories in beverages, because there is inadequate compensation by reducing other foods there is concern that the fructose in beverages which comes from the fructose or high fructose corn syrup may have additional detrimental effects. A new and emerging literature, first

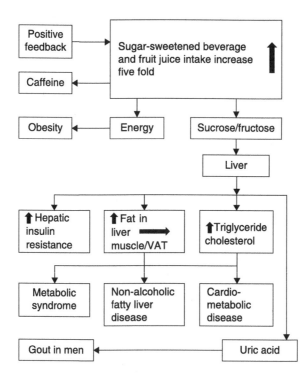

Figure 3.4 Model showing some potential consequences of increasing fructose and energy intake from sugar or high fructose corn syrup in beverages.

pushed by Bray *et al.*, (2004), has focused on the fructose in sugar and high fructose corn syrup as having separable metabolic consequences, from the glucose which also comes in sugar and HFCS. Fructose intake may affect cardio metabolic health as well as the liver and kidney.

Several short term clinical studies have provided insights into the metabolic consequences of ingesting fructose in sugar-sweetened beverages. Schall and Cohen showed in early studies comparing fructose, glucose, and sucrose that it is the fructose alone or in sucrose that increased triglycerides following a meal, but not glucose (Cohen and Schall, 1988). In another study there was an increase in body weight, blood pressure and inflammatory markers; in another an increase in triglycerides levels, particularly at night, a stimulation of de novo lipogenesis and an increase in visceral fat (Sorensen *et al.*, 2005). Stanhope and Havel have been two of those who have led research on this topic (Stanhope and Havel, 2008; Stanhope, 2009, 2012; Teff *et al.*, 2009; Stanhope *et al.*, 2011a, 2011b). In the final short term study, which compared milk, diet cola, a sugar-sweetened cola and water, the sugar-sweetened beverage increased liver fat, visceral fat, and triglycerides over the six months of beverage intake (Maersk *et al.*, 2012). This study suggests that consuming two 16 ounce sugar-containing beverages per day for six months can mimic many of the features of the metabolic syndrome and the non-alcoholic fatty liver disease (Maersk *et al.*, 2012). Many others have added to this literature that shows impact of fructose in initiating liver dysfunction and possibly leading to non-alcoholic fatty liver disease and the metabolic syndrome (Aeberli *et al.*, 2011).

Although studies on sugar sweetened beverages have shown in adequate caloric compensation this same conclusion, it applies equally to fruit juice. When sugar is consumed in solid food, caloric compensation appears to occur, but the effects of fructose are still present. It is the calories and fructose provided by HFCS and sucrose (table sugar) that create the cardio metabolic effects. Part of this metabolic response may be the fact that fructose, unlike glucose, does not stimulate insulin secretion or enhance leptin production.

3.4 Randomized clinical trials and longitudinal cohort studies link intake of sugar-sweetened beverages to the risk of obesity

Three recent publications – two randomized controlled trials (RCTs) and one longitudinal study – strongly suggest that calories from sugar-sweetened beverages do enhance weight gain. The two most noteworthy are the Boston (Ebbeling *et al.*, 2012) and Amsterdam (de Ruyter *et al.*, 2012) studies among children. In a study conducted in Boston, Ebbeling and colleagues showed that interventions designed to reduce consumption of sugar-sweetened beverages reduced weight gain mainly in the Hispanic subgroup of adolescents. After one year the control group in the Boston study gained significantly less weight than the group receiving the sugar-sweetened beverages. When the intervention was discontinued, the benefits on weight gain disappeared during an additional year of follow-up. A second randomized clinical trial was conducted on adolescents in The Netherlands. This study by de Ruyter and colleagues was unique in its double-blind design, large sample of normal-weight schoolchildren from 4 years 10 months to 11 years 11 months of age, and measurement of sucralose in urine as an additional compliance marker. One limitation was a 26% dropout rate. Nevertheless, the results clearly show that masked replacement of a sugar-containing beverage (104 kcal) with a sugar-free beverage significantly reduced weight gain and fat accumulation in normal-weight adolescents. This study went further than the Boston study and provided either 250 ml of low caloric sweetened beverage or a sugar-containing beverage providing 104 kcal to 641 youths over an 18 month period. The BMI, weight, and skinfold-thickness and fat mass showed significantly less increase in the low caloric beverage group. A third six-month randomized clinical trial in adults study had three treatment groups – low calorie beverage, water and normal beverage intake. It found a significantly greater likelihood of a 5% weight loss among the first two groups compared to the normal beverage group but all lost weight as this was part of an active weight loss regime (Tate *et al.*, 2012).

A final study in this group (Qi *et al.*, 2012) examined the interaction between the intake of sugar-sweetened beverages and a genetic-predisposition score that was calculated on the basis of 32 body-mass index (BMI) loci associated with obesity in women and men from two large prospective cohorts and in an independent replication cohort. This study provides strong evidence that there is a significant interaction between an important dietary factor – intake of sugar sweetened beverages – and a genetic-predisposition score, obesity, and the risk of obesity. But since they used a score calculated from multiple genetic variants, it is difficult to apply this to individuals.

Several meta-analyses have been undertaken on the effects of sugar-sweetened beverages on weight gain and risk of obesity. All were conducted prior to the randomized clinical trials described above. Two highlighted an important issue – the role of source of funding in affecting the results (Lesser *et al.*, 2007; Vartanian *et al.*, 2007). Hu and colleagues conducted a meta-analysis evaluating change in BMI per one-serving increase of sugar-sweetened beverages per day and found a significant positive association between beverage intake and weight gain (0.08, 95% CI: 0.03, −0.13 kg) (Malik *et al.*, 2009) among studies that did not adjust for total energy intake (Ludwig *et al.*, 2001; Berkey *et al.*, 2004; James *et al.*, 2004; Phillips *et al.*, 2004; Ebbeling *et al.*, 2006). Given the mediating role of sugar-sweetened beverages on caloric intake, many studies that control for SSB energy intake are likely to provide misleading results. In studies in adults, the effect was strongest in larger studies with longer durations of follow-up that used robust dietary assessment methods such as food frequency questionnaires rather than a single 24-hour diet recall, which is not able to capture patterns in dietary intake (Berkey *et al.*, 2004; Ludwig *et al.*, 2001). A variety of reviews support these results (Malik *et al.*, 2006; Olsen and Heitmann, 2009; Vartanian *et al.*, 2007).

Among adults, more epidemiological work has been undertaken. Cross-sectional studies are not optimal because of the high potential for intractable confounding and reverse causation. Prospective cohort studies tend to provide the most robust evidence despite a large degree of diversity between studies in terms of outcome measurements, size and duration of follow-up. Therefore greater emphasis should be placed on larger studies of longer duration which are better powered to detect an effect. In this literature, the longest and largest studies (Schulze *et al.*, 2004; Palmer *et al.*, 2008) show stronger and more consistent associations compared to smaller and shorter studies (Kvaavik *et al.*, 2004; French *et al.*, 1994). For example, in the study by Schulze *et al.* (2004) with over 50,000 nurses followed for two four-year periods (1991–1995 and 1995–1999), a higher consumption of sugar sweetened beverages was associated with a greater magnitude of weight gain. After adjustment for potential confounders, women who increased their beverage consumption from 1991 to 1995 and maintained a high level of intake gained on average 8.0 kg over the two periods while women who decreased SSB intake between 1991 and 1995 and maintained a low level of intake gained on average 2.8 kg over the two periods.

3.5   Fruit juice and weight gain

There are few large-scale studies with fruit juice, in contrast to the larger literature on sugar-sweetened beverages, and there have been no randomized clinical trials. The limited set of studies suggests that fruit juices are associated with the same cardio metabolic and weight problems as the sugar-sweetened beverage and provide virtually no health benefits except in unique, rare circumstances (Bazzano *et al.*, 2008; Sanigorski *et al.*, 2007; Mueller *et al.*, 2010). Fruit juice is the new focal point for some countries. As found in one study (Ng *et al.*, 2012), fruit juice concentrate is not subject to the same trade barriers and quotas as other sugars and carries a natural, healthy aura. Thus a large number of sugar-sweetened beverages are now sweetened with fruit juice concentrate, and fruit juices themselves are being pushed very hard as a natural healthy drink. In fact, in this same study, an exploration of detailed ingredients in the 400,000-plus products sold by consumer packaged goods companies in the United States found that 31% of sugar-sweetened beverages contained fruit juice concentrate and even 29% of so-called diet-sweetened beverages contained fruit juice concentrate.

3.6   Future trends

Scientific evidence of the adverse effects of sugar-sweetened beverages on weight gain and risk of obesity will increase steadily as more and more randomized controlled trials and other studies on this topic are completed. The mechanisms behind the effect of sugar-sweetened beverages on body weight and cardio metabolic risk will also grow with the coming years. The role of fructose in risk for cardio metabolic and hepatic injury will become clearer. Nevertheless, any caloric sweetener will carry risks for obesity and be particularly problematic when consumed as a beverage.

The food industry might begin to try to find ways to use glucose and other caloric sweeteners that are low in fructose but this will not affect the relationship between body weight sugar-sweetened beverages but might minimize some of the related cardio metabolic effects. However this is not the preferred option and the public health and medical community will increasingly promote water as the key hydrating beverage.

Limiting intake of SSBs is seen as the simplest first step in addressing global obesity. Several dozen countries have banned sugar-sweetened beverages in schools and a smaller number have banned fruit juice. A few countries have also limited use of mass media to promote sugar-sweetened beverages, particularly on TV. Importation is even limited in selected countries. In the public health world there is close to universal acceptance in the Americas and Europe of the need to limit sugar sweetened beverages. This is spreading to the Middle East and Africa and slowly to Asia. Ministries of Health in Israel, the Gulf States, selected Western European countries and elsewhere have promoted taxes on sugar-sweetened beverages. In the future we expect to see some successful taxes implemented and other regulations such as the portion size implemented in NYC focused on reducing intake of sugar-sweetened beverages. It will take many years before there is adequate evidence and successful education to begin to reduce fruit juice intake the way the push for sugar-sweetened beverage limitations are taking hold globally.

3.7   Sources of further information and advice

Knowledge is growing most rapidly in this area so there is no one reference book that will suffice. For data on sales country by country and by major beverage and food companies, there is the Euromonitor International data base (Euromonitor, 2011). Individual country data come from various individual dietary intake surveys. A useful scholarly work on sugar, its sources, roles, and health effects is Goran (2014).

References

Aeberli, I., Gerber, P. A., Hochuli, M., Kohler, S., Haile, S. R., *et al.* (2011), Low to moderate sugar-sweetened beverage consumption impairs glucose and lipid metabolism and promotes inflammation in healthy young men: a randomized controlled trial, *Am J Clin Nutr*, 94, 479–85.

Barquera, S., Hernández, L., Tolentino, M. L., Espinosa, J., Leroy, J., *et al.* (2008), Energy from beverages is on the rise among Mexican adolescents and adults, *J Nutr*, 138, 2454–61.

Barquera, S., Campirano, F., Bonvecchio, A., Hernández, L., Rivera, J. and Popkin, B. (2010), Caloric beverage consumption patterns in Mexican children, *Nutr J*, 9, 47–56.

Bazzano, L. A., Li, T. Y., Joshipura, K. J. and Hu, F. B. (2008), Intake of fruit, vegetables, and fruit juices and risk of diabetes in women, *Diabetes Care*, 31, 1311–17.

Berkey, C. S., Rockett, H. R., Field, A. E., Gillman, M. W. and Colditz, G. A. (2004), Sugar-added beverages and adolescent weight change, *Obes Res*, 12, 778–88.

Bray, G. A. (2007), How bad is fructose?, *Am J Clin Nutr*, 86, 895–6.

Bray, G. A. (2010), Fructose: pure, white, and deadly? Fructose, by any other name, is a health hazard, *J Diabetes Sci Technol*, 4, 1003–7.

Bray, G. A., Nielsen, S. J. and Popkin, B. M. (2004), Consumption of high-fructose corn syrup in beverages may play a role in the epidemic of obesity, *Am J Clin Nutr*, 79, 537–43.

Cohen, J. C. and Schall, R. (1988), Reassessing the effects of simple carbohydrates on the serum triglyceride responses to fat meals, *Am J Clin Nutr*, 48, 1031–4.

DellaValle, D. M., Roe, L. S. and Rolls, B. J. (2005), Does the consumption of caloric and non-caloric beverages with a meal affect energy intake?, *Appetite*, 44, 187–93.

de Ruyter, J. C., Olthof, M. R., Seidell, J. C. and Katan, M. B. (2012), A trial of sugar-free or sugar-sweetened beverages and body weight in children, *New Eng J Med*, 367, 1397–1406.

DiMeglio, D. P. and Mattes, R. D. (2000), Liquid versus solid carbohydrate: effects on food intake and body weight, *Int J Obes Relat Metab Disord*, 24, 794–800.

Duffey, K. J. and Popkin, B. M. (2008), High-fructose corn syrup: is this what's for dinner?, *Am J Clin Nutr*, 88, S1722–32.

Duffey, K. J., Huybrechts, I., Mouratidou, T., Libuda, L., Kersting, M., *et al.* (2011), Beverage consumption among European adolescents in the HELENA study, *Eur J Clin Nutr*, 66, 244–52.

Ebbeling, C. B., Feldman, H. A., Osganian, S. K., Chomitz, V. R., Ellenbogen, S. J. and Ludwig, D. S. (2006), Effects of decreasing sugar-sweetened beverage consumption on body weight in adolescents: a randomized, controlled pilot study, *Pediatrics*, 117, 673–80.

Ebbeling, C. B., Feldman, H. A., Chomitz, V. R., Antonelli, T. A., Gortmaker, S. L., *et al.* (2012), A randomized trial of sugar-sweetened beverages and adolescent body weight, *N Engl J Med*, 367, 1407–16.

Elliott, S. S., Keim, N. L., Stern, J. S., Teff, K. and Havel, P. J. (2002), Fructose, weight gain, and the insulin resistance syndrome, *Am J Clin Nutr*, 76, 911–22.

Euromonitor. (2011), *Euromonitor International* [Online]. Available: http://www.euromonitor.com/ [accessed February 9 2011].

Flood, J., Roe, L. and Rolls, B. (2006), The effect of increased beverage portion size on energy intake at a meal, *J Am Diet Assoc*, 106, 1984–90.

French, S. A., Jeffery, R. W., Forster, J. L., Mcgovern, P. G., Kelder, S. H. and Baxter, J. E. (1994), Predictors of weight change over two years among a population of working adults: the Healthy Worker Project, *Int J Obes Relat Metab Disord*, 18, 145–54.

Gladson. 'Gladson – Nutrition Database'. Retrieved January 21, 2011, from http://www.gladson.com/SERVICES/NutritionDatabase/tabid/89/Default.aspx.

Goran, M. I., Tappy, L., Le, K.A. and Ulijaszek, S. (editors) (2014), *Dietary Sugars and Health*, Abingdon, Taylor and Francis.

Homescan The Nielsen Co. The new ways we watch and buy. http://en-us.nielsen.com/. Accessed January 29, 2011.

James, J., Thomas, P., Cavan, D. and Kerr, D. (2004), Preventing childhood obesity by reducing consumption of carbonated drinks: cluster randomised controlled trial, *BMJ*, 328, 1237.

Kleiman, S., Ng, S. W. and Popkin, B. (2011), Drinking to our health: can beverage companies cut calories while maintaining profits?, *Obes Rev*, 13, 258–74.

Kvaavik, E., Meyer, H. E. and Tverdal, A. (2004), Food habits, physical activity and body mass index in relation to smoking status in 40–42 year old Norwegian women and men, *Prev Med*, 38, 1–5.

Lee, H.-S., Duffey, K.J. Kiyah J. and Popkin, B.M. (2012), South Korea's entry to the global food economy: shifts in consumption of food between 1998 and 2009, *Asia Pacific J Clin Nutr*, 21, 618–29.

Lesser, L. I., Ebbeling, C. B., Goozner, M., Wypij, D. and Ludwig, D. S. (2007), Relationship between funding source and conclusion among nutrition-related scientific articles, *PLoS Med*, 4, e5.

Ludwig, D. S., Peterson, K. E. and Gortmaker, S. L. (2001), Relation between consumption of sugar-sweetened drinks and childhood obesity: a prospective, observational analysis, *Lancet*, 357, 505–8.

Maersk, M., Belza, A., Stødkilde-Jørgensen, H., Ringgaard, S., Chabanova, E., *et al.* (2012), Sucrose-sweetened beverages increase fat storage in the liver, muscle, and visceral fat depot: a 6-mo randomized intervention study, *Am J Clin Nutr*, 95, 283–9.

Malik, V. S., Schulze, M. B. and Hu, F. B. (2006), Intake of sugar-sweetened beverages and weight gain: a systematic review, *Am J Clin Nutr*, 84, 274–88.

Malik, V. S., Willett, W. C. and Hu, F. B. (2009), Sugar-sweetened beverages and BMI in children and adolescents: reanalyses of a meta-analysis, *Am J Clin Nutr*, 89, 438–9; author reply 9–40.

Mattes, R. D. (1996), Dietary compensation by humans for supplemental energy provided as ethanol or carbohydrate in fluids, *Physiol Behav*, 59, 179–87.

Mattes, R. (2006), Fluid calories and energy balance: the good, the bad, and the uncertain, *Physiol Behav*, 89, 66–70.

Mintz, S. W. (1979), Time, sugar and sweetness, *Marxist Perspect*, 2, 56–73.

Mintz, S. (1986), *Sweetness and Power: The Place of Sugar in Modern History*, New York City, Penguin.

Mourao, D., Bressan, J., Campbell, W. and Mattes, R. (2007), Effects of food form on appetite and energy intake in lean and obese young adults, *Int J Obes (Lond)*, 31, 1688–95.

Mueller, N. T., Odegaard, A., Anderson, K., Yuan, J.-M., Gross, M., *et al.* (2010), Soft drink and juice consumption and risk of pancreatic cancer: the Singapore Chinese Health Study, *Cancer Epidemiol Biomarkers Prev*, 19, 447–55.

Ng, S. W., Mhurchu, C., Jebb, S. and Popkin, B. (2011), Patterns and trends of beverage consumption among children and adults in Great Britain, 1986–2009, *Br J Nutr* 20, 1–16.

Ng, S. W., Slining, M. M. and Popkin, B. M. (2012), Use of caloric and noncaloric sweeteners in US consumer packaged foods, 2005–2009, *J Acad Nutr Diet*, 112, 1828–34.

Olsen, N. J. and Heitmann, B. L. (2009), Intake of calorically sweetened beverages and obesity, *Obes Rev*, 10, 68–75.

Page, K. A., Chan, O., Arora, J., Belfort-Deaquiar, R., Dzuira, J., *et al.* (2013), Effects of fructose vs glucose on regional cerebral blood flow in brain regions involved with appetite and reward pathways, *JAMA*, 309, 63–70.

Palmer, J. R., Boggs, D. A., Krishnan, S., Hu, F. B., Singer, M. and Rosenberg, L. (2008), Sugar-sweetened beverages and incidence of type 2 diabetes mellitus in African American women, *Arch Intern Med*, 168, 1487–92.

Phillips, S. M., Bandini, L. G., Naumova, E. N., Cyr, H., Colclough, S., *et al.* (2004), Energy-dense snack food intake in adolescence: longitudinal relationship to weight and fatness, *Obes Res*, 12, 461–72.

Piernas C, N. S. P. B. (2013), Trends in purchases and consumption of foods and beverages containing caloric and low-calorie sweeteners over the last decade in the U.S. *Pediar Obes*, 8, 294–306.

Qi, Q., Chu, A. Y., Kang, J. H., Jensen, M. K., Curhan, G. C., *et al.* (2012), Sugar-sweetened beverages and genetic risk of obesity, *N Eng J Med*, 367, 1387–96.

Rolls, B. J., Kim, S. and Fedoroff, I. C. (1990), Effects of drinks sweetened with sucrose or aspartame on hunger, thirst and food intake in men, *Physiol Behav*, 48, 19–26.

Sanigorski, A. M., Bell, A. C. and Swinburn, B. A. (2007), Association of key foods and beverages with obesity in Australian schoolchildren, *Public Health Nutr*, 10, 152–7.

Schulze, M. B., Manson, J. E., Ludwig, D. S., Colditz, G. A., Stampfer, M. J., *et al.* (2004), Sugar-sweetened beverages, weight gain, and incidence of type 2 diabetes in young and middle-aged women, *JAMA*, 292, 927–34.

Sorensen, L., Raben, A., Stender, S. and Astrup, A. (2005), Effect of sucrose on inflammatory markers in overweight humans, *Am J Clin Nutr*, 82, 421–7.

Stanhope, K. L. (2009), Consuming fructose-sweetened, not glucose-sweetened, beverages increases visceral adiposity and lipids and decreases insulin sensitivity in overweight/obese humans, *J Clin Invest*, 119, 1322–34.

Stanhope, K. L. (2012), Role of fructose-containing sugars in the epidemics of obesity and metabolic syndrome, *Ann Rev Med*, 63, 329–43.

Stanhope, K. L. and Havel, P. J. (2008), Fructose consumption: potential mechanisms for its effects to increase visceral adiposity and induce dyslipidemia and insulin resistance, *Current Opin Lipidol*, 19, 16–24.

Stanhope, K. L., Bremer, A. A., Medici, V., Nakajima, K., Ito, Y., *et al.* (2011a), Consumption of fructose and high fructose corn syrup increase postprandial triglycerides, LDL-cholesterol, and apolipoprotein-b in young men and women, *J Clin Endocrinol Metabol*, 96, E1596–E605.

Stanhope, K. L., Griffen, S. C., Bremer, A. A., Vink, R. G., Schaefer, E. J., *et al.* (2011b), Metabolic responses to prolonged consumption of glucose- and fructose-sweetened beverages are not associated with postprandial or 24-h glucose and insulin excursions, *Am J Clin Nutr*, 94, 112–19.

Tate, D. F., Turner-Mcgrievy, G., Lyons, E., Stevens, J., Erickson, K., *et al.* (2012), Replacing caloric beverages with water or diet beverages for weight loss in adults: main results of the Choose Healthy Options Consciously Everyday (CHOICE) randomized clinical trial, *Am J Clin Nutr*, 95, 555–63.

Teff, K. L., Grudziak, J., Townsend, R. R., Dunn, T. N., Grant, R. W., *et al.* (2009), Endocrine and metabolic effects of consuming fructose- and glucose-sweetened beverages with meals in obese men and women: influence of insulin resistance on plasma triglyceride responses, *J Clin Endocrinol Metab*, 94, 1562–9.

U.S. Department of Agriculture (2012), My Pyramid Equivalents Database [Online]. Beltsville, MD. Available: http://www.ars.usda.gov/Services/docs.htm?docid=17558 [accessed Jan 31, 2012].

Vartanian, L. R., Schwartz, M. B. and Brownell, K. D. (2007), Effects of soft drink consumption on nutrition and health: a systematic review and meta-analysis, *Am J Public Health*, 97, 667–75.

Westrich, B. J., Buzzard, I. M., Gatewood, L. C. and Mcgovern, P. G. (1994), Accuracy and efficiency of estimating nutrient values in commercial food products using mathematical optimization, *J Food Composit Anal*, 7, 223–39.

Westrich, B. J., Altmann, M. A. and Potthoff, S. J. (1998), Minnesota's Nutrition Coordinating Center uses mathematical optimization to estimate food nutrient values, *Interfaces*, 28, 86–99.

Yudkin, J. (1964), Dietary fat and dietary sugar in relation to ischemic heart-disease and diabetes, *Lancet*, 2, 4.

Yudkin, J. (1972), *Sweet and Dangerous: The New Facts About the Sugar You Eat As a Cause of Heart Disease, Diabetes, and Other Killers*, David McKay Co.

The impact of fruit and vegetable intake on weight management

C. S. Diep, J. Baranowski, T. Baranowski
Baylor College of Medicine, Houston, TX, USA

4.1 Introduction

Fruit and vegetables (FV) are important sources of phytochemicals (Liu, 2003), dietary fiber (Slavin, 2005), and low energy density (Drewnowski *et al.*, 2004), and their consumption may be protective against obesity (Alinia *et al.*, 2009; Boeing *et al.*, 2012; Ledoux *et al.*, 2011; Newby, 2007, 2009; Rolls *et al.*, 2004; Tohill *et al.*, 2004). Despite these potential benefits of FV consumption on human health, rates of FV intake remain low throughout the world. This chapter reviews studies published in the past ten years on the effect of FV intake on weight management in obesity prevention research. Recommendations for future research on fruit, vegetable, and weight outcomes are offered.

4.2 Importance of fruits and vegetables (FV)

FV are essential components of a healthy diet. Increasing FV consumption reduces risk of hypertension, coronary heart disease, stroke, and other chronic diseases (Boeing *et al.*, 2012), and may protect against obesity (Alinia *et al.*, 2009; Boeing *et al.*, 2012; Ledoux *et al.*, 2011; Newby, 2007, 2009; Rolls *et al.*, 2004; Tohill *et al.*, 2004). In order to prevent chronic disease, the World Health Organization and Food and Agriculture Organization recommended daily consumption of 400 grams of FV, not including starchy tubers (World Health Organization, 2003). Unfortunately, 78% of respondents from 52 countries did not meet this recommendation in 2002–2003 (Hall *et al.*, 2009).

Many FV properties, including micronutrients and non-nutritive food constituents, make FV beneficial to promoting health and preventing chronic diseases (Boeing *et al.*, 2012). Some properties have been specifically linked to weight management and obesity prevention, including phytochemicals (Mirmiran *et al.*, 2012; Murthy *et al.*, 2009; Tucci, 2010; Vincent *et al.*, 2010; Williams *et al.*, 2013), fiber (Anderson *et al.*, 2009; Babio *et al.*, 2010; Slavin, 2005), and low energy density (Drewnowski *et al.*, 2004; Ledikwe *et al.*, 2006; Pérez-Escamilla *et al.*, 2012; Rolls *et al.*, 2004).

Managing and Preventing Obesity. http://dx.doi.org/10.1533/9781782420996.2.59

4.2.1 Phytochemicals

Phytochemicals, or 'plant chemicals', are bioactive non-nutrient plant compounds that provide a range of activities from inhibiting cancer cell proliferation to protecting against oxidative damage that prevent cardiovascular disease and multiple cancers (Gullett *et al.*, 2010; Heber, 2004; Johnson, 2007; Liu, 2003, 2004; Surh, 2003). For example, lycopene, found in cooked tomatoes, has antioxidant properties linked to decreased risk of some cancers (Heber, 2004). More than 5,000 phytochemicals have been identified, and many are still unknown (Liu, 2003).

Some phytochemicals (e.g., β-carotene, β-cryptoxanthin) have been linked to obesity prevention, although the evidence is not as strong (Mirmiran *et al.*, 2012; Murthy *et al.*, 2009; Tucci, 2010; Vincent *et al.*, 2010; Williams *et al.*, 2013). Higher dietary phytochemical indexes and some phytochemicals showed potentially promising effects on appetite and weight control (Mirmiran *et al.*, 2012; Tucci, 2010). For example, pinolenic acid, found in Korean pine nuts, may suppress appetite by triggering release of the satiety hormone cholecystokinin (Pasman *et al.*, 2008; Tucci, 2010). Research is needed to determine mechanisms, magnitude of effects, and confounders in the relationship between phytochemicals and weight.

4.2.2 Fiber

Fiber has been strongly linked to reduced risk of coronary heart disease, stroke, hypertension, diabetes, and obesity (Anderson *et al.*, 2009; Slavin, 2005). Fiber includes both dietary and functional fibers. The former are the indigestible carbohydrates and lignin intrinsic in plants (e.g., fructans in foods), while the latter are the isolated, indigestible carbohydrates that physiologically benefit humans and are added or provided as supplements (e.g., isolated, manufactured, or synthetic oligosaccharides) (Anderson *et al.*, 2009; Slavin, 2005). Based on recommendations from the Institute of Medicine of the U.S. National Academy of Sciences, adequate total fiber intake ranges from 19–38 grams per day depending on age, gender, and energy intake (Anderson *et al.*, 2009; Institute of Medicine, 2005; Slavin, 2005). However, fiber intake was consistently low in the United States, where mean dietary fiber intake in 2007–2008 was 15.9 grams per day (King *et al.*, 2012).

Dietary fiber intake is thought to protect against obesity by increasing satiety (Anderson *et al.*, 2009; Babio *et al.*, 2010; Slavin, 2005), especially with diets high in fruit, vegetables, nuts, legumes, and whole grains. This link was strongly supported by observational and epidemiological studies, although experimental and clinical trials had mixed findings (Babio *et al.*, 2010). The mechanisms of action remain debated and may be related to hormonal, intrinsic, and/or colonic effects (Slavin, 2005).

4.2.3 Energy density

Energy density is the amount of energy in a given weight of food, usually measured as kilocalories per gram or kilojoules per gram (Drewnowski *et al.*, 2004; Ledikwe *et al.*, 2006; Pérez-Escamilla *et al.*, 2012). Foods with higher energy density provide more energy per gram than do foods with lower energy density. Water content decreases energy density by adding weight to food without adding calories. Dietary fiber also decreases energy density by adding weight, but little energy. Dietary fat, on the other hand, increases energy density. Most FV have high water and fiber and low fat contents, making them low in energy density.

When added to diets (without sauces and added fats), FV reduce energy density and likely influence satiety, energy intake, and weight management (Drewnowski *et al.*, 2004; Ledikwe *et al.*, 2006; Pérez-Escamilla *et al.*, 2012; Rolls *et al.*, 2004). Laboratory and clinical studies showed a positive association among dietary energy density, energy intake, and weight gain in both adults and children (Drewnowski *et al.*, 2004; Pérez-Escamilla *et al.*, 2012), but longitudinal research is needed to strengthen these findings (Drewnowski *et al.*, 2004).

4.3   FV and obesity prevention

Many obesity prevention interventions have targeted FV intake. This section investigates the extent to which FV intake increased and enhanced obesity prevention.

4.3.1   Literature search methods

We searched electronic databases of Medline, CINAHL Plus with Full Text, and PubMed for English-language, peer-reviewed journal articles on FV and obesity prevention. Per editors' request, only articles published within the last ten years were included. Search terms included fruit, vegetable, and variations of obesity prevention terms (e.g., weight management). We also examined references of included articles for additional studies.

Inclusionary criteria were (a) written in English, (b) peer-reviewed research article published between 2003 and April 2013, (c) include FV consumption as a component of the program, and (d) present weight-related and FV findings on an obesity prevention or healthy weight management program. Studies were excluded if they (a) presented findings from an obesity treatment or weight management program for individuals who were overweight or obese or (b) were literature reviews.

For each article, we extracted information on research design, sample, country, program name, program duration, diet measurements, anthropometric measurements, analyses, effects on FV consumption, effects on weight outcomes, and FV by weight outcome interactions. We also assessed risk of bias in the studies based on Cochrane (Higgins and Altman, 2008) and PRISMA guidelines (Jüni *et al.*, 2001). Risk of bias items included random sequence generation (adequacy of randomization), allocation concealment, blinding of patients and data collectors, incomplete outcome data, selective outcome reporting, and other sources of bias. All articles were independently abstracted by two abstractors (CD and TB). Interabstractor agreement was 84%. All disagreements were discussed and/or rechecked by CD.

4.3.2   Literature search results

We screened 158 articles, of which 25 met inclusionary and exclusionary criteria and were included in the final sample (Figure 4.1). Over 40% of screened studies were excluded because they did not test an obesity prevention or healthy weight management program. An additional 30.4% did not present data on FV consumption or a weight-related outcome. Study details and findings of the final sample are provided in Table 4.1.

Of the included studies, a majority ($n=18$) were conducted in the United States, but there was also representation from Germany ($n=2$), England ($n=2$), New Zealand ($n=1$), the Netherlands ($n=1$), and Australia ($n=1$). Included programs lasted between three weeks to 2.5 years, and targeted children or adolescents ($n=11$), adults ($n=8$), or both children and adults ($n=6$). Each study tested a different program, although two programs were similar for different age groups. Most studies ($n=23$) employed a randomized controlled design. One had a one-group nonexperimental design and another had a nonrandomized control design.

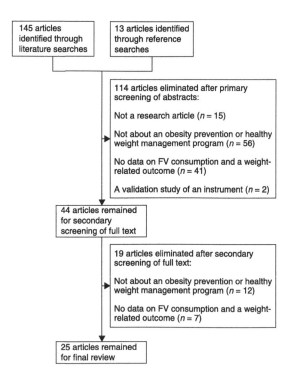

Figure 4.1 Literature search selection process for retrieving articles on FV and weight management.

Table 4.1 Summary of research studies' findings

First author	Pub Year	Title Primary	Effects on FV consumption	Effects on weight outcomes
Bayer, O	2009	Short- and mid-term effects of a setting based prevention program to reduce obesity risk factors in children: a cluster-randomized trial	(1) There was greater FV consumption in the intervention group both six and 18 months after initiation of the program. Significant adjustable odds ratios for high fruit consumption was 1.64 for sample 1, and for high fruit and vegetable consumption were 1.59 and 1.48, respectively, for sample 2 after 18 months. (2) Program's effects on FV consumption for normal weight versus overweight children were similar.	There was a strong trend to less overweight and obesity in the intervention group, but this was not statistically significant.
Branscum, P	2013	A true challenge for any superhero: an evaluation of a comic book obesity prevention program	FV consumption (in servings) significantly improved over time from pretest to posttest to follow-up for experimental (3.41 to 4.68 to 4.62 servings, respectively) and comparison (3.35 to 4.15 to 4.91 servings, respectively). The reported effect size (Cohen's f) was 0.20.	There were no significant differences for BMI percentile for the interaction (group-by-time).
Chen, JL	2010	Efficacy of a child-centered and family-based program in promoting healthy weight and healthy behaviors in Chinese American children: a randomized controlled study	Significantly more of the children in the intervention group increased FV intake over time (effect=0.306) than in the control group.	(1) Significantly more of the children in the intervention group decreased their BMI over time (effect=−0.150) than in the control group. (2) There were no statistical differences in waist-to-hip ratio between intervention and control.

(Continued overleaf)

Table 4.1 Continued

First author	Pub Year	Title Primary	Effects on FV consumption	Effects on weight outcomes
Chen, JL	2011	The efficacy of the web-based childhood obesity prevention program in Chinese American adolescents (Web ABC study)	Significantly more adolescents in intervention group increased FV intake (effect size=0.14).	Significantly more adolescents in intervention group decreased their waist-to-hip ratio (effect size=−0.01).
De Bock, F	2012	Positive impact of a pre-school-based nutritional intervention on children's fruit and vegetable intake: results of a cluster-randomized trial	There was a significant change in FV intake between pre-intervention and post-intervention (mean increase of 0.17 points on the 6-point ordinal scale for fruit consumption frequency and 0.22 points in vegetable consumption), unadjusted for other characteristics.	There were no significant effects on BMI, waist-to-height-ratio, or skinfold sum.
Foster, GD	2008	A policy-based school intervention to prevent overweight and obesity	Students in both intervention and control schools showed similar decreases in FV consumption after 2 years (unadjusted change = −1.05 FV per day for control and −1.09 for intervention); thus there was no difference between intervention and control.	(1) Significantly fewer children in the intervention schools than in control schools became overweight after 2 years (odds ratio=0.67). (2) There were no differences between intervention and control schools in obesity incidence. (3) Prevalence of overweight was lower in the intervention schools (odds ratio=0.65).
French, SA	2010	Worksite environment intervention to prevent obesity among metropolitan transit workers	FV intake increased significantly in intervention garages when compared to control garages (intervention effect=0.25).	Intervention effect on garage mean BMI change was not significant.

Gentile, DA	2009	Evaluation of a multiple ecological level child obesity prevention program: switch what you Do, View, and Chew	(1) There were significant differences in experimental and control for parent-reported FV servings per day at immediate post-intervention (Cohen's d = 1.36) and 6-months post intervention (Cohen's d = 1.01). (2) There were marginally significant differences in experimental and control for child-reported FV servings per day at immediate post-intervention (Cohen's d = 0.52) and significant differences at 6-months post intervention (Cohen's d = 0.26).	At both post-intervention and 6 months post-intervention, the mean BMI values were not significantly different between the treatment and control groups.
Gephart, EF	2013	Use of prevention and prevention plus weight management guidelines for youth with developmental disabilities living in group homes	The mean number of FV servings consumed daily increased significantly across the study period (2.92 at baseline to 4.13 at month 4).	There was a significant decrease in mean BMI percentile (56.39 at baseline to 52.23 at month 4), primarily from change in the healthy weight category (57.39 at baseline to 50.43 at month 4).
Gow, RW	2010	Preventing weight gain in first year college students: an online intervention to prevent the 'freshman fifteen'	There were no differences among groups in FV intake.	The combined intervention group had significantly lower BMI scores than the control group (means = 24.13 versus 24.56, respectively), but there were no differences between intervention, feedback, and control groups.

(Continued overleaf)

Table 4.1 Continued

First author	Pub Year	Title Primary	Effects on FV consumption	Effects on weight outcomes
Haire-Joshu, D	2008	High 5 for Kids: the impact of a home visiting program on fruit and vegetable intake of parents and their preschool children	(1) H5-KIDS parents significantly improved FV intake when compared to controls (adjusted intervention effect=0.20). (2) For preschoolers, combined FV servings increased in normal weight (adjusted intervention effect=0.34) but not overweight children relative to controls. Normal weight intervention children were more likely than controls to increase their FV intake.	
Hoffman, JA	2011	Decaying behavioral effects in a randomized, multi-year fruit and vegetable intake intervention	Children in the experimental group consumed more fruit compared with children in the control in Year 1 (mean of 45 grams versus 27, respectively) and Year 2 (34 vs. 23), and children in the experimental group consumed more vegetables than children in the control in Year 1 (17 grams versus 8), Year 2 (15 vs. 8), and Year 3 (16 versus 11). There were no differences in FV consumption at follow-up.	BMI did not differ between experimental and control group children during any post-intervention year.

Kennedy, BM	2009	The 'Rolling Store': an economical and environmental approach to the prevention of weight gain in African American women	In the intervention group, number of FV servings significantly increased (mean change of 1.0 fruit/fruit juice servings per day and 0.9 vegetable servings). There was also a significant mean difference between control and treatment groups in FV change. The control did not change mean fruit/fruit juice servings per day, and decreased 0.2 in vegetable servings.	Participants in intervention group, when compared to the control, lost significantly more weight (mean change of 1.1 kg in the control vs. −2.0 in the intervention) and BMI (0.4 in the control vs. −0.7 in the intervention).
Kim, Y	2010	Telephone intervention promoting weight-related health behaviors	Those in the SH+C group increased FV consumption from baseline to 6-month follow-up more than those in the SH group (mean change of 1.13 servings of FV per day for SH+C vs. 0.88 for SH).	(1) There was no significant difference in weight management between the SH and SH+C groups. (2) Among the overweight and obese participants, weight loss was significant in both SH and SH+C groups (1.23 kg change among overweight and 2.85 kg change among obese).
LaChausse, RG	2012	My Student Body: effects of an internet-based prevention program to decrease obesity among college students	Frequency of FV consumption increased for the online (MSB-Nutrition) group (mean of 2.67 to 3.37 for fruit and 2.40 to 2.80 for vegetable) but not for the other groups.	There was no change in BMI among participants in any group.

(Continued overleaf)

Table 4.1 Continued

First author	Pub Year	Title Primary	Effects on FV consumption	Effects on weight outcomes
Luszczynska, A	2009	Changing nutrition, physical activity and body weight among student nurses and midwives: effects of a planning intervention and self-efficacy beliefs	The intervention had a medium effect on FV consumption (Cohen's d=0.51).	Study groups did not differ in their BMI, but there were significant effects among overweight or obese participants in the treatment group ($\eta^2 = 0.06$).
Neumark-Sztainer, D	2009	'Ready. Set. ACTION!' A theater-based obesity prevention program for children: a feasibility study	According to preliminary analyses for impact evaluation, there were no statistical differences in FV consumption between intervention and control groups.	According to preliminary analyses for impact evaluation, there were no statistical differences in BMI between intervention and control groups.
Østbye, T	2012	Parent-focused change to prevent obesity in preschoolers: results from the KAN-DO study	The percentage of mothers eating 5 or more FV a day increased in the intervention when compared to the control (mean change of 8.4% vs. 0.0%, respectively).	Change in maternal weight was not statistically different between groups.
Rosenkranz, RR	2010	A group-randomized control-led trial for health promotion in Girl Scouts: healthier troops in a SNAP (Scouting Nutrition & Activity Program)	There were no significant main intervention effects for FV consumption.	There were no significant main intervention effects for girl or parent BMI.

Siegel, JM	2010	A worksite obesity intervention: results from a group-randomized trial	There was no significant difference between intervention and control groups for FV consumption.	(1) The intervention resulted in a significant change in BMI: school employees reduced their BMI in intervention schools (−0.14), whereas employees in control schools increased their BMI (+0.42). (2) There was no significant difference between intervention and control groups for waist-hip ratio.
Spiegel, SA	2006	Reducing overweight through a multidisciplinary school-based intervention	There was an increase in FV consumption in both groups, with a notably higher increase in the intervention group.	There were significant shifts in BMI in the intervention group, particularly a 2% reduction in overweight youth in the intervention group.
Taylor, RW	2007	APPLE Project: 2-y findings of a community-based obesity prevention program in primary school age children	Intervention children, when compared to control, consumed more servings of fruit (difference = 0.8 servings), but there was no effect on vegetables.	Mean BMI z score was significantly lower in intervention children than in control children by 0.09. However, prevalence of overweight was not different between groups.

(Continued overleaf)

Table 4.1 Continued

First author	Pub Year	Title Primary	Effects on FV consumption	Effects on weight outcomes
van Wier, MF	2009	Phone and e-mail counselling are effective for weight management in an overweight working population: a randomized controlled trial	There were no intervention effects on FV consumption.	The completers in the phone group and internet group had a significant weight loss (1.6 kg and 1.1 kg, respectively) and waist circumference loss (1.9 cm and 1.2 cm, respectively) in comparison to the control group. The phone group appeared to have larger changes than the internet group, but there were no statistically significant differences.
Warren, JM	2003	Evaluation of a pilot school programme aimed at the prevention of obesity in children	Overall, there was a significant increase in FV consumption. By group, there was a significant increase in fruit consumption in the Eat Smart (nutrition) (from 5.9 average weekly frequency to 6.6) and Be Smart (control) (from 5.1 to 6.6) groups.	There were no significant changes in overweight or obesity rates. There were also no significant differences in BMI between groups.
Zask, A	2012	Tooty Fruity Vegie: an obesity prevention intervention evaluation in Australian preschools	In comparison to controls, children in intervention preschools significantly had more FV serves in their lunch boxes (difference = 0.61 serves).	In comparison to controls, children in intervention preschools significantly had decrease in waist circumference growth (difference = −0.80) and reduction in BMI Z scores (difference = −0.15).

4.3.2.1   Risk of bias

For numerous studies, risk of bias and quality were difficult to measure because of unavailable or unclear information. Based on the information available, 10 studies were considered to have low risk of bias (Chen *et al.*, 2010, 2011; Gow *et al.*, 2010; Kennedy *et al.*, 2009; Kim *et al.*, 2010; LaChausse, 2012; Luszczynska and Haynes, 2009; Østbye *et al.*, 2012; Rosenkranz *et al.*, 2010; Zask *et al.*, 2012), nine had moderate risk (Bayer *et al.*, 2009; De Bock *et al.*, 2012; Gentile *et al.*, 2009; Gephart and Loman, 2013; Haire-Joshu *et al.*, 2008; Hoffman *et al.*, 2011; Neumark-Sztainer *et al.*, 2009; Siegel *et al.*, 2010; van Wier *et al.*, 2009), and six had high risk (Branscum *et al.*, 2013; Foster *et al.*, 2008; French *et al.*, 2010; Spiegel and Foulk, 2006; Taylor *et al.*, 2007; Warren *et al.*, 2003).

Nine studies reported randomization by a computer, random number tables, or permuted blocks. Of these nine studies, concealment of allocation sequence was unclear in six studies (making risk of selection bias unclear), was performed in one study (making risk of selection bias low), and was not performed in two studies (making risk of selection bias moderate). Fourteen studies did not specify their method of random sequence generation, of which five studies did not conceal alloc-ation sequence (making risk of selection bias high) and nine studies did not specify concealing allocation sequence (making risk of selection bias unclear). One study was nonrandomized and did not conceal allocation sequence, so risk of selection bias was high. The remaining study had only one group, so allocation concealment was not applicable. Most studies with no concealment of allocation sequence randomized their sample at the group (e.g., school) level, so recruiters were aware of participants' allocation during recruitment.

Thirteen studies did not specify whether data collectors or participants were blinded, so risks of performance and detection bias were unclear. Aside from these, three studies reported not blinding participants to group allocation, so risk of performance bias was high. In two of these three studies, the non-blinded participants provided outcome measures so risk of detection bias was also high, and in the third study, risk of detection bias was unclear. Two studies had low risk of performance bias because there was an objective outcome measure (e.g., lunch box audits) or parti-cipants were blinded, and detection bias was also low in both studies. Five studies indicated that study staff were blinded or that a third party (e.g., a research assistant) collected data, so risk of detection bias was low. Risk of performance bias in these studies was unclear. One study had an unclear risk of performance bias and a high risk of detection bias (the research team was not blinded). Lastly, in the remaining study, there was only one group, and blinding was not applicable.

Most studies reported missing data at follow-up. Eleven studies were judged to have low risk of attrition bias because retention rates were high (i.e., above 80%). Twelve studies had low retention rates, so they were considered to have high risk of attrition bias. In the remaining two studies, attrition rates were unclear. In addition, most studies appeared to report complete data, so there was low risk of reporting bias. For two studies, there was insufficient evidence to determine if there was selective reporting.

Other potential sources of bias were identified. In all but one study, the method of diet and/or weight assessment was self report. In addition, ten studies had limited statistical power because of small sample sizes. Other potential sources of bias were intervention and control groups not being equally matched at baseline, analyses not accounting for clustering at group levels in group randomized studies, and some studies not having a control group.

4.3.2.2 Effects on FV consumption

Nineteen of 25 studies reported positive effects on increasing fruit and/or vegetable consumption (Bayer *et al.*, 2009; Branscum *et al.*, 2013; Chen *et al.*, 2010, 2011; De Bock *et al.*, 2012; French *et al.*, 2010; Gentile *et al.*, 2009; Gephart and Loman, 2013; Haire-Joshu *et al.*, 2008; Hoffman *et al.*, 2011; Kennedy *et al.*, 2009; Kim *et al.*, 2010; LaChausse, 2012; Luszczynska and Haynes, 2009; Østbye *et al.*, 2012; Spiegel and Foulk, 2006; Taylor *et al.*, 2007; Warren *et al.*, 2003; Zask *et al.*, 2012), while five revealed no FV effects (Gow *et al.*, 2010; Neumark-Sztainer *et al.*, 2009; Rosenkranz *et al.*, 2010; Siegel *et al.*, 2010; van Wier *et al.*, 2009). One study detected decreased FV consumption (Foster *et al.*, 2008). There appeared to be similarities in FV consumption effects between studies with low risk, moderate risk, and high risk of bias.

When separated by target population (i.e., children or adolescents versus adults), there appeared to be more success in increasing FV consumption in children and adolescents than adults. Of the 17 children or adolescent interventions, 70.6% (n = 12) reported positive effects on FV consumption in children (Bayer *et al.*, 2009; Branscum *et al.*, 2013; Chen *et al.*, 2010; 2011; De Bock *et al.*, 2012; Gentile *et al.*, 2009; Gephart and Loman, 2013; Hoffman *et al.*, 2011; Spiegel and Foulk, 2006; Taylor *et al.*, 2007; Warren *et al.*, 2003; Zask *et al.*, 2012). Of the 14 interventions with adults, 57.1% (n = 8) reported positive effects in adults (French *et al.*, 2010; Gentile *et al.*, 2009; Haire-Joshu *et al.*, 2008; Kennedy *et al.*, 2009; Kim *et al.*, 2010; LaChausse, 2012; Luszczynska and Haynes, 2009; Østbye *et al.*, 2012).

4.3.2.3 Effects on weight outcomes

There were mixed results regarding effects on BMI, weight, or similar weight outcome. Thirteen studies (52.0%) reported statistically significant decreases in a weight outcome (Chen *et al.*, 2010, 2011; Foster *et al.*, 2008; Gephart and Loman, 2013; Gow *et al.*, 2010; Kennedy *et al.*, 2009; Kim *et al.*, 2010; Luszczynska and Haynes, 2009; Siegel *et al.*, 2010; Spiegel and Foulk, 2006; Taylor *et al.*, 2007; van Wier *et al.*, 2009; Zask *et al.*, 2012). There appeared to be similar weight outcome effects in children and adults.

When separated by risk of bias, there appeared to be most success in improving weight outcomes in studies with low risk of bias and least success in studies with moderate risk of bias. Seventy percent (n = 7) of studies with low risk of bias (Chen *et al.*, 2010, 2011; Gow *et al.*, 2010; Kennedy *et al.*, 2009; Kim *et al.*, 2010; Luszczynska and Haynes, 2009; Zask *et al.*, 2012), 33.3% (n = 3) with moderate risk (Gephart and Loman, 2013; Siegel *et al.*, 2010; van Wier *et al.*, 2009), and 50%

(n = 3) with high risk (Foster *et al.*, 2008; Spiegel and Foulk, 2006; Taylor *et al.*, 2007) reported statistically significant decreases in weight outcome.

4.3.2.4   Interaction between FV consumption and weight outcomes

Two studies statistically tested interactions between FV intake and weight outcomes. One study (Bayer *et al.*, 2009) performed cluster-randomized multivariate analysis to determine intervention effects in normal versus overweight subgroups. The study found similar effects on FV consumption for non-overweight and overweight children, suggesting that change in FV intake did not influence change in adiposity. In contrast, another study (Haire-Joshu *et al.*, 2008) found that normal weight intervention, when compared to control children, were 1.49 times more likely to increase their FV intake by at least half a serving per day (based on logistic regression analysis and baseline BMI). No results were reported on changes in weight outcomes.

Although none of the studies specifically tested whether the extent to which FV change contributed to adiposity change, for FV to have contributed to weight control, a study would have had to document a change in FV intake and enhanced weight control. Nine studies had effects on both FV consumption and weight outcomes (Chen *et al.*, 2010, 2011; Gephart and Loman, 2013; Kennedy *et al.*, 2009; Kim *et al.*, 2010; Luszczynska and Haynes, 2009; Spiegel and Foulk, 2006; Taylor *et al.*, 2007; Zask *et al.*, 2012); another ten studies reported effects on FV consumption, but not on weight outcomes (Bayer *et al.*, 2009; Branscum *et al.*, 2013; De Bock *et al.*, 2012; French *et al.*, 2010; Gentile *et al.*, 2009; Haire-Joshu *et al.*, 2008; Hoffman *et al.*, 2011; LaChausse, 2012; Østbye *et al.*, 2012; Warren *et al.*, 2003); and four reported effects on weight outcomes, but not FV consumption (Foster *et al.*, 2008; Gow *et al.*, 2010; Siegel *et al.*, 2010; van Wier *et al.*, 2009). Because none of the studies that reported changes in FV and weight used mediating variable analysis (Fairchild and MacKinnon, 2009) or controlled for other confounders to determine the overall effect of FV on weight, there are no clear, causal conclusions that can be made about the relationship between FV and weight management.

4.4   Future trends

This chapter aimed to identify studies of the impact of increased FV intake on weight management in obesity prevention research. Twenty-five articles were identified. No study specifically tested (as in a mediating variable analysis (Fairchild and MacKinnon, 2009)) whether increased FV intake contributed to obesity prevention or weight management. Only 36% of programs had effects on both FV consumption and a weight outcome. An additional 56% reported effects on either weight outcomes or FV consumption, but not both. Eight percent affected neither FV intake nor weight management.

Based on these findings, it is unclear whether increasing FV intake enhanced obesity prevention, which is consistent with prior reviews on FV and body weight/ weight management (Alinia *et al.*, 2009; Boeing *et al.*, 2012; Ledoux *et al.*, 2011;

Rolls *et al.*, 2004; Sherry, 2005; Tohill *et al.*, 2004). Most of the programs detecting an effect on weight also targeted factors other than FV (e.g., physical activity or other food consumption), so the effects on weight outcomes may have been related to multiple behavior changes. Isolating the specific effects of FV on weight outcomes from these studies was difficult, if not impossible. Thus, although it is important to have comprehensive and holistic programs, more research is needed on programs focused solely on FV to determine if targeting FV is effective in weight management programs. Relatedly, only two studies reported interactions between FV intake and weight outcomes, so it is unclear what the relationship is between FV and weight. Analyses are needed to examine this relationship by controlling for other aspects of diet or lifestyle.

Increased attention to reduced risk of bias is needed in future such studies. Although randomization was performed in most studies, the methods of random sequence generation and allocation concealment were not specified, making risk of selection bias unclear. In addition, more than half of studies did not indicate whether data collectors or participants were blinded, which has implications for detection and performance biases. Blinding study staff should be done whenever possible. Lastly, all but one study relied primarily on self-reported measures of diet and/or weight management. These sources of data may not be valid. More effort is needed to complement self-reported data with observations, biomarkers, or other more objective measures (Jia *et al.*, 2012).

Although this chapter and other similar reviews revealed weak evidence supporting the relationship between FV and weight management, it is important for future research, especially longitudinal studies, to continue investigating the specific effects of FV on weight, either through controlled experiments on only FV or using analyses that control for other confounders. Such research should clarify the role of FV in weight management, thus informing future obesity-related interventions and the extent to which they should target FV consumption. In addition, findings from this review do not negate the important contribution of FV to a healthy diet, and FV should continue to be a major focus in public health and medical efforts.

4.5   Sources of further information

Prior literature reviews have examined the relationship between FV and body weight/ weight management. For further information and advice, please consult these reviews.

Alinia, S., Hels, O. and Tetens, I. (2009).
Boeing, H., Bechthold, A., Bub, A., Ellinger, S., Haller, D., *et al.* (2012).
Ledoux, T.A., Hingle, M.D. and Baranowski, T. (2011).
Newby, P.K. (2007).
Newby, P. (2009).
Rolls, B.J., Ello-Martin, J. and Tohill, B.C. (2004).
Sherry, B. (2005).
Tohill, B.C., Seymour, J., Serdula, M., Kettel-Khan, L. and Rolls, B.J. (2004).

References

Alinia, S., Hels, O. and Tetens, I. (2009) 'The potential association between fruit intake and body weight – a review.', *Obes Rev*, 10, 639–647.

Anderson, J.W., Baird, P., Davis, R.H., Ferreri, S., Knudtson, M., *et al.* (2009) 'Health benefits of dietary fiber', *Nutr Rev*, 67, 188–205.

Babio, N., Balanza, R., Basulto, J., Bullo, M. and Salas-Salvado, J. (2010) 'Dietary fibre: Influence on body weight, glycemic control and plasma cholesterol profile', *Nutr Hosp*, 25, 327–340.

Bayer, O., von Kries, R., Strauss, A., Mitschek, C., Toschke, A.M., *et al.* (2009) 'Short- and mid-term effects of a setting based prevention program to reduce obesity risk factors in children: a cluster-randomized trial', *Clin Nutr*, 28, 122–128.

Boeing, H., Bechthold, A., Bub, A., Ellinger, S., Haller, D., *et al.* (2012) 'Critical review: vegetables and fruit in the prevention of chronic diseases', *Eur J Nutr*, 51, 637–663.

Branscum, P., Sharma, M., Wang, L.L., Wilson, B.R.A. and Rojas-Guyler, L. (2013) 'A true challenge for any superhero: an evaluation of a comic book obesity prevention program', *Fam Community Health*, 36, 63–76.

Chen, J.L., Weiss, S., Heyman, M.B. and Lustig, R.H. (2010) 'Efficacy of a child-centred and family-based program in promoting healthy weight and healthy behaviors in Chinese American children: a randomized controlled study', *J Public Health*, 32, 219–229.

Chen, J.L., Weiss, S., Heyman, M.B., Cooper, B. and Lustig, R.H. (2011) 'The efficacy of the web-based childhood obesity prevention program in Chinese American adolescents (Web ABC study)', *J Adolesc Health*, 49, 148–154.

De Bock, F., Breitenstein, L. and Fischer, J.E. (2012) 'Positive impact of a pre-school-based nutritional intervention on children's fruit and vegetable intake: results of a cluster-randomized trial', *Public Health Nutr*, 15, 466–475.

Drewnowski, A., Almiron-Roig, E., Marmonier, C. and Lluch, A. (2004) 'Dietary energy density and body weight: is there a relationship?', *Nutr Rev*, 62, 403–413.

Fairchild, A.J. and MacKinnon, D.P. (2009) 'A general model for testing mediation and moderation effects', *Prev Sci*, 10, 87–99.

Foster, G.D., Sherman, S., Borradaile, K.E., Grundy, K.M., Vander Veur, S., *et al.* (2008) 'A policy-based school intervention to prevent overweight and obesity', *Pediatrics*, 121, e794–802.

French, S.A., Harnack, L.J., Hannan, P.J., Mitchell, N.R., Gerlach, A.F. and Toomey, T.L. (2010) 'Worksite environment intervention to prevent obesity among metropolitan transit workers', *Prev Med*, 50, 180–185.

Gentile, D.A., Welk, G., Eisenmann, J.C., Reimer, R.A., Walsh, D.A., *et al.* (2009) 'Evaluation of a multiple ecological level child obesity prevention program: switch what you Do, View, and Chew', *BMC Med*, 7, 49.

Gephart, E.F. and Loman, D.G. (2013) 'Use of prevention and prevention plus weight management guidelines for youth with developmental disabilities living in group homes', *J Pediatr Health Care*, 27, 98–108.

Gow, R.W., Trace, S.E. and Mazzeo, S.E. (2010) 'Preventing weight gain in first year college students: an online intervention to prevent the "freshman fifteen" ', *Eat Behav*, 11, 33–39.

Gullett, N.P., Ruhul Amin, A., Bayraktar, S., Pezzuto, J.M., Shin, D.M., *et al.* (2010) 'Cancer prevention with natural compounds', *Semin Oncol*, 37, 258–281.

Haire-Joshu, D., Elliott, M.B., Caito, N.M., Hessler, K., Nanney, M.S., *et al.* (2008) 'High 5 for Kids: the impact of a home visiting program on fruit and vegetable intake of parents and their preschool children', *Prev Med*, 47, 77–82.

Hall, J.N., Moore, S., Harper, S.B. and Lynch, J.W. (2009) 'Global variability in fruit and vegetable consumption', *Am J Prev Med*, 36, 402–409.

Heber, D. (2004) 'Vegetables, fruits and phytoestrogens in the prevention of diseases', *J Postgrad Med*, 50, 145–149.

Higgins, J.P.T. and Altman, D.G. (2008) 'Assessing risk of bias in included studies', in Higgins JPT and Green S (eds.), *Cochrane Handbook for Systematic Reviews of Interventions*, West Sussex, England, John Wiley & Sons, 187–242.

Hoffman, J.A., Thompson, D.R., Franko, D.L., Power, T.J., Leff, S.S. and Stallings, V.A. (2011) 'Decaying behavioral effects in a randomized, multi-year fruit and vegetable intake intervention', *Prev Med*, 52, 370–375.

Institute of Medicine (2005) *Dietary Reference Intakes for Energy, Carbohydrate, Fiber, Fat, Fatty Acids, Cholesterol, Protein, and Amino Acids*, Washington, DC, The National Academies Press.

Jia, W., Yue, Y., Fernstrom, J.D., Zhang, Z., Yang, Y. and Sun, M. (2012) '3D localization of circular feature in 2D image and application to food volume estimation', *Conf Proc IEEE Eng Med Biol Soc*, 2012, 4545–4548.

Johnson, I.T. (2007) 'Phytochemicals and cancer', *Proc Nutr Soc*, 66, 207–215.

Jüni, P., Altman, D.G. and Egger, M. (2001) 'Systematic reviews in health care: assessing the quality of controlled clinical trials', *BMJ*, 323, 42–46.

Kennedy, B.M., Champagne, C.M., Ryan, D.H., Newton, R., Conish, B.K., *et al.*, Lower Mississippi Delta Nutrition Intervention Research and Initiative (2009) 'The "Rolling Store" an economical and environmental approach to the prevention of weight gain in African American women', *Ethn Dis*, 19, 7–12.

Kim, Y., Pike, J., Adams, H., Cross, D., Doyle, C. and Foreyt, J. (2010) 'Telephone intervention promoting weight-related health behaviors', *Prev Med*, 50, 112–117.

King, D.E., Mainous, A.G. and Lambourne, C.A. (2012) 'Trends in dietary fiber intake in the United States, 1999–2008', *J Acad Nutr Diet*, 112, 642–648.

LaChausse, R.G. (2012) 'My student body: effects of an internet-based prevention program to decrease obesity among college students', *J Am Coll Health*, 60, 324–330.

Ledikwe, J.H., Blanck, H.M., Khan, L.K., Serdula, M.K., Seymour, J.D., *et al.* (2006) 'Dietary energy density is associated with energy intake and weight status in US adults', *Am J Clin Nutr*, 83, 1362–1368.

Ledoux, T.A., Hingle, M.D. and Baranowski, T. (2011) 'Relationship of fruit and vegetable intake with adiposity: a systematic review', *Obes Rev*, 12, e143–150.

Liu, R.H. (2003) 'Health benefits of fruit and vegetables are from additive and synergistic combinations of phytochemicals', *Am J Clin Nutr*, 78, S517–520.

Liu, R.H. (2004) 'Potential synergy of phytochemicals in cancer prevention: mechanism of action', *J Nutr*, 134, S3479–3485.

Luszczynska, A. and Haynes, C. (2009) 'Changing nutrition, physical activity and body weight among student nurses and midwives: effects of a planning intervention and self-efficacy beliefs', *J Health Psychol*, 14, 1075–1084.

Mirmiran, P., Bahadoran, Z., Golzarand, M., Shiva, N. and Azizi, F. (2012) 'Association between dietary phytochemical index and 3-year changes in weight, waist circumference and body adiposity index in adults: Tehran Lipid and Glucose study', *Nutr Metab*, 9, 108.

Murthy, N.S., Mukherjee, S., Ray, G. and Ray, A. (2009) 'Dietary factors and cancer chemoprevention: an overview of obesity-related malignancies', *J Postgrad Med*, 55, 45–54.

Neumark-Sztainer, D., Haines, J., Robinson-O'Brien, R., Hannan, P.J., Robins, M., *et al.* (2009) ' "Ready. Set. ACTION!" A theater-based obesity prevention program for children: a feasibility study', *Health Educ Res*, 24, 407–420.

Newby, P.K. (2007) 'Are dietary intakes and eating behaviors related to childhood obesity? A comprehensive review of the evidence', *J Law Med Ethics*, 35, 35–60.

Newby, P. (2009) 'Plant foods and plant-based diets: Protective against childhood obesity?', *Am J Clin Nutr*, 89, S1572–1587.

Østbye, T., Krause, K.M., Stroo, M., Lovelady, C.A., Evenson, K.R., *et al.* (2012) 'Parent-focused change to prevent obesity in preschoolers: results from the KAN-DO study', *Prev Med*, 55, 188–195.

Pasman, W.J., Heimerikx, J., Rubingh, C.M., van den Berg, R., O'Shea, M., *et al.* (2008) 'The effect of Korean pine nut oil on in vitro CCK release, on appetite sensations and on gut hormones in post-menopausal overweight women', *Lipids Health Dis*, 7, 10.

Pérez-Escamilla, R., Obbagy, J.E., Altman, J.M., Essery, E.V., McGrane, M.M., *et al.* (2012) 'Dietary energy density and body weight in adults and children: a systematic review', *J Acad Nutr Diet*, 112, 671–684.

Rolls, B., Ello Martin, J. and Tohill, B. (2004) 'What can intervention studies tell us about the relationship between fruit and vegetable consumption and weight management?', *Nutr Rev*, 62, 1–17.

Rosenkranz, R.R., Behrens, T.K. and Dzewaltowski, D.A. (2010) 'A group-randomized controlled trial for health promotion in Girl Scouts: healthier troops in a SNAP (Scouting Nutrition & Activity Program)', *BMC Public Health*, 10, 81.

Sherry, B. (2005) 'Food behaviors and other strategies to prevent and treat pediatric overweight', *Int J Obes*, 29, S116–126.

Siegel, J.M., Prelip, M.L., Erausquin, J.T. and Kim, S.A. (2010) 'A worksite obesity intervention: results from a group-randomized trial', *Am J Public Health*, 100, 327–333.

Slavin, J.L. (2005) 'Dietary fiber and body weight', *Nutrition*, 21, 411–418.

Spiegel, S.A. and Foulk, D. (2006) 'Reducing overweight through a multidisciplinary school-based intervention', *Obesity*, 14, 88–96.

Surh, Y.J. (2003) 'Cancer chemoprevention with dietary phytochemicals', *Nat Rev Cancer*, 3, 768–780.

Taylor, R.W., McAuley, K.A., Barbezat, W., Strong, A., Williams, S.M. and Mann, J.I. (2007) 'APPLE Project: 2–y findings of a community-based obesity prevention program in primary school age children', *Am J Clin Nutr*, 86, 735–742.

Tohill, B.C., Seymour, J., Serdula, M., Kettel-Khan, L. and Rolls, B.J. (2004) 'What epidemiologic studies tell us about the relationship between fruit and vegetable consumption and body weight', *Nutr Rev*, 62, 365–374.

Tucci, S.A. (2010) 'Phytochemicals in the control of human appetite and body weight', *Pharmaceuticals*, 3, 748–763.

van Wier, M.F., Ariëns, G.A.M., Dekkers, J.C., Hendriksen, I.J.M., Smid, T. and van Mechelen, W. (2009) 'Phone and e-mail counselling are effective for weight management in an overweight working population: a randomized controlled trial', *BMC Public Health*, 9, 6.

Vincent, H.K., Bourguignon, C.M. and Taylor, A.G. (2010) 'Relationship of the dietary phytochemical index to weight gain, oxidative stress and inflammation in overweight young adults', *J Hum Nutr Diet*, 23, 20–29.

Warren, J.M., Henry, C.J.K., Lightowler, H.J., Bradshaw, S.M. and Perwaiz, S. (2003) 'Evaluation of a pilot school programme aimed at the prevention of obesity in children', *Health Promot Int*, 18, 287–296.

Williams, D.J., Edwards, D., Hamernig, I., Jian, L., James, A.P., *et al.* (2013) 'Vegetables containing phytochemicals with potential anti-obesity properties: a review', *Food Research International*, 52, 323–333.

World Health Organization (2003) *Diet, Nutrition and the Prevention of Chronic Diseases: Report of a joint WHO/FAO expert consultation*, Geneva, World Health Organization.

Zask, A., Adams, J.K., Brooks, L.O. and Hughes, D.F. (2012) 'Tooty Fruity Vegie: an obesity prevention intervention evaluation in Australian preschools', *Health Promot J Austr*, 23, 10–15.

High protein diets in obesity management and weight control

N. D. Luscombe-Marsh
CSIRO Animal, Food and Health Sciences, VIC, Australia

5.1   Introduction

There is no single diet that will help, or suit the lifestyle, of every individual. Some weight management diets are however much better than others because they are nutritionally balanced and produce sustained weight loss that is associated with greater metabolic improvements, including the substantial lowering of blood pressure and blood glucose, insulin, bad (i.e. low-density lipoprotein) cholesterol and triglycerides levels. In fact, some diets provide metabolic benefits that can be seen with as little as 5–10% loss of initial weight, proving that you do not have to become 'skinny' to enjoy better physical and mental health.

A persisting question, often asked, is what nutritionally balanced dietary pattern can help you to control your weight and improve your metabolic health? Research suggests a protein-rich (i.e. ~25–35% of daily energy requirements from mixed protein sources including plants, lean red and/or white meat, fish and dairy), low-fat, moderate carbohydrate eating plan is effective for the management of obesity, heart health and Type 2 diabetes. Much of this evidence has been underpinned by a program of high-quality research that has been performed at the Australian Commonwealth Scientific and Industrial Organisation (CSIRO) and backed by an extensive review of the scientific literature in this field. Many of these research findings have helped define the principles of the publicly acclaimed CSIRO Total Wellbeing Diet book series including *The CSIRO Total Wellbeing Diet* books 1 (Noakes, 2005) and 2 (Noakes, 2006) and the recipe book (CSIRO, 2010) which have been embraced by more than 800,000 Australians. As such, the findings from CSIRO scientists as well as others from international research teams from across Europe and the USA are influencing global management strategies for conditions related to overweight/obesity.

This chapter provides a brief background of popular higher-protein diets that are commonly used by the international dieting public and introduces the basic principles of the CSIRO Total Wellbeing Diet. It is also based on the latest international scientific evidence that demonstrates that small but consistent clinical benefits are achievable using dietary patterns that contain higher amounts of protein. Safety concerns that are often raised by clinicians about higher-protein dietary patterns are addressed briefly. The objective is to provide readers with the latest information to

Managing and Preventing Obesity. http://dx.doi.org/10.1533/9781782420996.2.79

shape their own opinion regarding the efficacy of a higher-protein dietary pattern for weight control and the management overweight/obesity and its associated disease.

5.2   Internationally popular higher-protein diets

Higher-protein diets have a long history (Denke, 2001) and the resurgence of their popularity in modern society presumably has been influenced by the marketing of books that promote varying types of higher-protein diets that promise rapid weight loss within seven days. Many people have also been encouraged to try higher-protein diets due to their poor experiences in failing to achieve and maintain clinically relevant weight loss using the more traditional modern standard-protein, high-carbohydrate, low-fat diets (Roberts, 2001). A major issue with the high-carbohydrate, low-fat diets is that people thought they could eat as much low-fat food as possible and still lose weight – they did not understand that a reduction in total energy intake was also critical. Moreover, high-carbohydrate diets are becoming increasingly controversial to use for the management of overweight/obesity, Type 2 diabetes and heart disease because a large proportion of people in Westernised countries typically consume refined carbohydrates that are quickly released into the bloodstream causing large spikes in blood glucose levels and high triglyceride levels (a form of blood fat); refined carbohydrates also are not as rich in other vital nutrients and tend to be combined with fat. These issues have led many in the scientific community to seriously question the validity of higher-carbohydrate diets for managing overweight/ obesity and its associated conditions. As such, there has been renewed interest in testing the effectiveness of alternative approaches such as higher-protein diets that replace varying amounts of carbohydrate.

The philosophy and principles of the several higher-protein diets that have been popular with the international dieting public over that last 40 years are summarised in Table 5.1. The listed diets fall into two different categories of higher-protein, low-carbohydrate diets that are referred to as: (i) very low-carbohydrate, high-protein concomitantly high in saturated fat (eg The 'Atkins' and 'Protein Power' diets; also termed *ketogenic* diets), and (ii) reduced-carbohydrate, high-protein diets that emphasise fat restriction (eg The 'Zone' and 'Sugar Busters'). While each of these higher-protein diets can assist people to lose weight, particularly those who are very disciplined with their food intake, several important points should be considered before recommending such diets to patients: (i) the initial weight loss achieved is predominately from the loss of water and lean muscle mass rather than from the loss of fat which is required for reducing disease risk factors; (ii) each of these particular dietary patterns rigidly restricts certain food groups and promotes the avoidance of many nutritious foods and do not achieve recommended allowances for all necessary macro- and micro- nutrients; and (iii) Atkins, Protein Power and the Stillman diets promote higher than recommended intakes of saturated fat (i.e. < 10% of total daily energy should come from saturated fat) which is associated strongly with increased risk factors (eg high triglycerides, total and low-density lipoprotein cholesterol, and

Table 5.1 Internationally popular higher-protein, low- to moderate-carbohydrate diets

	Atkins	Protein Power	Zone	Sugar Busters	Stillman
Philosophy	Too many carbohydrate causes obesity; ketosis leads to decreased hunger	Carbohydrates releases insulin in large quantities which contributes to obesity	Right food combinations leads to state at which body functions at peak performance; decreases hunger; increases weight loss and energy	Sugar is toxic and causes increased insulin levels which promotes fat storage	High-protein foods burn body fat; carbohydrates cause fat storage
Principle	Eat meat, fish, poultry, eggs, cheese, low-carb vegetables, butter, oil; no alcohol	Eat meat, fish, poultry, eggs, cheese, low-carb vegetables, butter, oil, salad dressing, moderate alcohol intake	Protein, fat and carbohydrates must be eaten in exact proportions at every meal (40/30/30); low glycaemic index foods; moderate alcohol intake	Eat protein and fat; low glycaemic index foods; olive oil, canola oil; moderate alcohol intake	Eat lean meats, skinless poultry, lean fish, eggs, cottage cheese, skim-milk cheeses; no alcohol
Composition	Protein 27%; carbohydrate 5%; fat 68% (saturated fat 26%)	Protein 26%; carbohydrate 16%; fat 54% (saturated fat 18%); alcohol 4%	Protein 34%; carbohydrate 36%; fat 29% (saturated fat 9%); alcohol 1%	Protein 27%; carbohydrate 52%; fat 21% (saturated fat 4%)	Protein 64%; carbohydrate 3%; fat 33% (saturated fat 13%)
Lose and maintain weight?	Yes but initial loss is mostly water. Promotes negative attitude to food groups. Difficult to maintain	Yes, via caloric restriction. Limited food choices; not practical for long term	Yes, via caloric restriction. Could achieve maintenance if followed carefully. Diet rigid	Yes, via caloric restriction. Limited food choices; not practical for long term	Yes, but mainly water lost; strict calorie counting; limited food choices; not practical for long term
Scientific evidence	No long-term validated studies	No long-term validated studies	No long-term validated studies	No long-term validated studies	No long-term validated studies
Compliance with AHA* protein criteria	No; does not achieve recommended allowance for macro- or micro-nutrients	No; does not achieve recommended allowance for macro- or micro-nutrients	Yes, but may be low in copper	No; does not achieve recommended allowance for micro-nutrients	No; does not achieve recommended allowance for macro- or micro-nutrients

*AHA denotes American Heart Association.
Source: Modified with permission from St. Jeor et al., 2001.

reduced high-density lipoprotein cholesterol and endothelial function). Despite the numerous limitations of diets like Atkins, Protein Power and Stillman, many people still insist on using them. Evidence regarding the efficacy and safety of higher-protein diets, particularly the very-low carbohydrate ketogenic style diets, for long-term management of obesity will be examined in section 5.4.

5.3   The Commonwealth Scientific and Industrial Research Organisation (CSIRO) Total Wellbeing Diet

The CSIRO Total Wellbeing Diet (TWD) is a higher-protein, nutritionally balanced 12 week weight-loss program (i.e. 30% energy restriction) followed by weight-main-tenance program that can be applied throughout all life stages. It is not a 'one diet fits all' program – rather, it is designed so it can be easily tailored to an individual's daily energy requirements to assist with achieving their personal weight-loss goals. The carbohydrate content and source are the common factors that differentiates the TWD from the more popular low-to-moderate carbohydrate and more traditional, high-carbohydrate, diets (Table 5.2); the diet contains low-to-moderate amounts of carbohydrates that release their energy slowly and maintain a lower blood glucose profile (i.e. low glycaemic index carbohydrates) (Barclay *et al.*, 2005).

Of course a reduction in the amount of carbohydrate must be offset by a moder-ate increase in another nutrient, and for the TWD approach, about 15% of the total energy originally derived from carbohydrate is replaced with protein. The rationale for increasing protein to assist with weight control is based on a range of research findings. Acute meal and short-term clinical studies have demonstrated that protein provides a greater feeling of fullness (or satisfaction) and reduces the feelings of hunger compared to a similar calorie load of carbohydrates, and energy intake at the next meal is reduced when individuals are allowed to eat freely (Westerterp-Plantenga *et al.*, 2009; Leidy and Racki, 2010). In addition, the energy cost of digest-ing, absorbing and storing protein in the body (termed the thermic effect of feeding) is much higher than that of either carbohydrate or fat (Westerterp-Plantenga *et al.*, 1999) and thus a higher-protein diet may result in a small increase in the energy being lost during this process. Higher-protein diets have also been associated with better retention of lean tissue mass (which includes muscle) during energy restric-tion (Piatti *et al.*, 1994) which has important implications for maintaining muscle mass and strength. Finally, protein-rich foods that come from mixed sources (i.e. lean red and white meat, seafood, dairy, eggs, nuts, seed and legumes) also provide many essential nutrients and minerals that are pivotal for the maintenance of health and vitality. For example, lean red meat (beef, pork and veal) is the richest source of highly-absorbed iron, and are also rich in zinc and good sources of omega-3 and vitamin B12 which play a key role in haemoglobin and antioxidant enzyme formation as well as immunity and protecting cognitive health. Seafood is an important source of omega-3 fats which protect the heart, and low-fat dairy is also rich in riboflavin (vitamin B2) and calcium. Eggs are also rich in essential vitamins (i.e. A, D, E and

Table 5.2 Amount and type of carbohydrate consumed in different diets

Diet	Amount of carbohydrate (g)	% energy (kj) from carbohydrate	Main type of carbohydrate	Amount of protein (g)	% energy (kj) from protein
High-carbohydrate diet (e.g. traditional weight-loss/ management diet)	>200	>55	Complex, low-glycaemic index	70–120	~15–20
Very-low carbohydrate (e.g. Atkins)	<100	<20	No guideline	No guideline	No guideline
Moderate to low-carbohydrate diet (e.g. TWD)	100–200	20–40	Complex, low-glycaemic index	90–140	~25–35
Average non-diet	~245	~45	Mixed	~70–120	~15–20

B-group) as well as iron, phosphorus and zinc, and are a good source of antioxidants and low in saturated fat.

While the TWD uses a highly-prescriptive daily meal plan that is designed around meeting the individuals' daily protein requirements first and foremost, it also includes plenty of whole grains, fruits and vegetables, and good fats (i.e. poly- and mono-unsaturated fats). The TWD approach also advocates that the dietary plan is followed in conjunction with about 30 minutes of moderate intensity physical activity, three times per week (this can be as simple as brisk walking). Evidence regarding the efficacy and safety of high-protein diets, including the TWD, for long-term management of obesity will be examined in section 5.4.

5.4 Evidence from meta-analyses and selected randomised control trials for the efficacy of higher-protein diets for weight control and metabolic health

5.4.1 Findings from meta-analyses of higher-protein diets followed for ≥ 1 year

Three recent meta-analyses have examined the short-term (i.e. < 1 year) effects of energy-restricted and/or ad-libitum, higher compared with lower protein diets (i.e. 16–45% vs. 5–23% of total energy from protein) on body weight management and cardio-metabolic outcomes (Santesso *et al.*, 2012; Wycherley *et al.*, 2012; Dong *et al.*, 2013). While these meta-analyses demonstrated that the magnitude of weight loss as well as improvements in several cardio-metabolic risk factors including triglycerides, HbA1c and blood pressure were of clinical relevance in obesity management, the true benefits of higher-protein diets should really be judged on their ability to sustain clinically significant weight loss over the longer-term – that is they must be able to prevent weight re-gain. The following discussion will therefore focus on the current evidence exploring whether increased dietary protein is a significant factor for long-term success in achieving and maintaining weight loss and cardio-metabolic risk reduction.

A recent meta-analysis that examined the effects of low fat diets (< 30% of intake as fat) that contained either higher- or lower-protein (≥ 25% vs. ≤ 20% of energy as protein) on long-term (i.e. ≥ 12 months) changes in body weight, body composition, and cardio-metabolic risk factors was performed by Schwingshackl and Hoffman (2013) and included fifteen high-quality RCTs. While the different dietary approaches achieved comparable improvements in weight, waist circumference, fat mass, blood lipids (i.e. total cholesterol, LDL-cholesterol, HDL-cholesterol, triglycerides), C-reactive protein, diastolic and systolic blood pressure, fasting glucose and glycosylated haemoglobin, the higher protein diet reduced fasting insulin concentrations more than the lower-protein diet. Furthermore, exclusion of studies that included people with Type 2 diabetes demonstrated that the high protein diet yielded a greater improvement in HDL-cholesterol (Schwingshackl and Hoffmann, 2013).

A second and more comprehensive meta-analysis was recently published by Clifton and coworkers (Clifton *et al.*, 2014). This analysis included 32 RCTs with 3492 individuals who were randomised to diets that differed in the percentage of protein and who were followed for more than 12 months. Very low-carbohydrate, ketogenic (i.e. Atkins style) and also low- to moderate-carbohydrate, higher-protein diets were included. The recommendation to consume a lower-carbohydrate, higher-protein diet when compared to the recommendation to consume a high-carbohydrate, lower-protein diet, was associated with better weight loss, but the effect size was small (i.e. ~0.4 kg). Of clinical importance, the weight loss was predominately loss of fat whereas changes in lean mass were not different between the two diets. Moreover, increasing protein intake by 5% or more was associated with a 3-fold greater reduction in fat mass (mean difference 0.9 kg vs. 0.3 kg) at 12 months when compared to diets with change in protein of <5%. Triglyceride and insulin concentrations were also reduced more potently following higher-protein diets, whereas improvements in fasting glucose concentrations, HbA1c, blood pressure and C-reactive protein were comparable for both diet patterns regardless of whether studies with or without Type 2 diabetes were included.

5.4.2   Findings from selected randomised control trials of higher-protein diets

It must be noted that neither of the previous meta-analyses included the findings from the pan-European multi-center, Diogenes study, which is the largest study to compare lower- versus higher-protein diets for weight-loss maintenance (Larsen *et al.*, 2010a, 2010b; Damsgaard *et al.*, 2013). This study included 938 adults and 253 children of these adults. The parents completed an initial 8-week energy restriction period. In the families where at least one parent lost 8% of their initial body weight (mean difference of −11.0 kg), their children were invited to join the parent to complete 26 weeks of weight maintenance on either a higher- or lower-protein (25% vs. 13% of daily energy as protein), ad libitum diet (Larsen *et al.*, 2010a, 2010b). In the adults who completed the study, the higher-protein diet led to less weight regain (mean difference of −0.93 kg) than the lower-protein diet (Larsen *et al.*, 2010b). The children who followed the higher-protein compared to lower-protein regimen displayed a greater reduction in waist circumference (mean difference of 2.7 cm) and LDL cholesterol (−0.25 mmol/L) (Damsgaard *et al.*, 2013). This study also demonstrated that the adults who consumed a diet with a combination of an increased protein-to-carbohydrate ratio with low-glycaemic index foods had beneficial effects on risk factors of the metabolic syndrome (Papadaki *et al.*, 2014).

5.4.3   Limitations in the current scientific literature

Limitations in the current scientific literature must be considered when deciding whether to recommend a higher-protein diet to a specific individual/patient population. Within the studies included in the various meta-analyses, the dropout rates ranged from 7–55% (average 30 ± 12%). This contributed to large amounts of missing data, but since only about half of these studies reported intention to treat analyses along with more complete results there was a high risk of bias in the interpretation of data. In addition, after the first six months, most of the studies displayed poor compliance to the prescribed programs regardless of dietary pattern. For example, Schwingshackl and colleagues found the higher protein diet groups reduced their protein content throughout the study, whereas the lower protein diet groups increased their protein content, meaning that both diet groups tended to turn back towards their habitual protein intakes recorded at baseline (Schwingshackl and Hoffmann, 2013). The lack of protein differential between diets was also supported by the urinary biomarker data reported in 9 of the 15 studies included in the Schwingshackl meta-analysis, and in 8 of the 32 included in the meta-analysis by Clifton et al., (Schwingshackl and Hoffmann, 2013; Clifton, 2014). Despite the limitations, an important finding from both the Diogenes study (Larsen et al., 2010a, 2010b) and Clifton and colleagues meta-analysis (Clifton, 2014) was that they are both indicative that an absolute increase in protein intake by as little as 5% has impact, albeit small, on the clinical management of body weight and cardio-metabolic health in the overweight and obese individuals.

5.5 Potential risks of high protein dietary patterns

Concern is often expressed by many people including general physicians and dietitians that higher-protein diets should not be advocated, particularly to people with pre-existing health conditions. Much of the concern is based on low-quality scientific evidence from cross sectional association studies have that have linked high animal protein intakes to higher risks for coronary heart (McGee et al., 1984) and renal (Pan et al., 2008; Fouque and Laville, 2009), disease, osteoporosis (Misra et al., 2011), and cancer (Cross et al., 2007; Alaejos et al., 2008; Hu et al., 2011), as well as with increased mortality (Noto et al., 2013). However, the number of high-quality RCTs is increasing and the evidence indicates that higher-protein dietary patterns are safe for people without pre-existing disease, especially when they contain plenty of whole grains, fruits and vegetables, lean cuts of meat, nuts/seeds and oils/fat that are high in poly- and mono-unsaturated fatty acids. For example, Clifton and colleagues compared the effects of a moderate- and standard-protein weight loss diet, over 12 months, on changes in renal function in 76 overweight and obese people with Type 2 diabetes with early stage renal disease (i.e. patients with an albumin : creatinine ratio from 3 to 30 mg/mmol) (Jesudason et al., 2013). The average difference in protein intake between diets was 19 ± 6 g/d and there was a comparable improvement in renal function with both diets (Jesudason et al., 2013). In addition, in healthy obese individuals, no deleterious effects of higher-protein diets were found over 1 to 2 years on any markers of inflammation, or renal, vascular or bone function (Brinkworth et al., 2010, Friedman et al., 2012). While no RCTs are available in humans to alleviate the concern that eating red meat, or increasing the total amount of protein in the diet, causes the onset and development of many types of cancers, other factors including age, smoking, being overweight/obese, having a family history of cancer, and being physically inactive, remain the strongest predictors for developing cancer (ASCO, 2012).

5.6   Strategies to improve compliance to higher protein diets

The findings from the meta-analyses discussed above also revealed multiple behavioral factors contribute to the adherence rate observed in dietary interventions. One factor that has been strongly identified as a predictor of high compliance with weight-loss and weight-maintenance programs is the attendance to dietary face-to-face structured, counselling sessions. For example, Layman *et al.* (2009), the studies conducted by CSIRO (Brinkworth *et al.*, 2004, 2009; Luscombe-Marsh *et al.*, 2005; Wycherley *et al.*, 2010) and studies conducted by Foster *et al.* (2010), all incorporated regular weekly/fortnightly/monthly dietary counselling sessions in their 12-month studies. While some studies reported a lower drop-out rate in the higher-compared with lower-protein group (ie 36 vs 55%, respectively) (Layman *et al.*, 2009), others have reported comparable drop-out rates of ~30% and attribute this to the intensive counselling program received by both groups (Brinkworth *et al.*, 2004, 2009; Luscombe-Marsh *et al.*, 2005; Wycherley *et al.*, 2010). Another factor that seems to improve adherence to long-term higher-protein diets is the incorporation of family-based dietary strategies which were incorporated in the Diogenes study (Larsen *et al.*, 2010a, 2010b; Damsgaard *et al.*, 2013). Additionally, the inclusion of regular physical activity into the program may amplify the beneficial effects of the diet, but to what extend remains unclear (Foster *et al.*, 2010; Friedman *et al.*, 2012).

5.7   Conclusions

The latest scientific evidence indicates that weight-loss and weight-maintenance diets containing 25–35% of daily energy from protein, and when followed for 1 to 2 years, may provide small but consistent improvements on body weight, body composition (i.e. enhance fat loss and preserve lean mass) as well as several key cardiometabolic risk factors. These improvements are above those that are seen with alternative lower-protein diets but notably the protein intakes consumed by many participants during research studies were on average only 5% greater than some people's habitual intakes at baseline. Also of significance, the beneficial effects observed with either of the dietary patterns were greater when highly-prescriptive daily meal plans were used (particularly over the initial 3 to 6 months), and when regular support was provided by a medical physician and dietitians. In conclusion, higher-protein diets containing mixed sources of protein (including lean red meat and limited process meat), in combination with plenty of whole grains, fruits, and vegetables, nuts/seeds and oils/fat that are high in poly- and mono-unsaturated fatty acids, represent a safe and effective dietary strategy to manage obesity, particularly in those without substantial existing disease. Supervision from a medical physician and an accredited dietitian should always be part of the management program.

References

Alaejos, M. S., Gonzalez, V. and Afonso, A. M. (2008). Exposure to heterocyclic aromatic amines from the consumption of cooked red meat and its effect on human cancer risk: a review. *Food Addit Contam Part A Chem Anal Control Expo Risk Assess,* 25, 2–24.

ASCO (2012). *The Role of Major Nutrients in Cancer Prevention.* Cancer.Net American Society of Clinical Oncology (ASCO). Available from http://www.cancer.net/navigating-cancer-care/prevention-and-healthy-living/diet-and-nutrition/role-major-nutrients-cancer-prevention.htm [Accessed 31 March 2014].

Barclay, A. W., Brand-Miller, J. C. and Wolever, T. M. (2005). Glycemic index, glycemic load, and glycemic response are not the same. *Diabetes Care,* 28, 1839–40.

Brinkworth, G. D., Buckley, J. D., Noakes, M. and Clifton, P. M. (2010). Renal function following long-term weight loss in individuals with abdominal obesity on a very-low-carbohydrate diet vs high-carbohydrate diet. *J Am Diet Assoc,* 110, 633–8.

Brinkworth, G. D., Noakes, M., Buckley, J. D., Keogh, J. B. and Clifton, P. M. (2009). Long-term effects of a very-low-carbohydrate weight loss diet compared with an isocaloric low-fat diet after 12 mo. *Am J Clin Nutr,* 90, 23–32.

Brinkworth, G. D., Noakes, M., Keogh, J. B., Luscombe, N. D., Wittert, G. A. and Clifton, P. M. (2004). Long-term effects of a high-protein, low-carbohydrate diet on weight control and cardiovascular risk markers in obese hyperinsulinemic subjects. *Int J Obesity,* 28, 661–670.

Clifton, C. D. and Keogh, J. B. (2014). Long term weight maintenance after advice to consume low carbohydrate, higher protein diets – a systematic review and meta analysis. *Nutrition, metabolism, and cardiovascular diseases,* 24, 224.

Cross, A. J., Leitzmann, M. F., Gail, M. H., Hollenbeck, A. R., Schatzkin, A. and Sinha, R. (2007). A prospective study of red and processed meat intake in relation to cancer risk. *Plos Med,* 4, e325.

CSIRO (2010). *The CSIRO Total Wellbeing Recipe Book,* Australia, Penguin.

Damsgaard, C. T., Papadaki, A., Jensen, S. M., Ritz, C., Dalskov, S. M. *et al.* (2013). Higher protein diets consumed ad libitum improve cardiovascular risk markers in children of overweight parents from eight European countries. *J Nutr,* 143, 810–17.

Denke, M. A. (2001). Metabolic effects of high-protein, low-carbohydrate diets. *Am J Cardiol,* 88, 59–61.

Dong, J. Y., Zhang, Z. L., Wang, P. Y. and Qin, L. Q. (2013). Effects of high-protein diets on body weight, glycaemic control, blood lipids and blood pressure in type 2 diabetes: meta-analysis of randomised controlled trials. *Br J Nutr,* 110, 781–9.

Foster, G. D., Wyatt, H. R., Hill, J. O., Makris, A. P., Rosenbaum, D. L. *et al.* (2010). Weight and metabolic outcomes after 2 years on a low-carbohydrate versus low-fat diet: a randomized trial. *Ann Intern Med,* 153, 147–57.

Fouque, D. and Laville, M. (2009). Low protein diets for chronic kidney disease in non diabetic adults. *Cochrane Database Syst Rev,* CD001892.

Friedman, A. N., Ogden, L. G., Foster, G. D., Klein, S., Stein, R. *et al.* (2012). Comparative effects of low-carbohydrate high-protein versus low-fat diets on the kidney. *Clin J Am Soc Nephrol,* 7, 1103–11.

Hu, J., La Vecchia, C., Morrison, H., Negri, E. and Mery, L., for Canadian Cancer Registries Epidemiology Research (2011). Salt, processed meat and the risk of cancer. *Eur J Cancer Prev*, 20, 132–9.

Jesudason, D. R., Pedersen, E. and Clifton, P. M. (2013). Weight-loss diets in people with type 2 diabetes and renal disease: a randomized controlled trial of the effect of different dietary protein amounts. *Am J Clin Nutr*, 98, 494–501.

Larsen, T. M., Dalskov, S., Van Baak, M., Jebb, S., Kafatos, A. *et al.* (2010a). The Diet, Obesity and Genes (Diogenes) Dietary Study in eight European countries – a comprehensive design for long-term intervention. *Obes Rev*, 11, 76–91.

Larsen, T. M., Dalskov, S. M., Van Baak, M., Jebb, S. A., Papadaki, A. *et al.* (2010b). Diets with high or low protein content and glycemic index for weight-loss maintenance. *N Engl J Med*, 363, 2102–13.

Layman, D. K., Evans, E. M., Erickson, D., Seyler, J., Weber, J. *et al.* (2009). A moderate-protein diet produces sustained weight loss and long-term changes in body composition and blood lipids in obese adults. *J Nutr*, 139, 514–21.

Leidy, H. J. and Racki, E. M. (2010). The addition of a protein-rich breakfast and its effects on acute appetite control and food intake in 'breakfast-skipping' adolescents. *Int J Obes (Lond)*, 34, 1125–33.

Luscombe-Marsh, N. D., Noakes, M., Wittert, G. A., Keogh, J. B., Foster, P. and Clifton, P. M. (2005). Carbohydrate-restricted diets high in either monounsaturated fat or protein are equally effective at promoting fat loss and improving blood lipids. *Am J Clin Nutr*, 81, 762–72.

McGee, D. L., Reed, D. M., Yano, K., Kagan, A. and Tillotson, J. (1984). Ten-year incidence of coronary heart disease in the Honolulu Heart Program. Relationship to nutrient intake. *Am J Epidemiol*, 119, 667–76.

Misra, D., Berry, S. D., Broe, K. E., Mclean, R. R., Cupples, L. A. *et al.* (2011). Does dietary protein reduce hip fracture risk in elders? The Framingham Osteoporosis Study. *Osteoporos Int*, 22, 345–9.

Noakes M, C. P. (2005). *The CSIRO Total Wellbeing Diet*, Australia, Penguin.

Noakes M, C. P. (2006). *The CSIRO Total Wellbeing Diet Book 2*, Australia, Penguin.

Noto, H., Goto, A., Tsujimoto, T. and Noda, M. (2013). Low-carbohydrate diets and all-cause mortality: a systematic review and meta-analysis of observational studies. *Plos One*, 8, e55030.

Pan, Y., Guo, L. L. and Jin, H. M. (2008). Low-protein diet for diabetic nephropathy: a meta-analysis of randomized controlled trials. *Am J Clin Nutr*, 88, 660–6.

Papadaki, A., Linardakis, M., Plada, M., Larsen, T. M., Damsgaard, C. T. *et al.* (2014). Impact of weight loss and maintenance with ad libitum diets varying in protein and glycemic index content on metabolic syndrome. *Nutrition*, 30, 410–17.

Piatti, P. M., Monti, F., Fermo, I., Baruffaldi, L., Nasser, R. *et al.* (1994). Hypocaloric high-protein diet improves glucose oxidation and spares lean body mass: comparison to hypo-caloric high-carbohydrate diet. *Metabolism*, 43, 1481–7.

Roberts, D. C. (2001). Quick weight loss: sorting fad from fact. *Med J Aust*, 175, 637–40.

Santesso, N., Akl, E. A., Bianchi, M., Mente, A., Mustafa, R. *et al.* (2012). Effects of higher-versus lower-protein diets on health outcomes: a systematic review and meta-analysis. *Eur J Clin Nutr*, 66, 780–8.

Schwingshackl, L. and Hoffmann, G. (2013). Long-term effects of low-fat diets either low or high in protein on cardiovascular and metabolic risk factors: a systematic review and meta-analysis. *Nutr J*, 12, 48.

St. Jeor, S. T., Howard, B. V., Prewitt, T. E., Bovee, V., Bazzarre, T. and Eckel, R. H., for the AHA Nutrition Committee (2001). Dietary protein and weight reduction: a statement for healthcare professionals from the Nutrition Committee of the Council on Nutrition, Physical Activity, and Metabolism of the American Heart Association. *Circulation*, 104(15), 1869–1874.

Westerterp-Plantenga, M. S., Lejeune, M. P. G. M., Smeets, A. J. P. G. and Luscombe-Marsh, N. D. (2009). Sex differences in energy homeostatis following a diet relatively high in protein exchanged with carbohydrate, assessed in a respiration chamber in humans. *Physiology & Behavior*, 97, 414–19.

Westerterp-Plantenga, M. S., Rolland, V., Wilson, S. A. and Westerterp, K. R. (1999). Satiety related to 24 h diet-induced thermogenesis during high protein/carbohydrate vs high fat diets measured in a respiration chamber. *Eur J Clin Nutr*, 53, 495–502.

Wycherley, T. P., Moran, L. J., Clifton, P. M., Noakes, M. and Brinkworth, G. D. (2012). Effects of energy-restricted high-protein, low-fat compared with standard-protein, low-fat diets: a meta-analysis of randomized controlled trials. *Am J Clin Nutr*, 96, 1281–98.

Wycherley, T. P., Noakes, M., Clifton, P. M., Cleanthous, X., Keogh, J. B. and Brinkworth, G. D. (2010). A high-protein diet with resistance exercise training improves weight loss and body composition in overweight and obese patients with type 2 diabetes. *Diabetes Care*, 33, 969–76.

Low-fat diets in obesity management and weight control

M. Hunsberger, G. Tognon, L. Lissner
University of Gothenburg, Gothenburg, Sweden

6.1 Introduction: overview of dietary fat and body weight

In the last part of the twentieth century, novel laboratory research convincingly demonstrated that a high-fat diet was extremely successful at fattening lab animals. As a consequence, there was a general movement towards fat-reduced diets and low-fat food products in anticipation of multiple health benefits including weight management. Counter intuitively, as low-fat products were increasingly consumed, the obesity epidemic accelerated, leading to wide speculations that the fat-reduced diet could actually have been a *cause* of the epidemic. Examination of the epidemiologic evidence available at the time, ranging from ecological to longitudinal studies in various populations, provided some support for the hypothesis that fat intake was positively associated with overweight, rather than the reverse. This chapter will present evidence, including animal studies, human trials and observational studies, that total dietary fat and specific subtypes may be associated with energy balance. Based on the large accumulation of early and recent literature on amount and type of fat intake in this context, our aim is to consider whether low-fat diets are a useful component of weight loss and maintenance.

6.2 Total fat: mechanisms for association with body weight regulation

The idea that dietary fat intake might be positively related to body weight is primarily based on the fact that fat is the most energy dense macronutrient. The energy density of high-fat food is thus believed to be a key mechanism for passive overconsumption and weight gain when compared to low-fat diets with higher proportions of carbohydrate and protein (Blundell, 1999). The potential impact of fatty foods on energy intake is not only attributed to energy density but also to the particularly palatable sensation fat stimulates in the mouth, sometimes referred to as mouth feel (Drewnowski, 1997). The above-mentioned supermarket or cafeteria diet, first described by Sclafani, supports this notion of fatty foods leading to overconsumption, as the cafeteria diet's palatability induces animals to forsake their animal chow in favor of this experimental diet (Sclafani, 1976). Specifically, in an attempt to fatten adult rats in a manner that mimicked human accumulation of body fat, animals were fed two different diets; the control group received rat chow and the experimental group received in addition to chow, Crisco fat (a brand of solid baking fat popular in the United States, introduced in 1911 by Proctor & Gamble Co., made entirely of vegetable oil), sweetened condensed milk, and a variety of readily available human foods such as chocolate chip cookies, salami, cheese, milk chocolate, and peanut butter. This 60 day experiment proved to be extremely effective in producing obesity, showing a 53% increase in weight. It may be noted that many of these foods were also high in sugar, salt, or both. In subsequent years, this type of diet has been widely used as a model to induce obesity in lab animals (Tschöp, 2001). Furthermore, a number of studies have indicated that fat is less satiating than carbohydrate and protein when compared on a calorie for calorie basis. However, it has also been demonstrated that passive overconsumption is not unique to high-fat diets despite other macronutrients being less satiating. When subjects are offered high-fat or high carbohydrate foods that have been altered to be equally energy dense, the fat-specific overeating phenomenon is eliminated (Astrup, 2001). Thus, through various mechanisms that are not all specific to dietary fat *per se*, overconsumption of palatable, fatty foods has been widely documented.

Another reason that dietary fat consumption might be associated with body fat is preferential storage. The priority between macronutrient oxidation and storage is determined by how much energy must be spent to either oxidize or store the nutrient in the fat tissue as well as by the availability of nutrient-specific body storage sites (Franz, 2000). In order to be stored in the adipose tissue, fatty acids need to be assembled into triglycerides with minimal energy cost. Conversely, alcohol, carbohydrates and proteins need to be oxidized to pyruvate, converted into fatty acids and then assembled into triglycerides, before being stored in the adipose tissue (Nelson and Cox, 2008). Alcohol and proteins have no specific body storage site while, albeit to a limited degree, carbohydrates can be stored as glycogen in both liver and muscle tissue with a limited impact on body fatness in part due to the highly hydrated nature of glycogen. Based on these considerations, alcohol has the highest priority for oxidation, followed by proteins and carbohydrates and finally fat. When a person fails to consume adequate protein, or is in negative nitrogen balance, lean tissue can be broken down for energy and one could consider this a storage site in times of inadequate calories but it is by no means the energy reservoir provided by body fat. In the context of obesity and weight regulation, it has been proposed that dietary fat is more likely to be stored as adipose tissue if there is an excess energy intake (Flatt, 1995).

6.2.1   Evidence from observational epidemiology

The observational evidence that dietary fat is related to obesity in human populations has been examined using a variety of epidemiological designs, from ecological studies in which a whole population is the unit of observation, to prospective studies of associations between dietary fat and subsequent weight gain in individuals (reviewed by Lissner and Heitmann, 1995). For instance, ecological studies often show a positive association between per-capita fat intake and national obesity prevalence. Other ecological studies have shown an opposite trend. In the United States overweight rose by 31% from 1976 to 1991 while fat intake adjusted for total calories dropped by 11% based on data extracted from five adult population surveys (Heini and Weinsier, 1997). More recently, a population study of US adults aged 20–74 years of age extracted from the National Health and Nutrition Examination Survey spanning 1971–2006 reported the prevalence of obesity increased from 11.9% to 33.4% in men and from 16.6% to 36.5% in women (Austin *et al.*, 2011). During this same period the percentage of energy from total fat and protein decreased while the percentage of total energy from carbohydrates increased (Austin *et al.*, 2011). This trend in macronutrient consumption was the same across all BMI groups (normal, overweight, and obese) (Austin *et al.*, 2011). These data have been interpreted as support for the notion that decreasing fat intake may be driving the obesity epidemic. However, these observations may be driven by the presence of other underlying factors that differ systematically between populations and may be the driving factors, a phenomenon sometimes referred to as the "ecological fallacy".

The next level of evidence is based on analyses of individual data, but only correlating obesity with dietary data at a single point in time. As previously mentioned, the literature has yielded a number of such cross-sectional studies suggesting that dietary fat intake is positively correlated with body weight. In contrast, prospective studies, in which a chronology is established between fat intake and subsequent weight gain, do not consistently confirm the positive association often seen in cross-sectional studies. It should be noted that prospective as well as cross-sectional observational data relating diet to obesity are fraught with measurement errors, and in this context it is acknowledged that observed associations are likely to be affected by a variety of reporting biases. This has made it difficult to use epidemiological data as a basis for determining the dietary fat content that is optimal for weight management.

Epidemiological studies have also been used to consider whether familial or genetic predisposition may explain some of the inconsistencies described above. Specifically the susceptibility to weight gain may be influenced by dietary factors such as fat intake particularly in those who are genetically predisposed to obesity (Heitmann *et al*, 2001). However, results from the Nurses' Health Study and the European Youth Heart Study showed no clear evidence that the association between dietary fat and weight gain was stronger among offspring of overweight parents, suggesting that familial or genetic susceptibility may not be the full explanation for divergent epidemiological evidence (Field *et al.*, 2007; Brixval *et al*, 2009). One possible mechanism for susceptibility to weight gain on a high-fat-diet may involve taste sensitivity which has a genetic basis (Reed *et al.*, 1997); genes regulating uncoupling proteins have also been suggested in this context (Fleury *et al.*, 1997). Nonetheless, it must be concluded that the epidemiological evidence that genetic factors modify the association between dietary fat and weight status remain inconclusive.

6.2.2   Evidence from randomized controlled feeding studies and dietary trials

A number of early short term feeding trials demonstrated that low-fat diets consumed on an *ad libitum* basis could promote weight loss. In contrast to the epidemiological approach, these studies were based on direct observation of energy intake and/or expenditure under controlled conditions. Among these, two feeding studies from Cornell University randomizing fat-manipulated diets showed promising results on energy balance (Lissner *et al.*, 1987; Kendall *et al.*, 1991); in one of these studies the subjects even preferred the seemingly similar low-fat diet (15–20% fat) over the high-fat diet (45–50% fat) on which they lost and gained weight respectively (Lissner *et al.*, 1987). Subsequent studies from Cambridge University strengthened the evidence for effects of fat-manipulated diets on energy balance, further implicating energy density as the specific mechanism, and also suggesting a possible synergy between the high- or low-fat and sedentary living conditions (Stubbs *et al.*, 1995a, 1995b, 1996).

To date, the largest trial exploring the relationship between fat intake and body weight is the Women's Health Initiative (WHI) (Howard *et al.*, 2006), which included more than 48,000 postmenopausal women followed for over seven years. Women were randomized to either a control or intervention group. The intervention group was encouraged to reduce total dietary fat intake to 20% while increasing intake of vegetables and fruit to five or more servings and grains (whole grains encouraged) to six or more servings daily. This group was further informed that the diet was not intended to promote weight loss and they were encouraged to maintain energy intake by replacing dietary fat with mainly carbohydrate (Howard *et al*, 2006). Women in the intervention group lost more weight in the first year (1.9 kg difference) and maintained a greater weight reduction than controls during an average 7.5 years follow-up, although the size of the difference diminished over time. Importantly, a significant dose-response between dietary fat intake and body weight change was demonstrated, in which the proportion of fat in the diet increased proportionally with body weight changes in both control and intervention subjects (Figure 6.1). While the authors did not explicitly conclude from their data that a reduction in fat is associated with weight loss, they did emphasize that the low-fat diet did not result in weight gain.

A great number of other studies have been published on this subject, as summarized in a recent systematic review and meta-analysis of randomized controlled trials as well as cohort studies (Hooper *et al.*, 2012). This comprehensive review included 33 randomized controlled trials (73,589 participants, most of who participated in the WHI study) and 10 cohort studies (107,756 participants) in adults as well as four trials in children and young people. The authors concluded that there is consistent evidence that reduction of total fat intake leads to small but statistically significant sustained reductions in body weight in adults and evidence suggests a similar result in children and young people. The exclusion of the WHI results from the systematic analysis did not eliminate the overall protective effect of a fat reduced diet. These studies demonstrate that reductions in caloric intake, particularly dietary fat, can assist with weight maintenance.

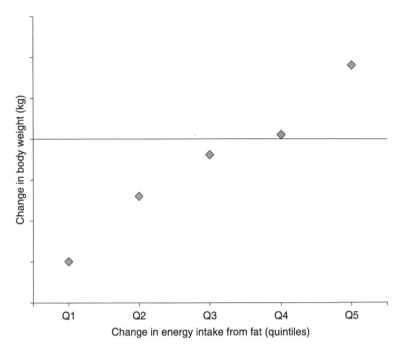

Figure 6.1 Dose-response between dietary fat intake and body weight change.

6.3 Type of fat: biological mechanisms for effects on energy balance

Most of the research described above has considered all types and sources of fat equally for their potential effects on energy regulation. As a preface to the next sections, we note that researchers have defined fat type differently in their invest-igations. These include specific fatty acid content, saturation or chain length characteristics, animal versus plant origins, and specific food sources. At the food level, the complex nature of fatty acid composition may be exemplified by pork fat which consists of 40% saturated fatty acids (SFA), 45% mono-unsaturated fatty acids (MUFA), and 15% polyunsaturated fatty acids (PUFA). This may be compared with olive oil which is 14% SFA, 74% MUFA, and 12% PUFA. Like other animal fats that are solid at room temperature, pork fat is often considered to be highly satur-ated when in fact MUFA is most predominant. In interpreting the emerging evidence on the role of dietary fat subtypes in relation to metabolism and weight regulation, it should be kept in mind that operationalization of the concept of fat quality has been highly variable in the available literature.

To assess the role of types of dietary fat in accumulation of adipose tissue or body fatness, it is useful to first review the biological mechanisms that regulate fat utiliz-ation and storage in the body and how unsaturated fats might differ from saturated fats biologically. Unsaturated fatty acids are, in general, more readily oxidized than SFA of similar chain length while chain length tends to be inversely associated to the oxidation rate (DeLany *et al.*, 2000). SFA has been shown to reduce lipolytic activity in adipocytes due to its impact on membrane fluidity thus limiting the ability to utilize stored fat (Awad and Chattopadhyay, 1986; Matsuo *et al*, 1995). Characteristics of fatty acid saturation also play a role in determining the differences in oxidation rates, including polarity, whereas polyunsaturated fats are more readily hydrolyzed (Perona *et al.*, 2000), with possible influences on expression of genes which encode for lipogenic enzymes, lipid oxidation proteins, fatty acid transport, and adipokines (Kersten, 2002; Khan and Vanden Heuvel, 2003; Sampath and Ntambi, 2005). Unsaturated fats also appear to be more effective than SFA in stimulating peroxisome proliferator-activated receptor α (*PPARα*), a ligand-activated transcription factor that regulates energy metabolism (Kliewer *et al.*, 1997).

Animal studies show that specific fatty acids differentially affect lipid metabolism and can influence the expression of genes related to lipogenesis (Moussavi *et al*, 2008; Hariri and Thibault, 2010; Lottenberg *et al.*, 2012). Studies of animal obesity have confirmed that consumption of different types of fat evoke different rates of weight change (Storlien *et al*, 1998) with differential impacts on fat distribution and body composition (Matsuo *et al*, 1995; Takeuchi *et al.*, 1995; Bell and Sherriff, 1997). In rodent models it has been shown that long-chain n-3 PUFA may reduce body fat mass by altering the expression of genes promoting fat oxidation and energy expenditure (Buckley and Howe, 2009). Moreover, a recent review summarizing studies on the association between n-6 fatty acid intake and obesity suggests that n-6 fatty acids might have pro-adipogenic properties (shown in both *in vitro* and in animal studies) as well as a possible role in the fetal programming of obesity (Muhlhauslera and Ailhaud, 2013).

Trans fatty acids (TFA) are unsaturated fatty acids (either MUFA or PUFA) containing at least one double bond in the *trans* configuration, while the usual configuration is the *cis*. TFA can be generated in the rumen, the first chamber of the stomach in ruminant animals, due to microbial fermentation (thus dairy products and meat naturally contain them) or through the industrial process of oil hydrogenation (Bhardwaj *et al*, 2011). The potential role of these fatty acids in weight gain has been the topic of a recent review (Thompson *et al*, 2011). However, results from both cell and rodent experimental studies concerning TFA's effects on glucose and lipid oxidation as well as body weight and body composition are conflicting (Thompson *et al*, 2011; Ochiai *et al.*, 2013). One randomized controlled trial in green monkeys, fed a diet containing 8% of energy from either TFA or MUFA for six years, resulted in a higher weight gain in the animals eating the TFA-rich diet when compared to the MUFA-rich diet (Kavanagh *et al.*, 2007). Moreover, computed tomography scan demonstrated that the differential gain in weight was due to a higher visceral fat deposition.

Special mention may be given to a particular class of TFA, the conjugated linoleic acids (CLA). CLA refer to a group of conjugated octadecadienoic acid isomers derived from linoleic acid, a fatty acid that contains 18 carbons and two double bonds in the *cis* configuration at the 9th and 12th carbons (Pariza *et al*, 2001). In addition to the natural presence in ruminant-derived products, supplements containing these fatty acids are also commercially available. Although chemically related, according to the Codex Alimentarius (www.codexalimentarius.org). What is commonly referred to as TFA does not include CLA (Wang, 2013). CLA was excluded due to its potential to reduce body weight and its anti-atherogenic properties (Kennedy *et al.*, 2010).

A full description of the different fat types that have been implicated in energy balance and imbalance is beyond the scope of this chapter. However, with this background, the next section will present selected evidence that fat type, as opposed to total fat intake, may be relevant for weight regulation in humans.

6.3.1   *Evidence from studies in humans*

Although the role of dietary fat subtypes on weight regulation in humans is not conclusive several human studies support the positive association between unsaturated fatty acids and fat oxidation. A short term intervention trial examined fat oxidation rates after a meal high in MUFA rather than SFA in men and found those on the high-MUFA diet experienced greater postprandial fatty acid oxidation rates (Piers *et al.*, 2002). Conversely, postprandial carbohydrate oxidation rate was significantly lower following the high-MUFA meals (Piers *et al.*, 2002). In another study of obese post-menopausal women, olive oil significantly promoted postprandial fat oxidation and stimulated dietary thermogenesis in abdominally obese post-menopausal women (Soares *et al.*, 2004). One interpretation of this finding was that this source of fat may be particularly beneficial to obese individuals.

In a 4-week trial with male subjects which examined replacement of dietary SFA with MUFA and PUFA, small but significant loss of body weight and fat mass were achieved without significant changes in total energy or fat intake (Piers *et al.*, 2003). Men on the SFA-rich diet gained fat mass particularly on the trunk rather than on the limbs, while on the MUFA-rich diet similar amounts of body fat were lost both from the trunk and from the limbs. Other studies using indirect calorimetry have indicated that PUFA is better oxidized than SFA in both normal weight and obese men (Jones *et al.*, 1992). Omega-3 fatty acids are a special type of PUFA essential to humans. While there are few studies of omega-3 and weight change, a recent review of the evidence in adults found that in four of the five studies that met inclusion criteria for review no change in body weight by dietary supplementation with n-3 PUFA was shown (Martinéz-Victoria and Yago, 2012). Interestingly though, in a study of children in the Project Viva cohort, a higher omega-6 to omega-3 ratio in umbilical cord blood phospholipids was associated with a higher subscapular skinfold thickness at the age of 3 suggesting that imbalances in omega-6 to omega-3 may alter adipose deposition (Donahue *et al.*, 2011).

TFA should also be considered for its role in energy balance and weight maintenance in humans; however, due to the cardiovascular risk that has been associated with TFA intake (Mozaffarian, 2006), assessing long-term effects in human trials is not possible for ethical reasons. Observational studies where TFA consumption was estimated through a food frequency questionnaire (FFQ) or food records have been performed and provide limited but consistent evidence of an association between TFA consumption and small weight gain and increases in waist circumference (Colditz *et al.*, 1990; Koh-Banerjee *et al.*, 2003; Wannamethee *et al.*, 2004; Field *et al.*, 2007; Oken *et al.*, 2007). It is important to note care must be taken when indirectly estimating TFA intake because of the potentially large variations in similar foods (Innis *et al* 1999) coupled with inconsistent findings. A recent Danish study found a weak inverse association with weight change and no association with changes in waist circumference (Hansen *et al.*, 2012). A small number of feeding studies investigating possible metabolic effects of TFA compared with SFA and MUFA reported conflicting results on possible effects on oxidation rate and appetite (Thompson and Williams, 2011). The lack of plausible biological mechanisms explaining different energy oxidation or deposition makes the association between TFA consumption and weight status at least questionable. The evidence supporting CLA health claims for the general population is lacking (EFSA, 2010).

While data on long-term associations between dietary fat composition and change in weight and/or body composition are limited, a recent study with participation from five European countries suggested that fish consumption (a source of PUFA) has no appreciable association with body-weight gain (Jakobsen *et al.*, 2013). Although changes in body composition and shape may occur without changes in weight, fish consumption was not associated with change in waist circumference (Jakobsen *et al.*, 2012).

In conclusion, there is evidence from *in vitro*, animal, and human studies that the fatty acid types are playing a role in energy balance but the complex nature of fatty acid composition makes it difficult to nuance the contribution of specific subtypes. One potential aspect confounding the evidence is the subtypes of unsaturated fats (e.g. n-6 vs. n-3 fatty acids and CLA) may play contrasting roles in energy regulation. In addition, there is a growing body of evidence that both type of fat and total fat intake play a role in adipose tissue deposition and by implication weight loss and maintenance, but to what extent is difficult to estimate.

6.4 Sustainability of weight loss on low-fat diets

Low-fat diets can potentially induce weight loss, but the evidence that they are the best way for an overweight person to lose weight and keep weight off is limited. Reducing energy for weight loss can be achieved through many strategies besides dietary fat reduction while the optimal proportion of fat for weight loss is not clear. In addition, there is not an established definition for 'low-fat', although several intervention studies have defined low-fat as 15–20% of energy from fat (Howard *et al.*, 2006; Hooper *et al.*, 2012). In fact, by their own definition, the WHI intervention group did not consume a 'low-fat diet' (Howard *et al.*, 2006). The WHI intervention did show a small but significant weight loss effect by lowering fat intake from a baseline average of 38.8% to 29.8% at follow-up, and by most accounts approximately 30% of calories from dietary fat would not be considered 'low-fat'. Particularly, the fact that there was an unmistakable dose-response between fat reduction and weight reduction in both WHI groups (Figure 6.1) underscores the notion that there can be benefits of a fat reduced diet that is not necessarily 'low-fat' by most definitions.

As noted previously, evidence indicates that diets high in energy density, independent of their fat content, are associated with greater intakes of energy (Vernarelli *et al.*, 2011). However, simply replacing dietary fat with another macronutrient does not necessarily decrease the density of the diet. If dietary fat is replaced by high sugar foods and drinks it is unlikely that these changes will lead to weight maintenance (Malik *et al.*, 2010). Today's highly processed fast foods provide a prime example of a modern diet that is both high in energy density and fat which might overcome the innate human ability to regulate food intake (Prentice and Jabb, 2003). Avoidance of this type of diet may have more important implications for weight management over long periods of time than fat reduction *per se*. However, even if differences in storage potential and oxidation rates probably exist between each macronutrient and the others, it is questionable whether they are relevant from a public health point of view or not. For instance, evidence that total energy is more important than reducing fat energy is provided by the 'Pounds Lost' trial where a reduction in total energy intake, rather than a particular macronutrient content of the diet, was the most important determinant of fat loss (de Souza *et al.*, 2012). For the purpose of weight loss, the low-fat diet consisting of 15–20% of calories from fat may even be detrimental to energy expenditure (Ebbeling *et al.*, 2012). In another study, the low-fat group had no weight loss advantage but higher attrition (Hession *et al.*, 2009). These findings may have important implications for long-term maintenance.

One source of evidence on weight maintenance comes from the National Weight Control Registry (NWCR) established in 1994 by Rena Wing and James O. Hill (NWCR, 2013). NWCR tracks greater than 10,000 people who have lost significant body weight and kept it off for long periods of time. A definition of weight maintenance proposed by Hill and Wing defines maintainers as 'individuals who have intentionally lost at least 10% of their body weight and kept it off at least one year' (Klem *et al.*, 1997). The NWCR reports that 98% of Registry participants report that they have modified their dietary intake in some way (NWCR, 2013). In an earlier publication, the most common dietary strategies for weight loss reported by Registry participants were to restrict certain foods (87.6%), limit quantities (44%), and count calories (43%) (Klem *et al.*, 1997; Wing and Phelan, 2005). To maintain weight loss the strategies included; consuming a low-calorie, low-fat diet, doing high levels of physical activity, weighing themselves frequently, and consuming breakfast daily (Wing and Phelan, 2005; Wyatt *et al.*, 2002). On average, members reported consuming 24% of their calories from fat (Wing and Phelan, 2005), a percentage that is in line with the United States Dietary Recommendations which advise adults aged 19 years and older to consume 20–35% of calories from fat (USDA, 2010). Restricting calories is important to weight loss, and restricting dietary fat can assist in reducing calories, yet 24% of calories from fat is not necessarily a low-fat diet.

A comprehensive meta-analysis provides further evidence. Based on studies from 1966 to 2008 examining the long-term effectiveness of diet-plus-exercise vs. diet-only interventions on weight loss, this meta-analysis reported weight loss after two or more years averaged 1.64 kg when a combination of dietary changes and increased physical activity were achieved (Wu *et al.*, 2009). Some of the dietary approaches cited include: calorie restriction to as low as 1000 calories; fat restriction to less than 30% of total intake; and increased fish, fruit, vegetables and fiber consumption while reducing saturated fat and sugar, although not an exhaustive list. Dropout rates ranged from 0% to 50% in the diet and exercise intervention groups and 0% to 65% in a diet-only intervention groups (Wu *et al.*, 2009). The highest dropout was experienced on the *Help Your Heart Eating Plan*, a United States study (Skender *et al.*, 1996). This diet consists of a low-cholesterol eating plan with energy intake of 30% from fat, 50% from carbohydrate, and 20% from protein with weekly brisk walking for 45 minutes 4–5 times per week at a level of vigorous but not strenuous activity (Skender *et al.*, 1996). The most severe dietary restriction included a low-calorie (800–1000 kcal/day), low-fat regimen (20% of calories from fat) during weeks one to eight; adjusting gradually up to 1200–1500 kcal/day at week sixteen (Wing *et al.*, 1998). Over the 14.5 month study duration, participants in the diet and exercise group lost an average of 7.9 kg whereas in the diet only group participants lost an average of 3.8 kg (Wing *et al.*, 1998). Findings from the Wu *et al.* (2009) meta-analysis demonstrate that long-term weight loss appears to be minimal across many years and many studies and the individuals that were most successful exercised in addition to controlling their dietary intake. Surprisingly, the study with the greatest dropout rate was one in which the dietary restriction was moderate and the physical activity included only vigorous walking (Skender *et al.*, 1996). From the current evidence it seems unlikely that that a low-fat diet alone or a low-fat diet combined exercise would promote long term weight loss.

6.5 Conclusions

Given the totality of the evidence, it may be concluded that fat-reduced diets are probably not causing weight gain and represent one of many actions that could contribute to obesity prevention. However, low-fat diets alone do not represent a long-term solution for the majority of individuals. In light of what we know about low-fat diets, most individuals maintain a diet that falls within the recommended dietary guideline of 20–35% of dietary intake from fat. Therefore, on the basis of available evidence, it may be more appropriate to discuss fat-reduced diets rather than low-fat diets.

We do not know if there is an optimal level of fat in the diet, or the optimal type of dietary fat for weight control, but evidence from both the National Weight Control Registry and the WHI cohort study suggest that fat intake in the range of 24–29% may be appropriate; this level is supported by the current US Dietary Recommendations (Howard *et al.*, 2006; USDA, 2010 NWCR, 2013). While not conclusive, current evidence suggests that fat quality may also be important. Fats are oxidized at different rates by different pathways and, for example, SFA may be oxidized less readily than MUFA and PUFA. However, the relevance to energy regulation or fat deposition is unclear. In the context of weight loss and maintenance, fat cannot be considered in isolation of other dietary, lifestyle, and environmental factors that may contribute independently and synergistically to energy balance in both the short- and long-term. In fact, an oversimplified energy balance model may be contributing to the confusion about low-fat diets and dietary fat in general. In light of this, public health scientists should consider the science of energy regulation more critically when making recommendations. Although dietary fat reduction at the population level occurred simultaneously with the surge in the obesity epidemic it cannot be concluded that they are causally related and more evidence points in the opposite direction. Fat and energy-reduced diets are clearly relevant to both weight loss and weight maintenance, but it is uncertain whether low-fat diets are necessary or sustainable over a lifetime.

6.6   Future trends

Trends in macronutrient intake have changed over time in response to public health messaging, food availability and advertising. This trend is visible in much of the Western world as an increasing number of individuals follow diets rich in lean protein, low in carbohydrate, and moderate to high in dietary fat. For instance, the diet known as hunter-gather, also known as Paleo or Caveman, is growing in popularity. A mid-2013 Google Trends search indicated that Paleo is surpassing low-carbohydrate, high-fat diets (also referred to as LCHF) (Google Trends, 2013). Both LCHF and Paleo are far more popular than low-carbohydrate or low-fat diets when interest over time is compared.

Given the growing evidence that focusing on specific types of fat rather than total fat may be helpful in understanding the mechanisms and long-term effects on weight loss and maintenance, it should be pointed out that the current popularity of the hunter-gatherer-like diets, which are associated with a greater intake of animal proteins, seem to have resulted in moving the population's animal fat intake and hence saturated fat intake in a direction that goes against current recommendations. The possible consequences of this shift towards more animal protein on cardiovascular diseases are being debated and over time will be documented in future epidemiological studies.

It must be emphasized that dietary fat cannot be considered in isolation. There is growing evidence that the fat–sugar combination and the fat–salt combination, as well as the salt, sugar, and fat combination, may be as highly palatable in humans as it was in the original cafeteria diet.

For instance, experimental studies in young children who are overweight have observed an enhanced preference for sweet, fat, and in particular both sweet and fat in combination (Lanfer et al., 2011). It has been proposed that an abundance of modern foods are formulated not to satisfy hunger but instead to stimulate the reward pathways in the brain (Kessler, 2009). In his book, Kessler (2009), the former commissioner of the Food and Drug Administration and the person responsible for heading the charge against big tobacco companies, identified salt, sugar and fat as the foods primarily responsible for inducing overeating and causing excessive weight gain. He describes these foods as hyperstimulating and theorizes that some individuals are conditioned to be *hypereaters*, overriding the biological mechanisms, and eating for appetite rather than hunger (Kessler, 2009). Michael Moss, an investigative reporter with the *New York Times*, builds on the ideas presented by Kessler in his book *Fat, Sugar, Salt: How the Food Companies Hooked Us* (Moss, 2013). Moss discusses the food industries manipulation of foods that capitalize on consumers' cravings, essentially producing addictive foods. Therefore, our current food supply may make it difficult to sustain the type of low-fat and low-sugar diets that could potentially prevent excess calorie intake.

In response to concerns about over consumption, some governments are discussing or implementing taxes on foods and beverages. France, Finland, Denmark, Britain, Ireland, and Romania have all either instituted food taxes or are in discussions (Daley, 2013). Hungary has imposed taxes on salt, sugar and the ingredients in energy drinks in an effort to raise revenue and raise public awareness regarding unhealthy foods (Holt, 2011). We will likely see further food taxation, however it is notable that Denmark quickly abandoned its fat tax on foodstuffs exceeding 2.3% saturated fat content. The consequence of the Danish policy not only led to purchasing of cheaper, lower quality, and occasionally less fatty alternatives but also drove some consumers to neighboring countries (Germany and Sweden) to shop for their favorite foods (Bomsdorf, 2012).

6.7   Sources of further information and advice

Resources that may be of interest to readers include the United States Dietary Guidelines issued by the United States Department of Agriculture with a most recent release in 2010 (available at: http://www.cnpp.usda.gov/dietaryguidelines.htm) and the new Nordic Nutrition Recommendations, released in 2013, which focus on the whole diet (available at http://www.norden.org/en/news-and-events/news/new-nordic-nutrition-recommendations-2013-focus-on-the-whole-diet).

To learn more about the Women's Health Initiative we refer readers to https://cleo.whi.org/SitePages/Home.aspx and the National Weight Council Registry (USA) http://www.nwcr.ws/; both of which are discussed in the text.

Readers looking for dietary trends may be interested in searching Google Trends themselves for international and national diet trends (at http://www.google.com/trends), exploring trends in the United States at the Economic Resource Service (http://www.ers.usda.gov/data-products.aspx) and European trends at the European Food Safety Authority (http://www.efsa.europa.eu/).

Further, with the popularity of Apps for iPhone and Android, readers may find value in knowing three of the most popular dietary tracking tools: The Eatery, My Fitness Pal and My Plate Calorie Tracker by Livestrong. The Eatery is available free of charge for iPhone and iPod touch and works using a built-in camera and notes.

Users take a photo of every meal eaten and add an optional note about the meal and then rate it on a scale from fit to fat. Each meal, along with the user rating, is then added to what has been eaten. My Fitness Pal is free and compatible with iPhone, Android, BlackBerry, and Windows phones. My Fitness Pal remembers what users have eaten and have done most often in the past, and makes it easy for users to add those foods and activities again to a log. My Plate Calorie Tracker by Livestrong offers a free version and an upgraded version for 2.99 USD which is compatible with iPhone, Android, BlackBerry, and Windows phones. My Plate includes both foods and fitness items for tracking calorie intake and calories expended. It also remembers both recently eaten and frequently eaten foods.

References

Astrup A (2001), 'The role of dietary fat in the prevention and treatment of obesity. Efficacy and safety of low-fat diets.', *Int J Obes Relat Metab Disord*, vol. 25, (Suppl 1), pp. S46–50.

Austin GL, Ogden LG and O'Hill J (2011), 'Trends in carbohydrate, fat, and protein intakes and association with energy intake in normal-weight, overweight, and obese individuals: 1971–2006', *Am J Clin Nutr*, vol. 93, no. 4, pp. 836–843.

Awad AB and Chattopadhyay JP (1986), 'Effect of dietary saturated fatty acids on hormone-sensitive lipolysis in rat adipocytes', *J Nutr*, vol. 116, no. 6, pp. 1088–94.

Bell RR, Spencer MJ and Sherriff JL (1997), 'Voluntary exercise and monounsaturated canola oil reduce fat gain in mice fed diets high in fat', *J Nutr*, vol. 127, no. 10, pp. 2006–10.

Bhardwaj S, Passi SJ and Misra A (2011), 'Overview of trans fatty acids: biochemistry and health effects.', *Diabetes Metab Syndr*, vol. 5, no. 3, pp. 161–4.

Blundell JE and Stubbs RJ (1999), 'High and low carbohydrate and fat intakes: limits imposed by appetite and palatability and their implications for energy balance', *Eur J Clin Nutr*, vol. 53, (Suppl 1), pp. S148–65.

Bomsdorf C (2012), 'Denmark scraps much-maligned 'Fat Tax' after a year', *The Wall Street Journal*, November 12. Available at: http://online.wsj.com/OF6z9G

Brixval CS, Andersen LB and Heitmann BL (2009), 'Fat intake and weight development from 9 to 16 years of age', *Obesity Facts*, vol. 3, pp. 166–170.

Buckley JD and Howe PR (2009), 'Anti-obesity effects of long-chain omega-3 polyunsaturated fatty acids', *Obes Rev*, vol. 10, no. 6, pp. 648–59.

Codex Alimentarius. www.codexalimentarius.org. Accessed Sept 12, 2014.

Colditz GA, Willett WC, Stampfer MJ, London SJ, Segal MR and Speizer FE (1990), 'Patterns of weight change and their relation to diet in a cohort of healthy women', *Am J Clin Nutr*, vol. 51, no. 6, pp. 1100–5.

Daley S (2013), 'Hungary tries a dash of taxes to promote healthier eating habits', *New York Times*, March 2. Available at: http://nyti.ms/1gzWKs8

de Souza RJ, Bray G A, Carey VJ, Hall KD, LeBoff MS, *et al.* (2012), 'Effects of 4 weight-loss diets differing in fat, protein, and carbohydrate on fat mass, lean mass, visceral adipose tissue, and hepatic fat: results from the POUNDS LOST trial', *Am J Clin Nutr*, vol. 95, no. 3, pp. 614–25.

DeLany JP, Windhauser MM, Champagne CM and Bray GA (2000), 'Differential oxidation of individual dietary fatty acids in humans', *Am J Clin Nutr*, vol. 72, no. 4, pp. 905–11.

Donahue SMA, Rifas-Shiman SL, Gold DR, Jouni ZE, Gillman MW and Oken E (2011), 'Prenatal fatty acid status and child adiposity at age 3 y: results from a US pregnancy cohort', *Am J Clin Nutr*, vol. 93, pp. 780–8.

Drewnowski A (1997), 'Taste preferences and food intake', *Annu Rev Nutr*, vol. 17, pp. 237–53.

Ebbeling CB, Swain JF, Feldman HA, Wong WW, Hachey DL, *et al.* (2012), 'Effects of dietary composition on energy expenditure during weight-loss maintenance', *JAMA*, vol. 307, no. 24, pp. 2627–34.

EFSA (European Food Safety Authority) (2010), 'EFSA Panel on Dietetic Products, Nutrition and Allergies (NDA); Scientific Opinion on the substantiation of health claims related to conjugated linoleic acid (CLA) isomers and contribution to the maintenance or achievement of a normal body weight (ID 686, 726, 1516, 1518, 2892, 3165), increase in lean body mass (ID 498, 731), increase in insulin sensitivity (ID 1517), protection of DNA, proteins and lipids from oxidative damage (ID 564, 1937), and contribution to immune defences by stimulation of production of protective antibodies in response to vaccination (ID 687, 1519) pursuant to Article 13(1) of Regulation (EC) No1924/2006', *EFSA Journal*, vol. 8, no. 10, p. 26.

Field AE, Willett WC, Lissner L and Colditz GA (2007), 'Dietary fat and weight gain among women in the Nurses' Health Study', *Obesity (Silver Spring)*, vol. 15, no. 4, pp. 967–76.

Flatt JP (1995), 'Use and storage of carbohydrate and fat', *Am J Clin Nutr*, vol. 61, no. 4 (Suppl), pp. S952–9.

Fleury C, Neverova M, Collins S, Raimbault S, Champigny O, *et al.* (1997), 'Uncoupling protein-2: a novel gene linked to obesity and hyperinsulinemia', *Nat Genet*, vol. 15, no. 3, pp. 269–72.

Franz MJ (2000), 'Protein Controversies in Diabetes', *Diabetes Spectrum*, vol. 13, no. 3, p. 132.

Google Trends. Available from: http://bit.ly/1vWbuMy

Hansen CP, Berentzen TL, Halkjær J, Tjønneland A, Sørensen TI, *et al.* (2012), 'Intake of ruminant trans fatty acids and changes in body weight and waist circumference', *Eur J Clin Nutr*, vol. 66, no. 10, pp. 1104–9.

Hariri N and Thibault L (2010), 'High-fat diet-induced obesity in animal models', *Nutr Res Rev*, vol. 23, no. 2, pp. 270–99.

Heini AF and Weinsier RL (1997), 'Divergent trends in obesity and fat intake patterns: the American paradox', *Am J Med*, vol. 102, no. 3, pp. 259–64.

Heitmann BL (2001), 'Fat in the diet and obesity', in *International Textbook of Obesity*, ed. P Björntrop, John Wiley & Sons Ltd, Chichester, pp. 137–43.

Hession M, Rolland C, Kulkarni U, Wise A and Broom J (2009), 'Systematic review of randomized controlled trials of low-carbohydrate vs. low-fat/low-calorie diets in the management of obesity and its comorbidities', *Obes Rev*, vol. 10, no. 1, pp. 36–50.

Holt E (2011), 'Hungary to introduce broad range of fat taxes', *The Lancet*, vol. 378, no. 9793, p. 755.

Hooper L, Abdelhamid A, Moore HJ, Douthwaite W, Skeaff CM and Summerbell CD (2012), 'Effect of reducing total fat intake on body weight: systematic review and meta-analysis of randomised controlled trials and cohort studies', *BMJ*, vol. 345, p. e7666.

Howard BV, Manson JE, Stefanick ML, Beresford SA, Frank G, *et al.* (2006), 'Low-fat dietary pattern and weight change over 7 years: the Women's Health Initiative Dietary Modification Trial', *JAMA*, vol. 295, no. 1, pp. 39–49.

Innis SM, Green TJ and Halsey TK (1999), 'Variability in the trans fatty acid content of foods within a food category: implications for estimation of dietary trans fatty acid intakes', *J Am Coll Nutr*, vol. 18, no. 3, pp. 255–60.

Jakobsen MU, Dethlefsen C, Due KM, May AM, Romaguera D, *et al.* (2013), 'Fish consumption and subsequent change in body weight in European women and men', *Br J Nutr*, vol. 109, no. 2, pp. 353–62.

Jakobsen MU, Due KM, Dethlefsen C, Halkjaer J, Holst C, *et al.* (2012), 'Fish consumption does not prevent increase in waist circumference in European women and men', *Br J Nutr*, vol. 108, no. 5, pp. 924–31.

Jones PJ, Ridgen JE, Phang PT and Birmingham CL (1992), 'Influence of dietary fat polyunsaturated to saturated ratio on energy substrate utilization in obesity', *Metabolism*, vol. 41, no. 4, pp. 396–401.

Kavanagh K, Jones KL, Sawyer J, Kelley K, Carr JJ, *et al.* (2007) 'Trans fat diet induces abdominal obesity and changes in insulin sensitivity in monkeys', *Obesity (Silver Spring)*, vol. 15, no. 7, pp. 1675–84.

Kendall A, Levitsky DA, Strupp BJ and Lissner L. (1991), 'Weight loss on a low-fat diet: consequence of the imprecision of the control of food intake in humans', *Am J Clin Nutr*, vol. 53, no. 5, pp. 1124–9.

Kennedy A, Martinez K, Schmidt S, Mandrup S, LaPoint K and McIntosh M (2010), 'Antiobesity mechanisms of action of conjugated linoleic acid', *J Nutr Biochem*, vol. 21, no. 3, pp. 171–9.

Kersten S (2002), 'Peroxisome proliferator activated receptors and obesity', *Eur J Pharmacol*, vol. 440, no. 2–3, pp. 223–34.

Kessler D (2009), *The end of overeating*, Rodale Books Emmaus, Pennsylvania, USA.

Khan SA and Vanden Heuvel JP (2003), 'Role of nuclear receptors in the regulation of gene expression by dietary fatty acids (review)', *J Nutr Biochem*, vol. 14, no. 10, pp. 554–67.

Klem ML, Wing RR, McGuire MT, Seagle HM and Hill JO (1997), 'A descriptive study of individuals successful at long-term maintenance of substantial weight loss', *Am J Clin Nutr*, vol. 66, no. 2, pp. 239–46.

Kliewer SA, Sundseth SS, Jones SA, Brown PJ, Wisely GB, *et al.* (1997), 'Fatty acids and eicosanoids regulate gene expression through direct interactions with peroxisome proliferator-activated receptors alpha and gamma', *Proc Natl Acad Sci USA*, vol. 94, no. 9, pp. 4318–23.

Koh-Banerjee P, Chu NF, Spiegelman D, Rosner B, Colditz G, *et al.* (2003), 'Prospective study of the association of changes in dietary intake, physical activity, alcohol consumption, and smoking with 9-y gain in waist circumference among 16 587 US men', *Am J Clin Nutr*, vol. 78, no. 4, pp. 719–27.

Lanfer A, Knof K, Barba G, Veidebaum T, Papoutsou S, *et al.*, on behalf of the IDEFICS consortium (2011), 'Taste preferences in association with dietary habits and weight status in European children: results from the IDEFICS study', *International Journal of Obesity*, vol. 36, no. 1, pp. 27–34.

Lissner L and Heitmann BL (1995), 'Dietary fat and obesity: evidence from epidemiology', *Eur J Clin Nutr*, vol. 49, no. 2, pp. 79–90.

Lissner L, Levitsky DA, Strupp BJ, Kalkwarf HJ and Roe DA (1987), 'Dietary fat and the regulation of energy intake in human subjects', *Am J Clin Nutr*, vol. 46, no. 6, pp. 886–92.

Lottenberg AM, Afonso Mda S, Lavrador MS, Machado RM and Nakandakare ER (2012), 'The role of dietary fatty acids in the pathology of metabolic syndrome', *J Nutr Biochem*, vol. 23, no. 9, pp. 1027–40.

Malik VS, Popkin BM, Bray GA, Despres JP, Willett WC and Hu FB (2010), 'Sugar-sweetened beverages and risk of metabolic syndrome and type 2 diabetes: a meta-analysis', *Diabetes Care*, vol. 33, no. 11, pp. 2477–83.

Martínez-Victoria E and Yago MD (2012), 'Omega 3 polyunsaturated fatty acids and body weight', *Br J Nutr*, vol. 107 (Suppl 2), pp. S107–16.

Matsuo T, Sumida H and Suzuki M (1995), 'Beef tallow diet decreases beta-adrenergic receptor binding and lipolytic activities in different adipose tissues of rat', *Metabolism*, vol. 44, no. 10, pp. 1271–7.

Moss M (2013), *Salt Sugar Fat: How the Food Giants Hooked Us*, Random House, New York, USA.

Moussavi N, Gavino V and Receveur O (2008), 'Could the quality of dietary fat, and not just its quantity, be related to risk of obesity?', *Obesity*, vol. 16, no. 1, pp. 7–15.

Mozaffarian D (2006), Trans fatty acids. Effects on systematic inflammation and endothelial function. Atherosclerosis supplements. doi:10.10.16/j.atherosclerosissup.2006.04.007

Muhlhausler BS and Ailhaud GP (2013), 'Omega-6 polyunsaturated fatty acids and the early origins of obesity', *Curr Opin Endocrinol Diabetes Obes*, vol. 20, no. 1, pp. 56–61.

National Weight Control Registry. Available from: http://www.nwcr.ws/. Accessed, Sept 5, 2014.

Nelson DL and Cox MM (2008), *Lehninger Principles of Biochemistry*, 5th edn, Macmillan, New York.

Nutrient Data Laboratory. Available from: http://ndb.nal.usda.gov/ndb/search/list.

Ochiai M, Fujii K, Takeuchi H and Matsuo T (2013), 'Effects of dietary trans fatty acids on fat accumulation and metabolic rate in rat', *J Oleo Sci*, vol. 62, no. 2, pp. 57–64.

Oken E, Taveras EM, Popoola FA, Rich-Edwards JW and Gillman MW (2007), 'Television, walking, and diet: associations with postpartum weight retention', *Am J Prev Med*, vol. 32, no. 4, pp. 305–11.

Pariza MW, Park Y and Cook ME (2001), 'The biologically active isomers of conjugated linoleic acid', *Prog Lipid Res*, vol. 40, no. 4, pp. 283–98.

Perona JS, Portillo MP, Teresa Macarulla M, Tueros AI and Ruiz-Gutiérrez V (2000), 'Influence of different dietary fats on triacylglycerol deposition in rat adipose tissue', *Br J Nutr*, vol. 84, no. 5, pp. 765–74.

Piers LS, Walker KZ, Stoney RM, Soares MJ and O'Dea K (2002), 'The influence of the type of dietary fat on postprandial fat oxidation rates: monounsaturated (olive oil) vs saturated fat (cream)', *Int J Obes Relat Metab Disord*, vol. 26, no. 6, pp. 814–21.

Piers LS, Walker KZ, Stoney RM, Soares MJ and O'Dea K (2003), 'Substitution of saturated with monounsaturated fat in a 4-week diet affects body weight and composition of over-weight and obese men', *Br J Nutr*, vol. 90, no. 3, pp. 717–27.

Prentice AM and Jebb SA (2003), 'Fast foods, energy density and obesity: a possible mechanistic link', *Obes Rev*, vol. 4, no. 4, pp. 187–94.

Reed DR, Bachmanov AA, Beauchamp GK, Tordoff MG and Price RA (1997), 'Heritable variation in food preferences and their contribution to obesity', *Behav Genet*, vol. 27, no. 4, pp. 373–87.

Sampath H and Ntambi JM (2005), 'Polyunsaturated fatty acid regulation of genes of lipid metabolism', *Annu Rev Nutr*, vol. 25, pp. 317–40.

Sclafani A and Springer D (1976), 'Dietary obesity in adult rats: similarities to hypothalamic and human obesity syndromes', *Physiol Behav*, vol. 17, no. 3, pp. 461–71.

Skender ML, Goodrick GK, Del Junco DJ, Reeves RS, Darnell L, *et al.* (1996), 'Comparison of 2-year weight loss trends in behavioral treatments of obesity: diet, exercise, and combination interventions', *J Am Diet Assoc*, vol. 96, no. 4, pp. 342–6.

Soares MJ, Cummings SJ, Mamo JC, Kenrick M and Piers LS (2004), 'The acute effects of olive oil v. cream on postprandial thermogenesis and substrate oxidation in postmenopausal women', *Br J Nutr*, vol. 91, no. 2, pp. 245–52.

Storlien LH, Hulbert AJ and Else PL (1998), 'Polyunsaturated fatty acids, membrane function and metabolic diseases such as diabetes and obesity', *Curr Opin Clin Nutr Metab Care*, vol. 1, no. 6, pp. 559–63.

Stubbs RJ, Harbron CG, Murgatroyd PR and Prentice AM (1995a), 'Covert manipulation of dietary fat and energy density: effect on substrate flux and food intake in men eating ad libitum', *Am J Clin Nutr*, vol. 62, no. 2, pp. 316–29.

Stubbs RJ, Harbron CG and Prentice AM (1996), 'Covert manipulation of the dietary fat to carbohydrate ratio of isoenergetically dense diets: effect on food intake in feeding men ad libitum', *Int J Obes Relat Metab Disord*, vol. 20, no. 7, pp. 651–60.

Stubbs RJ, Ritz P, Coward WA and Prentice AM (1995b), 'Covert manipulation of the ratio of dietary fat to carbohydrate and energy density: effect on food intake and energy balance in free-living men eating ad libitum', *Am J Clin Nutr*, vol. 62, no. 2, pp. 330–7.

Takeuchi H, Matsuo T, Tokuyama K, Shimomura Y and Suzuki M (1995), 'Diet-induced thermogenesis is lower in rats fed a lard diet than in those fed a high oleic acid safflower oil diet, a safflower oil diet or a linseed oil diet', *J Nutr*, vol. 125, no. 4, pp. 950–5.

Thompson AK, Minihane AM and Williams CM (2011), 'Trans fatty acids and weight gain.', *Int J Obes (Lond)*, vol. 35, no. 5, pp. 315–24.

Tschöp M and Heiman ML (2001), 'Rodent obesity models: an overview', *Exp Clin Endocrinol Diabetes*, vol. 109, no. 6, pp. 307–19.

USDA 2010, *Dietary Guidelines for Americans, 2010*, HaH Services, Goverment Printing Office, Washington DC.

Vernarelli JA, Mitchell DC, Hartman TJ and Rolls BJ (2011), 'Dietary energy density is associated with body weight status and vegetable intake in U.S. children', *J Nutr*, vol. 141, no. 12, pp. 2204–10.

Wang Y and Proctor SD (2013), 'Current issues surrounding the definition of trans-fatty acids: implications for health, industry and food labels', *Br J Nutr*, vol. 110, no. 8, pp. 1369–83.

Wannamethee SG, Field AE, Colditz GA and Rimm EB (2004), 'Alcohol intake and 8-year weight gain in women: a prospective study', *Obes Res*, vol. 12, no. 9, pp. 1386–96.

Wing RR and Phelan S (2005), 'Long-term weight loss maintenance', *Am J Clin Nutr*, vol. 82, (Suppl 1), pp. S222–5.

Wing RR, Venditti E, Jakicic JM, Polley BA and Lang W (1998), 'Lifestyle intervention in overweight individuals with a family history of diabetes', *Diabetes Care*, vol. 21, no. 3, pp. 350–9.

Wu T, Gao X, Chen M and van Dam RM (2009), 'Long-term effectiveness of diet-plus-exercise interventions vs. diet-only interventions for weight loss: a meta-analysis', *Obes Rev*, vol. 10, no. 3, pp. 313–23.

Wyatt HR, Grunwald GK, Mosca CL, Klem ML, Wing RR and Hill JO (2002), 'Long-term weight loss and breakfast in subjects in the National Weight Control Registry', *Obes Res*, vol. 10, no. 2, pp. 78–82.

The 'Mediterranean diet' and weight management

7

M. Bes-Rastrollo, M. A. Martinez-Gonzalez
University of Navarra, Navarra, Spain

7.1 Introduction: the Mediterranean diet and other dietary patterns in the context of obesity

In recent years, scientific societies and institutional reviews have recommended low-fat-diets as the most suitable approach to promote both health and weight loss [1].

Long-term adherence to low-fat diets tends to be very limited [2], and a weight gain relapse usually occurs after 6–12 months of follow-up [3, 4]. In addition, with low-fat diets, long-term vegetable intake is reduced in parallel with the associated restriction in use of vegetable oils usually recommended for achieving a low-fat intake. Low-fat diets are also poor in several micronutrients and may require multivitamin supplements [5, 6].

Alternative classical approaches for weight loss in obesity are those restricting carbohydrates. Low-carbohydrate, high-protein, high-fat diets (referred to as low-carbohydrate diets) have been compared to low-fat, energy-restricted diets. A meta-analysis of five trials with 447 participants suggested that a low-carbohydrate diet is a feasible alternative to a low-fat diet for achieving weight loss, and may also have favorable metabolic effects after a 6-month follow-up [7]. However, the weight loss capacity of low-carbohydrate diets, as well as the improvements they induce in blood pressure, glucose metabolism, and the lipid profile were lost after a 12-month follow-up [7]. Only one randomized controlled trial has been conducted comparing weight loss and metabolic outcomes after a 2-year follow-up with a low-carbohydrate diet or a low-fat diet, and no between-group differences in weight, body composition or bone mineral density were found [8]. Low-carbohydrate diets are usually rich in saturated fatty acids, which explain why these diets are associated with LDL cholesterol elevations [7]. Usually, low-carbohydrate diets are low in fiber, poor in calcium, potassium, magnesium, and iron, and deficient in some vitamins [9]. Subjects on these diets frequently report halitosis and constipation, which are linked to their poor intake of whole-grain cereals, potatoes, vegetables, legumes, and fruits [9].

The relative success of a dietary pattern to induce a loss of body weight has been more frequently ascribed to calorie restriction, length of treatment, and, especially to participant compliance and long-term adherence to the prescribed diet. These aspects are more relevant than the relative proportion of macronutrients in the diet [10–12].

Managing and Preventing Obesity. http://dx.doi.org/10.1533/9781782420996.2.109

For this reason, weight reduction diets that differ substantially from the usual dietary pattern in the proportion of macronutrient contents are: (1) difficult to follow for years and (2) their safety has not been well documented. Due to these facts, they seem unsuitable for the prevention of chronic diseases. The potential long-term risks associated with low-fat diets and low-carbohydrate diets are unknown. Moreover the efficacy of these dietary patterns has never been tested in long-term randomized controlled trials assessing hard clinical endpoints (i.e., the incidence or mortality from cardiovascular events or cancer).

The sole randomized trial that has addressed the long-term effect of an intensive weight-loss lifestyle program in obese adults on cardiovascular disease and mortality is the Look AHEAD trial [13]. This study included only diabetic subjects and used a low-fat diet (<30% of total energy intake with <10% from saturated fat) combined with a physical activity program. The study was stopped after 9.6 years of median follow-up because of the lack of effect of the intervention on cardiovascular events. Although participants in the intervention group of the Look AHEAD trial lost an average of 5% of total body weight, they regained weight, and the differences compared to control progressively waned during the long follow-up period. These results support the view that long-term compliance and sustainability of low-fat diets are suboptimal and that nutritional quality should be a higher priority than reducing fat intake [14].

In light of these findings, the dietary control of overweight and obesity for cardiovascular disease prevention should be based on long-established, healthy, and palatable dietary patterns. One dietary paradigm that may be beneficial when implemented within an intensive weight-loss intervention is a traditional Mediterranean-type diet (MeDiet), relatively rich in fat from natural vegetable sources (virgin olive oil, nuts), and including an abundance of minimally processed plant-foods (vegetables, fruits, whole grains, legumes), low meat consumption, but moderate amounts of fish and wine, usually consumed with meals.

7.2   Definition of a Mediterranean dietary pattern

A dietary pattern based on the traditional Mediterranean diet is becoming increasingly recognized for its health benefits, particularly in relation to cardiovascular diseases [15, 16]. A Mediterranean diet encourages consumption of plant-based foods and is rich in olive oil. The variety of palatable foods in this dietary pattern fosters adherence and long-term sustainability. In contrast to low-fat diets, the Mediterranean diet has passed the tests of long-term sustainability, effectiveness [15] and nutritional quality [17, 18]. Even if other dietary approaches prove efficacious in achieving weight loss, a low-calorie Mediterranean diet may still be considered the most appropriate approach for achieving weight loss and reducing cardiovascular disease risk at the same time.

The term 'Mediterranean diet' is commonly defined as the historical dietary pattern consumed by the population of the Mediterranean regions in the 1950s and 1960s. It came to prominence because it was associated with extremely low rates of coronary heart disease and mortality in the Seven Countries Study; an ecological study undertaken in the 1950s by Professor Ancel Keys. Many additional epidemiological assessments since this pioneer study have identified the health benefits associated with this dietary pattern.

Although there is not a unique 'Mediterranean diet' and there are variations in the components of the traditional Mediterranean diet both between and within Mediterranean countries, a commonly traditional 'Mediterranean diet' consists of:

- high consumption of plant-based foods: fruit, vegetables, legumes, nuts and seeds, and whole grain cereals;
- olive oil as the main source of dietary lipids used to cook, to fry, to dress salads, etc.;
- frequent but moderate consumption of wine (especially red), usually with meals;
- consumption of fresh fish and seafood;
- moderate to low consumption of dairy products (especially yogurt and cheese), poultry, and eggs;
- low consumption of red and processed meat.

Another typical characteristic is the use of seasonally fresh and locally grown foods, which are minimally processed.

The production of the MeDiet pyramid in 1995 which graphically highlighted the frequency of consumption of each food group has helped increase public recognition of this dietary approach [19]. Recently, a group of scientists presented a consensual renewed communication tool for the general public, health professionals and stakeholders incorporating others aspects of the Mediterranean diet culture and lifestyle elements such as moderation, socialization, seasonability, physical activity, and adequate rest [20]. In 2010 the Mediterranean Diet was recognized as an Intangible Cultural Heritage of Humanity by UNESCO [21].

There are several food scores or indices that have been developed to help evaluate the adherence of a population to the MeDiet pattern of eating [22]. The most commonly used measure in epidemiological studies is the Mediterranean Dietary Score (MDS) proposed by Professor Trichopoulou. Originally, this MDS included only eight components to define MeDiet: high ratio of mono-unsaturated/saturated fatty acids, high intake of grains, high intake of fruit and nuts, high intake of vegetables, low intake of meat and meat products, and moderate intake of milk and dairy products. Subsequently, the same group of researchers added high intake of fish into the MDS [23]. The MDS currently used assigns a score of 0 or 1 according to the daily intake of each of the nine components. Sex-specific medians of the sample are used to define cut-off points against which individual consumption is compared. For each of the six protective components (fatty acid ratio, legumes, grains, fruits, vegetables, or fish) participants receive one point if their intake is over the sample median. Participants received one point if the intake is below the median for the two non-protective components (dairy products or meat). For alcohol the median consumption levels are not used but instead one point is scored if consumption is 10–50 g/day for men or 5–25 g/day for women. If participants meet all the characteristics of the Mediterranean diet, their MDS is the highest (nine points), reflecting maximum adherence. If they met none of the characteristics the MDS is the minimum (zero), reflecting no adherence at all.

In order to have a feasible, reliable and fast tool to evaluate adherence to the Mediterranean diet, the PREDIMED group developed a 14-item score for rapid estimation of adherence to the Mediterranean diet which is also very useful in clinical practice [24]. The PREDIMED 14-item score was an adaptation of a previously validated 9-item index [25]. This tool is useful to assess adherence to the MeDiet and to allow for immediate feedback to participants. It is composed of the questions shown in Table 7.1.

The 14-score PREDIMED screener shows reasonable agreement with the information gathered from the full-length food-frequency questionnaire and it is a good predictor for metabolic syndrome and its components [26], cardiovascular risk factors [27], or obesity indexes such as body mass index, waist circumference, and waist-to-height ratio [28].

Table 7.1 Defining adherence to the Mediterranean diet: PREDIMED 14-item score

	Frequency*
1. Do you use olive oil as the principal source of fat for cooking?	Yes
2. How much olive oil do you consume per day (including that used in frying, salads, meals eaten away from home, etc.)?	≥ 4 Tablespoon†
3. How many servings of vegetables do you consume per day? Count garnish and side servings as ½ point; a full serving is 200 g.	≥ 2
4. How many pieces of fruit (including fresh-squeezed juice) do you consume per day?	≥ 3
5. How many servings of red meat, hamburger, or sausages do you consume per day? A full serving is 100–150 g.	< 1
6. How many servings (12 g) of butter, margarine, or cream do you consume per day?	< 1
7. How many carbonated and/or sugar-sweetened beverages do you consume per day?	< 1
8. Do you drink wine? How much do you consume per week?	≥ 7 glasses ‡
9. How many servings (150 g) of pulses do you consume per week?	≥ 3
10. How many servings of fish/seafood do you consume per week?	$>= 3$
11. How many times do you consume commercial (not homemade) pastry such as cookies or cake per week?	< 2
12. How many times do you consume nuts per week? (1 serving = 30 g)	$>= 3$
13. Do you prefer to eat chicken, turkey, or rabbit instead of beef, pork, hamburgers, or sausages?	Yes
14. How many times per week do you consume boiled vegetables, pasta, rice, or other dishes with 'sofrito' (a sauce of tomato, garlic, onion, and leeks sauted in olive oil?	$>= 2$

* Criterion to score 1 point. Otherwise, 0 recorded
† 1 tablespoon = 13.5 g
‡ 1 glass = 100 ml

Source: Predimed web page (www.predimed.es) in the sections: Investigators Tools (http://www.predimed.es/investigators-tools.html); Quantitative score of adherence to the Mediterranean diet (http://www.unav.es/departamento/preventiva/files/file/documentos/predimed/14puntos.pdf).

7.3 Epidemiological evidence on Mediterranean diet and weight management

Taking into account the high percentage of energy from fat in the MeDiet, the promotion of this dietary pattern has generated some concerns about the possible risks of weight gain or obesity. However, the results of meta-analyses support the opposite conclusion, suggesting that a MeDiet might have a potential role in preventing weight gain and obesity in the long-term [29, 30].

Since cross-sectional studies do not define causality, we will focus on the results from large prospective epidemiologic studies with adequate control of confounding together with randomized trials.

7.3.1 Prospective observational studies

One of the first prospective studies was conducted as a component of the SUN Project in 2006 [31]. In a cohort of 6,319 Spanish university graduates, those with the highest adherence to the MeDiet exhibited a lower weight gain during an average follow-up of two years, although differences did not remain statistically significant after adjusting for potential confounders. In a more recent and updated analysis [32] conducted also with the SUN Project including 10,376 participants followed-up for a mean period of 5.7 years (sd: 2.2) (therefore with higher statistical power), adherence to the MeDiet was significantly associated with reduced weight gain: those participants with the highest baseline adherence exhibited the lowest weight gain (adjusted odds ratio of gaining 5 kg or more during the first four years of follow-up was 0.76; 95% CI: 0.64–0.90). In addition, when the association between a MeDiet and metabolic syndrome was assessed in the SUN cohort, those participants with the highest MeDiet adherence exhibited the lowest waist circumference after 6 years of follow-up [33].

Results from the EPIC-Spain cohort in 2006 [34] with a sample of 17,238 women and 10,589 men free of obesity at baseline showed that a higher adherence to the MeDiet was associated with lower risk of developing obesity after an average follow-up of 3.3 years. For women the risk was reduced by 31% (odds ratio: 0.69; 95% CI: 0.54–0.89), and for men by 32% (odds ratio: 0.68; 95% CI: 0.53–0.89).

In 2009, investigators from the ATTICA Study [35] did not find any significant association between adherence to the MeDiet and the incidence of overweight/obesity after assessing 1,528 women and 1,514 men in Greece. Similar non-significant results were found in a Chinese general population (n = 1,010) followed-up for 5.9 years [36]. By contrast, also in 2009 results from the Framinghan Heart Study Offspring revealed that a higher adherence to a Mediterranean-style dietary pattern was associated with lower waist circumference in 2,730 participants with a median age of 54 years followed-up for a mean time of 7 years [37].

One year later, in 2010, results from the EPIC-PANACEA cohort [38] with a very large sample size of 270,384 women and 373,803 men aged between 25 and 70 years showed that individuals with a high adherence to the MeDiet were 10% (95% CI: 4–18%) less likely to develop overweight or obesity than those with a low adherence to the MeDiet. The authors concluded that promoting a MeDiet as a model of healthy eating may help to slow down weight gain and prevent the development of obesity.

Results from the SUVIMAX study [39] reported that male participants with higher adherence to a MeDiet presented lower weight gain after 13 years of follow-up (the odds ratio for obesity for 1 standard deviation increase in MeDiet was 0.72; 95% CI: 0.59–0.88). However, for women the inverse association was not statistically significant.

More recently, data from a population-based survey conducted in Girona (Spain) (n = 3,058 men and women aged 25–74 years) showed that a high adherence to the MeDiet was associated with a statistically significant lower fat gain and lower incidence of abdominal obesity within 10 years, although the last association was not statistically significant [40].

7.3.2 Intervention studies

In 2001 McManus and colleagues [2] published the results of a randomized prospective 18-month trial in a free-living sample of 101 overweight men and women evaluating a MeDiet with moderate fat intake (35% of energy) versus a standard low-fat diet for weight loss. Those allocated to a MeDiet reduced body weight to a greater extent (between-group difference in weight change was 7.0 kg (95% CI: 5.3–8.7)) and achieved better adherence to the prescribed diet than those allocated to the low-fat diet (p < 0.002).

Two years later, Esposito et al. [41] found that 120 obese pre-menopausal patients on a low-energy Mediterranean-style diet with increased physical activity, attained a greater body weight reduction after two years than the control group which only received general information. Similarly, 279 post-menopausal women with type 2 diabetes in the USA allocated to a Mediterranean Lifestyle Program had a larger decrease in BMI compared to those in the control group after 6 months of follow-up [42]. Results from 34 Spanish overweight patients (18–63 years) with hypercholesterolemia showed that the isocaloric substitution of a diet rich in saturated fat by a diet high in mono-unsaturated fat produced a statistically significant reduction in body fat, although there were no differences in BMI, weight, or waist to hip ratio [43]. Around the same time, Esposito and colleagues [44] published the results of a randomized trial conducted in 180 Italian patients with metabolic syndrome (defined according to ATPIII criteria) to assess the effect of a Mediterranean-style diet compared to a control group that followed a prudent diet (50–60% of carbohydrates, 15–20% proteins, <30% total fat). They found that body weight decreased more in patients in the intervention group (−4 kg vs −1.2 kg; p < 0.001) after two years of follow-up.

In 2005, results from the Medi-RIVAGE study in France [45] (n = 212 patients with at least one CVD risk factor) showed a reduction in BMI after the 3-month dietary intervention with a MeDiet, however the differences versus a low-fat diet were not statistically significant. Similarly, results from a study of 101 German patients with coronary artery disease showed no differences in BMI after one year of intervention when compared to those in the control group who received written information about a healthy diet [46]. Results from the first three months follow-up of the larger PREDIMED trial (with 772 participants) showed that those allocated to a MeDiet, rich in virgin olive oil or nuts, exhibited no differences in body weight or BMI in comparison to those allocated to low-fat diet [47].

In 2008, Shai and colleagues [48] reported the results of their 2-year trial of 322 obese subjects randomized to three groups: a restricted-calorie low-fat diet, restricted-calorie MeDiet and non-restricted-calorie low-carbohydrate diet. They reported that a low-carbohydrate or a MeDiet restricted in calories were effective alternatives to a low-fat diet for weight loss. However, a trial with 202 survivors of myocardial infarction who were randomized to either a MeDiet or a low-fat diet (with a control group of usual-care) found that an active intervention with either a low-fat or a MeDiet significantly benefited these patients [49]. Elhayany and others [50] reported the results of a trial with 259 overweight diabetic patients allocated to one of three diets: low-carbohydrate Mediterranean, a traditional MeDiet, and 2003 American Diabetes Association (ADA) guidelines. After a 12-month follow-up they found significantly better weight losses and improved HDL levels among those allocated to a low-carbohydrate Mediterranean diet compared to the traditional MeDiet and ADA diet.

The consistent finding is that intervention studies that used a MeDiet with an energy restriction showed a reduction in body weight and beneficial effects regarding cardiovascular risk factors.

There are several mechanisms that may explain the beneficial effects of MeDiet on weight gain. The MeDiet provides a large quantity of dietary fiber increasing satiety and satiation through mechanisms, such as prolonged mastication and increased gastric retention [51]. At the same time the MeDiet has a low-energy density [51] and a low glycaemic load [29] compared with many other dietary patterns. These characteristics, together with its high water content, are likely to play a role in the prevention of weight gain.

So far, there has not been a meta-analysis that summarizes all the presented results, probably due to the heterogeneity between studies. Inconsistent results might be explained by the use of different scores to evaluate MeDiet, the adjustment for different confounding factors, lack of statistical power in some studies, and the use of different populations. It is important to note that no study concluded that a MeDiet was associated with higher weight gain or increased risk of obesity. All the results pointed towards an inverse association. Therefore, it seems that the high levels of obesity in the European Mediterranean countries might be explained by the recent departures from the traditional MeDiet in these countries [52], as well as a tendency to adopt more sedentary lifestyles [53]. Therefore, this dietary pattern should be promoted as it has many potential health benefits, including weight control.

7.4 Dietary and lifestyle intervention based on Mediterranean diet

Most experts agree that a feasible weight loss objective is a 10% reduction of body weight in 6 months, with weight losses of 0.5–1 kg per week. This should be based on a caloric restriction of 500–1000 kcal per day in comparison to the usual diet.

The European Research Council (ERC) has funded the ongoing PREDIMED-Plus trial [54] and the protocol of the PREDIMED-Plus (see www.predimedplus.com)

is presented below as an example of how to institute an energy-restricted MeDiet in practice. Many aspects of diet quality may affect body weight and risk of obesity-related disease to a greater extent than might be expected on the basis of macronutrient quantity [55, 56]. Two groups of foods (A and B) should be clearly differentiated in the education of participants:

A. Traditional eating patterns based on whole or minimally processed foods, such as the Mediterranean diet, incorporate most of the protective but few of the adverse individual dietary factors. The consumption of virgin olive oil, tree nuts, fruits and vegetables, salads, whole grains, fiber-rich foods and low-fat yogurts have been consistently related to weight loss or lower weight gain [55, 57].
B. On the contrary, sugar-sweetened beverages, fast food, refined grain products (especially white bread), white rice, pasta (excluding whole-grain pasta), French fries, potatoes, trans-fat (often present in commercial bakery goods), sweets, cakes, pies, sugar, precooked meals, sausages or cold cuts of processed meats, and patés have been consistently associated with weight gain [55, 58].

Therefore, the main focus of the intensive intervention will be in the overall quality of the diet aiming to avoid foods of the B group and to replace them with foods of the A group.

In addition, a reduction of 600 kcal in energy intake (or about 30% of estimated energy requirements) from the estimated energy requirements (based on the calculated basal metabolic rate of each individual and his/her physical activity) can be incorporated into the plan.

7.4.1 Energy-restricted Mediterranean diet

The energy-restricted Mediterranean diet should be planned by considering a reduction in the level of meat, carbohydrates, fruit juices, and sugary beverages and other foods of the B group as shown in Table 7.2 and expanded upon below.

1. A reduction in calories of 500 to 1,000 kcal/ day will help achieve a weight loss of 0.5 to 1 kg/week. Alcohol provides unneeded calories and displaces more nutritious foods. Alcohol consumption not only increases the number of calories in a diet but has been associated with obesity in epidemiological studies as well as in experimental studies. The impact of alcohol calories on a person's overall caloric intake needs to be assessed and appropriately controlled.
2. Fat restriction should focus on animal foods. Olive oil and nuts should be the preferred sources of fat.
3. Alcohol consumption will be no more than 2 glasses of wine/day for males and 1 glass for females.
4. Protein should be derived from plant sources and lean sources of animal protein.
5. Solid, minimally processed and fiber-rich carbohydrates with low glycemic index from different vegetables, fruits, and whole grains are good sources of vitamins, minerals, and fiber. A diet rich in soluble fiber, including oat bran, legumes, barley, and most fruits and vegetables may be effective in reducing blood cholesterol levels. A diet high in all types of fiber may also aid in weight management by promoting satiety at lower levels of calorie and fat intake.
6. During weight loss, attention should be given to maintaining an adequate intake of vitamins and minerals. Maintenance of the recommended calcium intakes of 1,000 to 1,500 mg/day is especially important for women who may be at risk of osteoporosis.

Table 7.2 **Energy-restricted Mediterranean diet**

Nutrient	Recommended intake
Calories[1]	Approximately 600 kcal/day (about 30%) reduction from usual intake
Total fat[2]	35–40 percent of total calories
Saturated fatty acids	8 to 10 percent of total calories
Mono-unsaturated fatty acids	Up to 20 percent of total calories
Polyunsaturated fatty acids	Up to 10 percent of total calories
Cholesterol	<300 mg/day
Protein[4]	Approximately 20 percent of total calories
Carbohydrate[5]	>40–45 percent or more of total calories of low glycemic index
Sodium chloride	No more than 100 mmol per day (approximately 2.4 g of sodium or approximately 6 g of sodium chloride)
Calcium[6]	1,000 to 1,500 mg
Dietary fiber[5]	30–35 g

Note: superscript numbers refer to the text.

Participants should receive counselling to progressively increase their compliance with the following dietary goals:

1. Use of virgin olive oil (exclusively the virgin variety) for cooking, dressing salads and as a spread.
2. Consumption of fruits ≥2 portions per day.
3. Consumption of vegetables ≥2 portions per day (at least 1 portion raw or as salad).
4. Reduction of white bread to ≤1 serving/day (1 serving = 75 g).
5. Use of whole grain products ≥5 times per week.
6. Less than one serving (1 serving = 100–150 g) of red meat, hamburger, or meat products (ham, sausage, etc.) per week.
7. Less than 1 serving of butter or cream per week (1 serving = 12 g).
8. Consumption of less than one sweet/carbonated beverage per week.
9. Consumption of three or more servings of legumes per week (1 serving = 150 g).
10. Consumption of 3 or more servings of fish or shellfish per week (1 serving: 100–150 g fish, or 4–5 units or 200 g shellfish).
11. Consumption of less than 3 commercial sweets or pastries (not homemade), such as cakes, cookies, biscuits, or custard per week.
12. Consumption of one or more servings of nuts (including peanuts) per week (1 serving = 30 g).
13. Consumption of chicken, turkey or rabbit meat instead of veal, pork, hamburger or sausage.
14. Use of *sofrito* (sauce made with tomato and onion, leek, and garlic, simmered with olive oil) more than 2 times per week.
15. Not adding sugar to beverages (coffee, tea), but replace it with non-caloric artificial sweeteners.

16. Consumption of pasta or rice less than 3 servings per week (unless they are whole grain products).

17. Consumption of wine with meals: 7–14 glasses (100 mL) per week in men and 4–8 glasses per week in women.

7.4.2 Exercise recommendations

Participants should be encouraged to gradually increase their level of physical activity to reach at least 45 minutes per day after 6 months of intervention. This physical activity intervention should include both aerobic activities, mainly brisk walking (or any equivalent physical activity of moderate intensity), and resistance training. These recommendations can be adapted to the preferences and convenience of the participant using replacements based on the same amount of METS-h/day.

7.5 Conclusions and future trends

In summary, a MeDiet is characterized by abundance of vegetarian foods, fresh and minimally processed, fresh fruit as the daily typical dessert, and only occasionally consumption of sweets. Numerous studies have shown that this is a healthy eating pattern that successfully combines pleasant taste and quality food with positive health benefits and has a large potential for long-term sustainability. However, there is a need of large randomized trials of longer duration to assess the effect of a MeDiet restricted in calories on weight management and its effect on hard clinical endpoints. This is the objective of the PREDIMED-Plus, a multicenter randomized trial in Spain which aims to recruit 6,000 participants. Its final results are expected in 2020.

7.6 Sources of further information and advice

Websites

Web of the PREDIMED clinical trial: www.predimed.es (with lists of publications, and educational tools used in the study).

Web of the PREDIMED-Plus clinical trial: www.predimedplus.com (with the protocol of the PREDIMED-Plus clinical trial).

Web Fundación Dieta Mediterránea: www.dietamediterranea.com (with the updated pyramid of the Mediterranean Diet and weekly MeDiet recipes in Spanish).

Web of Oldways: www.oldwayspt.org (a nonprofit food and nutrition education organization, inspiring good health through heritage by promoting traditional foods).

Books

Hu FB. *Obesity Epidemiology*. New York: Oxford University Press, 2008.

Zacharias E. *The Mediterranean Diet: a clinician's guide for patient care*. New York: Springer-Verlag Gmbh, 2012.

Willett WC, Skerret PJ. Eat, *Drink, and Be Healthy: The Harvard Medical School Guide to Healthy Eating.* New York: Free Press, 2005.

References

1. NHLBI/NHI. *The Practical Guide: identification, evaluation, and treatment of overweight and obesity in adults.* NIH Publication Number 00-4084, 2000.
2. McManus K, Antinoro L, Sacks F; A randomized controlled trial of a moderate-fat, low-energy diet compared with a low fat, low-energy diet for weight loss in overweight adults. *Int J Obes Relat Metab Disord,* 2001; 25:1503–11.
3. Barte JC, ter Bogt NC, Bogers RP, Teixeira PJ, Blissmer B, Mori TA, Bemelmans WJ. Maintenance of weight loss after lifestyle interventions for overweight and obesity, a systematic review. *Obes Rev,* 2010; 11:899–906.
4. Turk MW, Yang K, Hravnak M, Sereika SM, Ewing LJ, Burke LE. Randomized clinical trials of weight loss maintenance: a review. *J Cardiovasc Nurs,* 2009; 24:58–80.
5. Dwyer JT, Allison DB, Coates PM. Dietary supplements in weight reduction. *J Am Diet Assoc,* 2005; 105 (5 Suppl 1):S80–6.
6. Xanthakos SA. Nutritional deficiencies in obesity and after bariatric surgery. *Pediatr Clin North Am,* 2009; 56:1105–21.
7. Nordmann AJ, Nordmann A, Briel M, *et al.,* Effects of low-carbohydrate vs low fat diets on weight loss and cardiovascular risk factors: a meta-analysis of randomized controlled trials. *Arch Intern Med,* 2006; 166:285–93.
8. Foster GD, Wyatt HR, Hill JO, Makris AP, Rosenbaum DL, *et al.,* Weight and metabolic outcomes after 2 years on a low-carbohydrate versus low-fat diet: a randomized trial. *Ann Intern Med,* 2010; 153:147–57.
9. Foreyt JP, Salas-Salvado J, Caballero B, Bulló M, Gifford KD, *et al.,* Weight-reducing diets: are there any differences? *Nutr Rev,* 2009; 67 (Suppl 1): S99–101.
10. Bravata DM, Sanders L, Huang J, *et al.,* Efficacy and safety of low-carbohydrate diets: a systematic review. *JAMA,* 2003; 289:1837–50.
11. Dansinger ML, Gleason JA, Griffith JL, Selker HP, Schaefer EJ. Comparison of the Atkins, Ornish, Weight Watchers, and Zone diets for weight loss and heart disease risk reduction: a randomized trial. *JAMA,* 2005; 293:43–53.
12. Sacks FM, Bray GA, Carey VJ, Smith SR, Ryan DH, *et al.,* Comparison of weight-loss diets with different compositions of fat, protein, and carbohydrates. *N Engl J Med,* 2009; 360:859–73.
13. Look AHEAD Research Group, Wing RR, Bolin P, Brancati FL, *et al.,* Cardiovascular effects of intensive lifestyle intervention in type 2 diabetes. *N Engl J Med,* 2013; 369:145–54.
14. Després JP, Poirier P. Looking back at Look AHEAD—giving lifestyle a chance. *Nat Rev Cardiol,* 2013; 10:184–6.
15. Estruch R, Ros E, Salas-Salvado J, Covas MI, Corella D, Aros F, *et al.,* Primary prevention of cardiovascular disease with a Mediterranean diet. *N Engl J Med,* 2013; 368:1279–90.
16. Martinez-Gonzalez MA, Bes-Rastrollo M. Dietary patterns, Mediterranean diet, and cardiovascular disease. *Curr Opin Lipidol,* 2014; 25:20–6.
17. Serra-Majem L, Bes-Rastrollo M, Román-Viñas B, Pfrimer K, Gilabert R, Sánchez-Villegas A, Martínez-González MA. Dietary patterns and nutritional adequacy in a Mediterranean country. *Br J Nutr,* 2009; 101(Suppl. 2):S21–28.

18. Maillot M, Issa C, Vieux F, Lairon D, Darmon N. The shortest way to reach nutritional goals is to adopt Mediterranean food choices: evidence from computer-generated personalized diets. *Am J Clin Nutr*, 2011; 94:1127–37.

19. Willett WC, Sacks F, Trichopoulou A, Drescher G, Ferro-Luzzi, Helsing E, Trichopoulos D. Mediterranean diet pyramid: a cultural model for healthy eating. *Am J clin Nutr*, 1995; 61(Suppl):S1402–6.

20. Bach-Faig A, Berry EM, Lairon D, Reguant J, Trichopoulou A, Dernini S, *et al.*, Mediterranean diet pyramid today. Science and cultural updates. *Public Health Nutr*, 2011; 14:2274–84.

21. UNESCO. Convention for the safeguarding of the intangible cultural heritage: http://www.unesco.org/culture/ich/index.php?RL=00394 (accessed August 2013).

22. Bach A, Serra-Majem L, Carrasco JL, Roman B, Ngo J, Bertomeu I, Obrador I. The use of indexes evaluating the adhrence to the Mediterranean diet in epidemiological studies: a review. *Public Health Nutr*, 2006; 9:132–46.

23. Trichopoulou A, Costacou T, Bamia C, Trichopoulos D. Adherence to a Mediterranean diet and survival in a Greek population. *N Engl J Med*, 2003; 348:2599–608.

24. Schroder H, Fito M, Estruch R, Martinez-Gonzalez MA, Corella D, Salas-Salvado J, *et al.*, A short screener is valid for assessing Mediterranean diet adherence among older Spanish men and women. *J Nutr*, 2011; 141:1140–5.

25. Martinez-Gonzalez MA, Fernandez-Jarne E, Serrano-Martinez M, Wright M, Gomez-Gracia E. Development of a short dietary intake questionnaire for the quantitative estimation of adherence to a cordioprotective Mediterranean diet. *Eur J Clin Nutr*, 2004; 58:1550–2.

26. Babio N, Bullo M, Basora J, Martinez-Gonzalez MA, Fernandez-Ballart J, Marquez-Sandoval F, *et al.*, Adherence to the Mediterranean diet and risk of metabolic syndrome and its components. *Nutr Metab Cardiovasc Dis*, 2009; 19:563–70.

27. Sanchez-Tainta A, Estruch R, Bullo M, Corella D, Gomez-Gracia E, Fiol M, *et al.*, Adherence to a Mediterranean-type diet and reduced prevalence of clustered cardiovascular risk factors in a cohort of 3,204 high-risk patients. *Eur J Cardiovasc Rehabil*, 2008; 15:589–93.

28. Martinez-Gonzalez MA, Garcia-Arellano A, Toledo E, Salas-Salvado J, Buil-Cosiales P, Corella D, *et al.*, A 14-item Mediterranean diet assessment tool and obesity indexes among high-risk subjects: the PREDIMED trial. *PLoS One*, 2012; 7:e43134.

29. Buckland G, Bach A, Serra-Majem L. Obesity and the Mediterranean diet: a systematic review of observational and intervention studies. *Obes Reviews*, 2008; 9:582–93.

30. Kastorini CM, Milionis HJ, Goudevenos JA, Panagiotakos DB. Mediterranean diet and coronary heart disease: Is obesity a link? A systematic review. *Nutr Metab Cardiovasc Dis*, 2010; 20:536–51.

31. Sanchez-Villegas A, Bes-Rastrollo M, Martinez-Gonzalez MA, Serra-Majem L. Adherence to a Mediterranean dietary pattern and weight gain in a follow-up study: the SUN cohort. *Int J Obes (Lond)*, 2006; 30:350–8.

32. Beunza JJ, Toledo E, Hu FB, Bes-Rastrollo M, Serrano-Martinez M, Sanchez-Villegas A, *et al.*, Adherence to the Mediterranean diet, long-term weight change, and incident overweight or obesity: the Sesguimiento Universidad de Navarra (SUN) cohort. *Am J Clin Nutr*, 2010; 92:1–8.

33. Tortosa A, Bes-Rastrollo M, Sanchez-Villegas A, Basterra-Gortari FJ, Nunez-Cordoba JM, Martinez-Gonzalez MA. Mediterranean diet inversely associated with the incidence of metabolic syndrome: the SUN prospective cohort. *Diabetes Care*, 2007; 30:2957–9.

34. Mendez MA, Popkin BM, Jaksyn P, Berenguer A, Tormo MJ, Sanchez MJ, et al., Adherence to a Mediterranean diet is associates with reduced 3-year incidence of obesity. J Nutr, 2006; 136:2934–8.

35. Yannakoulia M, Panagiotakos D, Pitsavos C, Lentzas Y, Chrysohoou C, Skoumas I, et al., Five-year incidence of obesity and its determinants: the ATTICA study. Public Health Nutr, 2008; 12:36–43.

36. Woo J, Cheung B, Ho S, Sham A, Lam TH. Influence of dietary pattern on the development of overweight in a Chinese population. Eur J Clin Nutr, 2008; 62:480–7.

37. Rumawas ME, Meigs JB, Dwyer JT, McKeown NM, Jacques PF. Mediterranean-style dietary pattern, reduced risk of metabolic syndrome traits, and incidence in the Framingham Offspring Cohort. Am J Clin Nutr, 2009; 90:1608–14.

38. Romaguera D, Norat T, Vergnaud AC, Mouw T, May AM, Agudo A, et al., Mediterranean dietary patterns and prospective weight change in participants of the EPIC-PANACEA project. Am J Clin Nutr, 2010; 92:912–21.

39. Lassale C, Fezeu L, Andreeva VA, Hercberg S, Kengne AP, Czernichow S, et al., Association between dietary scores and 13-year weight change and obesity risk in a French prospective cohort. Int J Obes, 2012; 36:1455–62.

40. Funtikova AN, Benitez-Arciniega AA, Gomez SF, Fito M, Elosua R, Schroder H. Mediterranean diet impact on changes in abdominal fat and 10-year incidence of abominal obesity in a Spanish population. Brit J Nutr, 2014; 111:1481–7.

41. Esposito K, Pontillo A, Di Palo C, Giugliano G, Masella M, Marfella R, et al., Effect of weight loss and lifestyle changes on vascular inflammatory markeres in obese women: a randomized trial. JAMA, 2003; 289:1799–804.

42. Toobert DJ, Glasgow RE, Strycker LA, Barrera M Jr, Radcliffe JL, Wander RC, et al., Biologic and quality-of-life outcomes from the Mediterranean Lifestyle Program: a randomized clinical trial. Diabetes Care, 2003; 26:2288–93.

43. Fernandez de la Puebla RA, Fuentes F, Perez-Martinez P, Sanchez E, Paniagua JA, Lopez-Miranda J, et al., A reduction in dietary saturated fat decreases body fat content in overweight, hypercholesterolemic males. Nutr Metab Cardiovasc Dis, 2003; 13:273–7.

44. Esposito K, Marfella R, Ciotola M, Di Palo C, Giugliano F, Giugliano G, et al., Effect of a Mediterranean-style diet on endothelial dysfunction and markers of vascular inflammation in the metabolic syndrome: a randomized trial. JAMA, 2004; 292:1440–6.

45. Vincent-Baudry S, Defoort C, Gerber M, Bernard MC, Verger P, Helal O, et al., The Medi-RIVAGE study: reduction of cardiovascular disease risk factors after a 3-mo intervention with a Mediterranean-type diet or a low-fat diet. Am J Clin Nutr, 2005; 82:964–71.

46. Michalsen A, Lehmann N, Pithan C, Knoblausch NT, Mocbus S, Kannenberg F, et al., Mediterranean diet has no effect on markers of inlammatin and metabolic risk factors in patients with coronary artery disease. Eur J Clin Nutr, 2006; 60:478–85.

47. Estruch R, Martinez-Gonzalez MA, Corella D, Salas-Salvado J, Ruiz-Gutierrez V, Covas MI, et al., Effects of a Mediterranean-style diet on cardiovascular risk factors: a randomized trial. Ann Intern Med, 2006; 145:1–11.

48. Shai I, Schwarzfuchs D, Henkin Y, Shahar DR, Witkow S, Greenberg I, et al., Weight loss with a low-carbohydrate, Mediterranean, or low-fat diet. N Engl J Med, 2008; 359:229–41.

49. Tuttle KR, Shuler LA, Packard DP, Milton JE, Daratha KB, Bibus DM, et al., Comparison of low-fat versus Mediterranean-style dietary intervention after firs myocardial infarction (from the Heart Institute of Spokane Diet Intervention and Evaluation Trial). Am J Cardiol, 2008; 101:1523–30.

50. Elhayany A, Lustman A, Abel R, Attal-Singer J, Vinker S. A low carbohydrate Mediterranean diet improves cardiovascular risk factors and diabetes control among overweight patients with type 2 diabetes mellitus: a 1-year prospective randomized intervention study. *Diabetes Obes Metab*, 2010; 12:204–9.
51. Schroder H. Protective mechanisms of the Mediterranean diet in obesity and type 2 diabetes. *J Nutr Biochem*, 2007; 18:149–60.
52. Serra-Majem L, Helsing E. Changing patterns of fat intake in Mediterranean countries. *Eur J Clin Nutr*, 1993; 47(Suppl):S13–20.
53. Martinez-Gonzalez MA, Martinez JA, Hu FB, Gibney MJ, Kearney J. Physical inactivity, sedentary lifestyle and obesity in the European Union. *Int J Obes Relat Metab Disord*, 1999; 11:1192–201.
54. Advanced Research Grant (2014–2019) to Prof. Miguel A. Martinez-Gonzalez. Contract: 'Long-term effects of an energy-restricted Mediterranean diet on mortality and cardiovascular disease. The PREDIMED-PLUS STUDY'. Grant agreement no.: 340918. Duration: 60 months.
55. Mozaffarian D, Hao T, Rimm EB, Willett WC, Hu FB. Changes in diet and lifestyle and long-term weight gain in women and men. *N Engl J Med*, 2011; 364:2392–404.
56. Ludwig DS. Weight loss strategies for adolescents: a 14-year-old struggling to lose weight. *JAMA*, 2012; 307:498–508.
57. Martinez-González MA, Bes-Rastrollo M. Nut consumption, weight gain and obesity: Epidemiological evidence. *Nutr Metab Cardiovasc Dis*, 2011; 21(Suppl 1):S40–5.
58. Schulze MB, Fung TT, Manson JE, Willett WC, Hu FB. Dietary patterns and changes in body weight in women. Obesity (Silver Spring). 2006; 14:1444–53.

Breastfeeding and weight in mothers and infants

J. L. Baker

Institute of Preventive Medicine and University of Copenhagen, Denmark

8.1 Introduction

The worldwide obesity epidemic means that too many women enter into pregnancy carrying extra weight which puts their health and that of their unborn child at risk.[1,2] The risks associated with pregravid overweight and obesity (body mass index [BMI] 25.0–29.9 kg/m^2 and $\geq$30 kg/m^2, respectively) are further exacerbated by excessive gestational weight gain, which is particularly common in women from Australia,[3] Europe[4–6] and North America.[7–9] Furthermore, excessive gestational weight gain increases the risk of developing overweight and obesity in women who were at a healthy weight prior to pregnancy.[10,11] Overall, reproduction is associated with a net weight gain, averaging 0.5 to 4.0 kg at one year postpartum.[12] Nonetheless, there is great variability with 14–20% of women retaining >4.5 kg one year postpartum.[12] Returning to prepregnancy weight is a goal that most women have.[12,13] Although this goal is achievable for many women, the optimal intervention to help them succeed has yet to be identified.[12,13]

One attractive intervention is the promotion of breastfeeding as it provides numerous health benefits for the mother–infant dyad.[14,15] Breastfeeding is the optimal form of infant nutrition,[16] and its energetic cost to the mother theoretically contributes to maternal postpartum weight loss.[14] Additionally, evidence suggests that breastfed infants have a lower risk of being obese throughout life as compared with formula-fed infants.[15] This chapter will focus on the potential effects of breastfeeding on maternal postpartum weight change and upon on the infants' risk of obesity across the lifespan.

8.1.1 Definition of breastfeeding

Breastfeeding varies in its intensity, how it is practiced and in its duration. Breastfeeding is characterized by the degree to which the infant receives human milk as the sole source of nutrition. It ranges from exclusive (human milk only) to none (non-human milk only). Within this spectrum lies the categories of predominant/full (human milk is the primary form of nutrition) to any/partial (the infant receives human milk to any degree).[17] Milk expression for use by bottle or cup feeding is another method (breast milk feeding) and it is gaining in popularity in America and

Australia in particular.[18] It is worth remembering that even exclusively breastfed infants will, at some point, transition away from human milk as the primary source of nutrition. Since 2001, the World Health Organization (WHO) has recommended six months of exclusive breastfeeding and at least two years of partial breastfeeding.[19] Worldwide, however, few women achieve this target.[20]

8.1.2   Predictors of breastfeeding success

Social, psychosocial and biological factors contribute to breastfeeding success. Women with higher socio-economic status, older age, higher levels of education, supportive partners and who do not smoke are more likely to succeed.[14] Several psychosocial constructs also predict which women will be successful at breastfeeding. Success is associated with expressing an intention to breastfeed, having confidence in the ability to breastfeed, and believing that breastfeeding has health benefits.[14,21] Further, the biological factor of a woman's prepregnant weight is also associated with breastfeeding success. Compared with normal-weight women, women who are overweight or obese prior to conception are less successful at initiating breastfeeding and continue to do so for shorter durations.[22–24] In a large study of Danish women Baker et al.,[25] found that the risk of terminating any breastfeeding sooner than a normal-weight woman was 12% higher among overweight women and was 24 to 39% higher across class I to class III obesity (BMI 30.0–34.9 kg/m^2 and $\geq$ 40.0 kg/m^2, respectivlely). It is noteworthy that this study was conducted among women who had successfully initiated breastfeeding and were living in a social context that is supportive of breastfeeding. These findings have also been identified in other populations and ethnic groups.[23,24,26]

8.2   Energetic cost of breastfeeding

During pregnancy, a woman's body undergoes physiological and metabolic changes that lead to the accumulation of energy stores, particularly as visceral (intra-abdominal) fat.[27] After childbirth, shifts in hormone concentrations permit lactation to occur. Until 4 to 5 months of age, exclusively breastfed infants consume 750 to 800 g/day of human milk (range: 450 to 1200 g/day).[14] Thereafter, milk intakes vary even more due to changes in how the infants are fed once exclusive breastfeeding ceases. The energetic costs of milk production by the mother are estimated at 2021 to 2250 kJ/day.[28]

Breastfeeding women can compensate for the increased energy needs by increasing their energy intake, reducing their physical activity and/or mobilising body fat reserves.[28] Available evidence from affluent countries suggests that fat mobilisation is not the primary method used to cover the extra energy demands, particularly in the early postpartum period (through approximately 12 weeks).[29] Even though fat reserves can be mobilised during breastfeeding, the amount is highly variable among women and across its duration.[30] Breastfeeding has a modest energetic cost, and a plausible biological relation with weight loss, but it is a behaviour that occurs in the context of a wide range of environmental factors that influence its potential for enhancing the return to prepregnancy weight.

8.3   Postpartum weight change

Postpartum weight change is the difference between a woman's prepregnancy weight and her weight at some point after childbirth. A consensus is lacking on which is the appropriate time point to focus on. Some studies examine weight change within a few weeks after the birth whereas others examine it decades later. In particular with longer term follow-ups, disentangling the effects of age-related weight gain versus pregnancy weight retention is a challenge. Postpartum weight change has many determinants which differ in terms of if and when they are modifiable (i.e. ante-, peri- or postpartum). Of the identified risk factors, gestational weight gain has one of the strongest associations with postpartum weight retention.[10] Simply put, the more a woman gains, the more she is likely to retain. Additionally it is known that the effects of gestational weight gain vary by a woman's prepregnancy BMI, with overweight and obese women having the highest risk of retaining this weight.[31] Other factors of importance include a woman's age, ethnicity, parity, socioeconomic status, educational level, psychosocial burden, diet and physical activity levels.[10,31,32] The behaviour of breastfeeding, which has the advantage of being modified postpartum, also has associations with postpartum weight change, although the results are conflicting.[14]

8.3.1   *Very short term weight change (0 to 3 months)*

Studies examining associations between breastfeeding and weight change in the very short term typically find small or no associations.[29,33] During this period, weight loss has a physiologic basis as the woman's body loses the fluids gained during pregnancy (intra- and extra-cellular water, blood, plasma).[10] The relationship among energy intake, physical activity and body fat mobilisation constantly shifts during these months, and this affects how much weight women can potentially lose through breast-feeding.[29] In these early months, formula feeding mothers often lose more weight than breastfeeding mothers. Several studies have shown that compared to mothers who breastfeed, mothers who feed formula consume approximately 2931 kJ/day less during these early postpartum months, which may partially explain this finding.[34] Additionally when the breastfeeding demands are high in these early months, physical activity levels may be reduced.[29] The combination of energy intake and physical activity levels may explain why breastfeeding does not help reduce weight during this period.

8.3.2   *Short term weight change (0 to 6 months)*

When weight change during the first 6 months postpartum is examined, some, but not all, studies find that breastfeeding is associated with weight loss.[33] The rates of weight loss are generally higher in the first 4–6 months among breastfeeding women than during subsequent months.[14] Typically women from developed countries lose approximately 0.8 kg/month during these first 6 months.[30] In a study of Danish women, the association between breastfeeding and postpartum weight change at 6 months was investigated in the context of prepregnancy BMI, gestational weight gain and breastfeeding (using a scaled measure that captured its intensity and duration).[35] In this investigation Baker et al.,[35] found postpartum weight retention was reduced by 0.06 to 0.09 kg per week of breastfeeding among all women except those with prepregnancy BMI values ≥ 35.0 kg/m^2. Another large study on Norwegian women that accounted for similar factors found that each additional month of full breastfeeding reduced maternal weight at 6 months by 0.05 kg per month.[36] Interestingly, this study found that the greatest benefit for this weight loss occurred among women with low incomes.[36]

8.3.3   Long term weight change (6 months to 3 years)

In studies that examine the effects of breastfeeding on weight retention in this period postpartum, the results are again inconsistent.[33] In American populations, breastfeeding has been associated with reduced weight loss at 1 year postpartum in Michigan,[37] and rural upstate New York,[38] but it showed no association with weight loss in a study of overweight and obese women from a more racially diverse population in North Carolina.[39] In the North Carolina study, however, 'junk food' intake and a lack of physical activity were the strongest predictors of weight retention and gain, highlighting the importance of diet and activity in weight change. In an Australian population, investigators found that each additional week of breastfeeding (irrespective of the intensity) reduced weight retention at 1 year by 0.04 kg.[40]

At 18 months postpartum, an effect of breastfeeding was detected only for women who had fully breastfed for 6 months and then continued with any breastfeeding for an addition 6 months in the aforementioned Danish study.[35] Similar results were found in the previously described Norwegian study; each additional month of full breastfeeding reduced maternal weight at 18 months by 0.1 kg per month; partial breastfeeding did not have an effect.[36] These results suggest that breastfeeding needs to be intense and sustained to have a lasting effect. A 3-year follow up study of American women did not detect an effect.[41]

8.3.4   Very long-term weight change (beyond 3 years)

Further, some studies have investigated very long term effects, and the results are equivocal as well. Among Brazilian women, compared to those who breastfed for 6 to 11.9 months, those who breastfed for <1 month or for ≥ 12 months had less favourable anthropometric measures when followed-up 5 or more years later.[42] These associations suggest that characteristics associated with the reasons for continuing or terminating breastfeeding underlie the association. A study of American women found that compared to women who breastfed to any extent ≥ 12 weeks, women who never breastfed had a 3.73 kg greater weight change between 6 months post-partum and 5 or more years later.[43] A Danish study that examined weight change at 7 years postpartum found that the duration of breastfeeding had a small effect on weight loss, suggesting that the effects of breastfeeding may persist.[44] In a Swedish study, compared to women who remained normal-weight 15 years post-partum, those who became overweight had breastfed for shorter durations and/or less intensively.[45]

8.4 Breastfeeding benefits for infants

The period from birth to one year of age is the most rapid time of growth among humans; healthy infants generally triple their birth weight and settle into a postnatal growth trajectory.[46] Given this rapid growth, infants are vulnerable to nutritional and environmental influences.[47,48] Breastfeeding confers numerous health benefits to the infant during this time including a reduction in the risk of certain infections and diseases.[15] Further, a large body of evidence indicates that breastfeeding may reduce the risk of developing overweight and obesity during childhood, adolescence and even adulthood.[15,49–53] Therefore, breastfeeding may also help with preventing over-weight and obesity in the next generation.

8.4.1 Breastfeeding and infant growth

During infancy, it is well-established that breastfed infants in developed countries are leaner than those who were formula fed at one year of age.[54] Breastfeeding may contribute to differences in growth through several pathways. Breast milk composition changes during a single feed,[55] it contains a wide range of bioactive constituents (which are still being identified),[56] and it changes throughout the first year of infant life.[56–58] Formula cannot mimic the constantly changing composition of human milk. Formula has a higher protein concentration than breast milk, and this may result in greater accumulation of weight during the first years of life as compared with breastfed infants.[59] Evidence from several studies suggests that breast-fed infants eat to satiety.[46,47] In contrast, formula-fed infants are often encouraged to finish the bottle and to eat beyond satiety, and thus consume more energy.[60] Additionally, formula fed infants are likely to receive complementary foods sooner than breastfed infants.[61–63] Once an infant receives one type of solid (or semi-solid) food, others follow quickly thereafter.[61] The result is that breast fed and formula-fed infants are also exposed to entirely different feeding patterns.[60,64,65] Further, breastfeeding is dynamic; mothers continue breastfeeding infants if they are growing well and provide signals that they are satisfied whereas women are likely to discontinue it if these needs are not met. Studies may attribute the faster rate of growth to formula feeding rather than to the faster growth in the child that led to the end of breastfeeding in the first place (so-called 'reverse causality').[66] The totality of these differences in milk composition, bioactive factors, feeding patterns and the reasons for maternal feeding choices may contribute to differences in growth between breastfed and formula-fed infants.

8.4.2 Breastfeeding and later obesity

In the infancy period, many studies find that breastfed infants grow faster than formula fed infants during certain months,[51] but by one year of age there are often no differences between the groups.[51,54,67] In this period, the other factors that contribute to breastfeeding and infant growth must be considered simultaneously to disentangle the effects of breastfeeding. In a study of Danish mothers and infants it was found that higher maternal prepregnancy BMI values, shorter durations of any breastfeeding, and the earlier introduction of complementary foods were jointly associated with increased infant weight gain during the first year of life.[68] This study by Baker et al.,[25] estimated that compared to the infant of a woman who was normal-weight before pregnancy, breastfed for longer than 20 weeks and introduced to complementary foods after 16 weeks (government recommendations at the time) the infant of a woman who was obese before pregnancy, breastfed for <20 weeks and introduced to complementary foods at <16 weeks would gain 10 % (726 g) more weight during the first year of life. It is plausible that these effects may persist and translate into an increased risk of obesity later in childhood.

An investigation by Arenz et al.,[53] combined results from nine studies on breastfeeding and childhood obesity (baseline measure at >1 year of age) that adjusted for other factors and found a reduced odds of obesity among children who had been breastfed compared with those who had not (adjusted odds ratio [OR]: 0.78, 95% confidence interval [CI]: 0.71, 0.85). A different investigation by Owen et al.,[51] that combined results from 28 published studies (baseline measures primarily in children) found that there was a lower odds of obesity among those who had ever been breastfed compared to those who were formula-fed (OR =0.87, 95% CI: 0.85, 0.89). When these analyses accounted for socioeconomic status, parental BMI and maternal smoking, the odds of obesity between ever breastfed and formula-fed were reduced to 0.93 (95% CI: 0.88, 0.99),[51] thus demonstrating the importance of these other factors on the development of obesity.

Although the majority of studies focus on the effects of breastfeeding in reducing obesity in children, there is evidence that the effects may persist into adolescence and adulthood. The investigation by Owen et al.,[51] identified that the odds of obesity among breastfed versus formula fed changed little across age; the ORs were 0.50 (95% CI: 0.26, 0.94) among infants, 0.90 (95% CI: 0.87, 0.92) among young children, 0.66 (95% CI: 0.60, 0.72) among older children and 0.80 (95% CI: 0.71, 0.91) among adults. From these studies it is evident that breastfeeding, no matter what the extent, is associated with a reduced odds of obesity, especially in children and adolescents.

Of interest, however, are the effects of the duration and exclusivity of breastfeeding as 'ever breastfed' encompasses a wide range of behaviours. When the duration of breastfeeding was examined in relation to the later risk of obesity, Harder et al.,[69] combined results from 17 studies (baseline measurements from infancy through adolescence) and identified a dose–response relationship. The duration of breastfeeding was inversely related with the risk of later overweight and the effect was present from 1 through 9 months of breastfeeding, after which the effect levelled off.[69] When the degree of exclusivity was examined, the dose–response association strengthened, although it was limited to estimates from only two original studies.[69] Similarly, Owen *et al.*,[51] found that exclusive breastfeeding had a stronger protective against later obesity compared with formula feeding (OR: 0.76, 95% CI: 0.70, 0.83).

8.5   Commentary on studies into the effect of breastfeeding on the weight of mothers and infants

Results from the studies described here and elsewhere[33] suggest that although breast-feeding has the capacity to contribute to postpartum weight loss in women, the effect sizes are inconsistent and modest. Similarly, the available evidence suggests that breastfeeding has a consistent but a very modest protective effect against developing obesity throughout the lifecourse.

The potential impact of breastfeeding on postpartum weight change and obesity throughout the lifecourse of the infant must be considered in the context of the other factors that contribute to breastfeeding. For example, it remains a possibility that the link between breastfeeding and maternal weight loss is not due to breastfeeding *per se* but to the weight-loss promoting effects of the other factors that breastfeeding is associated with (e.g. lower prepregnancy BMI, higher socioeconomic status, etc.). Further, as few studies account for the influence of intentional dieting and physical activity, the effects of these behaviours are intertwined with the effects attributed to the method of feeding used. Similarly, the link between breastfeeding and a reduced risk of obesity in the lifetime of the infant may be attributable to the environment associated with breastfeeding mothers that has many other factors that are protect-ive against obesity.[70] Additionally, few studies in this area account for the entirety of the infant feeding pattern and rely upon reports of breastfeeding exclusivity to indicate when complementary foods are introduced; this is not necessarily precise. Nonetheless, as breastfeeding has numerous other health benefits for the mother and infant,[31] it is a healthy behaviour to promote. The caveat is that women must be counselled as to what effects of weight loss they can realistically expect.

8.6   Future trends

Evidence is beginning to emerge that effects of breastfeeding on postpartum weight change are only part of the picture; it is becoming apparent that breastfeeding has favourable effects on maternal body composition. In a follow-up of women on an average of seven years postpartum, it was found that compared to women who had breastfed their infant(s) for ≥3 months after every birth, women who had never breastfed had a greater amount of visceral adiposity.[71] These results tie in with a body of emerging evidence that breastfeeding has a positive impact on a woman's future metabolic profile.[72]

Similarly, long-term investigations are beginning to reveal whether breastfeeding favourably impacts the metabolic profile and body composition throughout the life of the infant. To date, the findings are largely equivocal,[15] but as follow-up periods are extended and investigations occur among infants from prospective birth cohorts in the 1990s and 2000s, these may become better elucidated. Additionally, there is an emerging awareness of the importance of the overall feeding pattern for later health. Studies are beginning to investigate the effects of complementary foods in addition to breastfeeding on the later risk of obesity.[73,74] And finally, investigations are now explicitly considering whether infants receive milk directly from the breast or expressed milk and the subsequent effects on infant health and growth, which is important given the increase in this mode of feeding.[75]

8.7   Sources of further information and advice

Two reports from the United States Institute of Medicine ('Nutrition during lacta-tion'[14] and 'Weight gain during pregnancy: re-examining the guidelines'[10]) are a substantial source of reference material for the topics covered in this chapter. With regards to the effects of breastfeeding on postpartum weight change, the excellent review by Neville et al.,[33] is recommended reading. Although not explicitly addressed in this chapter, a description of the effectiveness of different interventions for post-partum weight loss can be found in the most recent Cochrane review on this topic.[12] A useful and concise overview of the benefits of breastfeeding for infant health (includ-ing the later risks of obesity) is provided in the report by Ip et al.,[15] And finally, the studies by Arenz et al.,[53] and Owen et al.,[51] provide the best summary of the associations between breastfeeding and obesity across the lifecourse.

References

1. Sebire NJ, Jolly M, Harris JP, Wadsworth J, et al., Maternal obesity and pregnancy outcome: a study of 287,213 pregnancies in London. Int J Obes Relat Metab Disord 2001; 25:1175–82.
2. Nohr EA, Timpson NJ, Andersen CS, Davey Smith G, Olsen J, Sørensen TIA. Severe obesity in young women and reproductive health: the Danish National Birth Cohort. PLoS One 2009; 4:e8444.
3. de Jersey SJ, Nicholson JM, Callaway LK, Daniels LA. A prospective study of pregnancy weight gain in Australian women. Aust N Z J Obstet Gynaecol 2012; 52:545–51.
4. Holowko N, Mishra G, Koupil I. Social inequality in excessive gestational weight gain. Int J Obes (Lond) 2014; 38:91–6.
5. Gaillard R, Durmus B, Hofman A, Mackenbach JP, Steegers EA, Jaddoe VW. Risk factors and outcomes of maternal obesity and excessive weight gain during pregnancy. Obesity (Silver Spring) 2013; 21:1046–55.

6. Rode L, Kjaergaard H, Ottesen B, Damm P, Hegaard HK. Association between gestational weight gain according to body mass index and postpartum weight in a large cohort of Danish women. *Matern Child Health J* 2012; 16:406–13.

7. Dalenius K, Brindley P, Smith B, Reinold C, Grummer-Strawn L. *Pregnancy Nutrition Surveillance 2010 Report*. Atlanta: U.S. Department of Health and Human Services, Centers for Disease Control and Prevention; 2012.

8. Kowal C, Kuk J, Tamim H. Characteristics of weight gain in pregnancy among Canadian women. *Matern Child Health J* 2012; 16:668–76.

9. Reyes E, Martinez N, Parra A, Castillo-Mora A, Ortega-Gonzalez C. Early intensive obstetric and medical nutrition care is associated with decreased prepregnancy obesity impact on perinatal outcomes. *Gynecol Obstet Invest* 2012; 73:75–81.

10. Rasmussen KM, Yaktine AL, for Institute of Medicine (U.S.), Committee to Reexamine IOM Pregnancy Weight Guidelines. *Weight Gain During Pregnancy: reexamining the guidelines*. Washington, D.C.: National Academies Press; 2009.

11. Nohr EA, Vaeth M, Baker JL, Sørensen TIA, Olsen J, Rasmussen KM. Combined associations of prepregnancy body mass index and gestational weight gain with the outcome of pregnancy. *Am J Clin Nutr* 2008; 87:1750–9.

12. Amorim Adegboye AR, Linne YM. Diet or exercise, or both, for weight reduction in women after childbirth. *Cochrane Database Syst Rev* 2013; 7:CD005627.

13. van der Pligt P, Willcox J, Hesketh KD, Ball K, *et al.*, Systematic review of lifestyle interventions to limit postpartum weight retention: implications for future opportunities to prevent maternal overweight and obesity following childbirth. *Obes Rev* 2013; 14:792–805.

14. Institute of Medicine (U.S.), Subcommittee on Nutrition during Lactation, United States. Health Resources and Services Administration. *Nutrition during lactation*. Washington, D.C.: National Academies Press; 1991.

15. Ip S, Chung M, Raman G, Chew P, *et al.*, Breastfeeding and Maternal and Infant Health Outcomes in Developed Countries. *Evidence Report/Technology Assessment No. 153* (prepared by Tufts-New England Medical Center Evidence-based Practice Center, under Contract No. 290–02–0022). Rockville, MD: Agency for Healthcare Research and Quality; 2007 April.

16. World Health Organization. *Global Strategy for Infant and Young Child Feeding: the optimal duration of exclusive breastfeeding*. Geneva: World Health Organization; 2001.

17. World Health Organization. *Indicators for Assessing Breast-Feeding Practices*. Geneva, Switzerland; 1991.

18. Johns HM, Forster DA, Amir LH, McLachlan HL. Prevalence and outcomes of breast milk expressing in women with healthy term infants: a systematic review. *BMC Pregnancy Childbirth* 2013; 13:212.

19. World Health Organization. Dept. of Nutrition for Health and Development. *Report of the Expert Consultation of the Optimal Duration of Exclusive Breastfeeding, Geneva, Switzerland, 28–30 March 2001*. Geneva: World Health Organization; 2001.

20. Cai X, Wardlaw T, Brown DW. Global trends in exclusive breastfeeding. *Int Breastfeed J* 2012; 7:12.

21. Kronborg H, Vaeth M. The influence of psychosocial factors on the duration of breastfeeding. *Scand J Public Health* 2004; 32:210–16.

22. Hilson JA, Rasmussen KM, Kjolhede CL. Maternal obesity and breast-feeding success in a rural population of white women. *Am J Clin Nutr* 1997; 66:1371–8.

23. Li R, Jewell S, Grummer-Strawn L. Maternal obesity and breast-feeding practices. *Am J Clin Nutr* 2003; 77:931–6.

24. Donath SM, Amir LH. Does maternal obesity adversely affect breastfeeding initiation and duration? *J Paediatr Child Health* 2000; 36:482–6.

25. Baker JL, Michaelsen KF, Sørensen TIA, Rasmussen KM. High prepregnant body mass index is associated with early termination of full and any breastfeeding in Danish women. *Am J Clin Nutr* 2007; 86:404–11.

26. Wojcicki JM. Maternal prepregnancy body mass index and initiation and duration of breastfeeding: a review of the literature. *J Womens Health (Larchmt)* 2011; 20:341–7.

27. Lawrence RA, Lawrence RM. *Breastfeeding: a guide for the medical profession*, 5th edn. St. Louis: Mosby; 1999.

28. Institute of Medicine (U.S.). Panel on Macronutrients, Institute of Medicine (U.S.). Standing Committee on the Scientific Evaluation of Dietary Reference Intakes. *Dietary Reference Intakes for Energy, Carbohydrate, Fiber, Fat, Fatty Acids, Cholesterol, Protein, and Amino Acids*. Washington, D.C.: National Academies Press; 2002.

29. Lovelady C. Balancing exercise and food intake with lactation to promote post-partum weight loss. *Proc Nutr Soc* 2011; 70:181–4.

30. Butte NF, Hopkinson JM. Body composition changes during lactation are highly variable among women. *J Nutr* 1998; 128:381S–5S.

31. Viswanathan M, Siega-Riz A, Moos M-K, Deierlein A, et al., *Outcomes of Maternal Weight Gain, Evidence Report/Technology Assessment No. 168* (prepared by RTI International–University of North Carolina Evidence-based Practice Center under Contract No. 290-02-0016.). Rockville, MD: Agency for Healthcare Research and Quality; 2008.

32. Pedersen P, Baker JL, Henriksen TB, Lissner L, et al., Influence of psychosocial factors on postpartum weight retention. *Obesity (Silver Spring)* 2011; 19:639–46.

33. Neville CE, McKinley MC, Holmes VA, Spence D, Woodside JV. The relationship between breastfeeding and postpartum weight change-a systematic review and critical evaluation. *Int J Obes (Lond)* 2013; Epub ahead of print 29 July.

34. Stuebe AM, Rich-Edwards JW. The reset hypothesis: lactation and maternal metabolism. *Am J Perinatol* 2009; 26:81–8.

35. Baker JL, Gamborg M, Heitmann BL, Lissner L, Sørensen TIA, Rasmussen KM. Breastfeeding reduces postpartum weight retention. *Am J Clin Nutr* 2008; 88:1543–51.

36. Brandhagen M, Lissner L, Brantsaeter AL, Meltzer HM, et al., Breast-feeding in relation to weight retention up to 36 months postpartum in the Norwegian Mother and Child Cohort Study: modification by socio-economic status? *Public Health Nutr* 2013; Epub ahead of print 6 August.

37. Janney CA, Zhang D, Sowers M. Lactation and weight retention. *Am J Clin Nutr* 1997; 66:1116–24.

38. Olson CM, Strawderman MS, Hinton PS, Pearson TA. Gestational weight gain and postpartum behaviors associated with weight change from early pregnancy to 1 y postpartum. *Int J Obes Relat Metab Disord* 2003; 27:117–27.

39. Østbye T, Peterson BL, Krause KM, Swamy GK, Lovelady CA. Predictors of postpartum weight change among overweight and obese women: results from the Active Mothers Postpartum study. *J Womens Health (Larchmt)* 2012; 21:215–22.

40. Martin JE, Hure AJ, Macdonald-Wicks L, Smith R, Collins CE. Predictors of post-partum weight retention in a prospective longitudinal study. *Matern Child Nutr* 2012; Epub ahead of print 13 September.

41. Sichieri R, Field AE, Rich-Edwards J, Willett WC. Prospective assessment of exclusive breastfeeding in relation to weight change in women. *Int J Obes Relat Metab Disord* 2003; 27:815–20.

42. Gigante DP, Victora CG, Barros FC. Breast-feeding has a limited long-term effect on anthropometry and body composition of Brazilian mothers. *J Nutr* 2001; 131:78–84.

43. Rooney BL, Schauberger CW. Excess pregnancy weight gain and long-term obesity: one decade later. *Obstet Gynecol* 2002; 100:245–52.

44. Kirkegaard H, Stovring H, Rasmussen KM, Abrams B, Sorensen T, Nohr EA. How do pregnancy-related weight changes and breastfeeding relate to maternal weight and BMI-adjusted waist circumference 7 y after delivery? Results from a path analysis. *Am J Clin Nutr* 2014; 99:312–19.

45. Linne Y, Dye L, Barkeling B, Rossner S. Weight development over time in parous women – the SPAWN study – 15 years follow-up. *Int J Obes Relat Metab Disord* 2003; 27:1516–22.

46. Falkner FT, Tanner JM. *Human Growth: A Comprehensive Treatise*, 2nd edn. New York: Plenum Press; 1986.

47. Dietz WH. Critical periods in childhood for the development of obesity. *Am J Clin Nutr* 1994; 59:955–9.

48. Gillman MW. The first months of life: a critical period for development of obesity. *Am J Clin Nutr* 2008; 87:1587–9.

49. Horta BL, Bahl R, Martines JC, Victora CG. *Evidence of the Long-term Effects of Breastfeeding: systemic review and meta-analyses*. Geneva: World Health Organization; 2007.

50. Lawrence RA. Does breastfeeding protect against overweight and obesity in children? A review. *Childhood Obesity* 2010; 6:193–7.

51. Owen CG, Martin RM, Whincup PH, Smith GD, Cook DG. Effect of infant feeding on the risk of obesity across the life course: a quantitative review of published evidence. *Pediatrics* 2005; 115:1367–77.

52. Owen CG, Martin RM, Whincup PH, Davey-Smith G, Gillman MW, Cook DG. The effect of breastfeeding on mean body mass index throughout life: a quantitative review of published and unpublished observational evidence. *Am J Clin Nutr* 2005; 82:1298–307.

53. Arenz S, Ruckerl R, Koletzko B, von Kries R. Breast-feeding and childhood obesity – a systematic review. *Int J Obes Relat Metab Disord* 2004; 28:1247–56.

54. Kramer MS, Guo T, Platt RW, Vanilovich I, *et al.*, Feeding effects on growth during infancy. *J Pediatr* 2004; 145:600–5.

55. Neville MC, Keller RP, Seacat J, Casey CE, Allen JC, Archer P. Studies on human lactation. I. Within-feed and between-breast variation in selected components of human milk. *Am J Clin Nutr* 1984; 40:635–46.

56. Ballard O, Morrow AL. Human milk composition: nutrients and bioactive factors. *Pediatr Clin North Am* 2013; 60:49–74.

57. Allen JC, Keller RP, Archer P, Neville MC. Studies in human lactation: milk composition and daily secretion rates of macronutrients in the first year of lactation. *Am J Clin Nutr* 1991; 54:69–80.

58. Mitoulas LR, Kent JC, Cox DB, Owens RA, Sherriff JL, Hartmann PE. Variation in fat, lactose and protein in human milk over 24ïh and throughout the first year of lactation. *Br J Nutr* 2002; 88:29–37.

59. Koletzko B, von Kries R, Closa R, Escribano J, *et al.*, Lower protein in infant formula is associated with lower weight up to age 2 y: a randomized clinical trial. *Am J Clin Nutr* 2009; 89:1836–45.

60. Stunkard AJ, Berkowitz RI, Stallings VA, Schoeller DA. Energy intake, not energy output, is a determinant of body size in infants. *Am J Clin Nutr* 1999; 69:524–30.

61. Skinner JD, Carruth BR, Houck K, Moran J 3rd, *et al.*, Transitions in infant feeding during the first year of life. *J Am Coll Nutr* 1997; 16:209–15.
62. Shukla A, Forsyth HA, Anderson CM, Marwah SM. Infantile overnutrition in the first year of life: a field study in Dudley, Worcestershire. *Br Med J* 1972; 4:507–15.
63. D'Souza SW, Black P. A study of infant growth in relation to the type of feeding. *Early Hum Dev* 1979; 3:245–55.
64. Nielsen GA, Thomsen BL, Michaelsen KF. Influence of breastfeeding and complementary food on growth between 5 and 10 months. *Acta Paediatr* 1998; 87:911–7.
65. Dewey KG, Cohen RJ, Brown KH, Rivera LL. Age of introduction of complementary foods and growth of term, low-birth-weight, breast-fed infants: a randomized intervention study in Honduras. *Am J Clin Nutr* 1999; 69:679–86.
66. Kramer MS, Moodie EE, Platt RW. Infant feeding and growth: can we answer the causal question? *Epidemiology* 2012; 23:790–4.
67. Durmus B, van Rossem L, Duijts L, Arends LR, *et al.*, Breast-feeding and growth in children until the age of 3 years: the Generation R Study. *Br J Nutr* 2011; 105:1704–11.
68. Baker JL, Michaelsen KF, Rasmussen KM, Sørensen TIA. Maternal prepregnant body mass index, duration of breastfeeding, and timing of complementary food introduction are associated with infant weight gain. *Am J Clin Nutr* 2004; 80:1579–88.
69. Harder T, Bergmann R, Kallischnigg G, Plagemann A. Duration of breastfeeding and risk of overweight: a meta-analysis. *Am J Epidemiol* 2005; 162:397–403.
70. Butte NF. The role of breastfeeding in obesity. *Pediatr Clin North Am* 2001; 48:189–98.
71. McClure CK, Catov J, Ness R, Schwarz EB. Maternal visceral adiposity by consistency of lactation. *Matern Child Health J* 2012; 16:316–21.
72. Gunderson EP. Impact of breastfeeding on maternal metabolism: implications for women with gestational diabetes. *Curr Diab Rep* 2014; 14:460.
73. Schack-Nielsen L, Sørensen TIA, Mortensen EL, Michaelsen KF. Late introduction of complementary feeding, rather than duration of breastfeeding, may protect against adult overweight. *Am J Clin Nutr* 2010; 91:619–27.
74. Pearce J, Taylor MA, Langley-Evans SC. Timing of the introduction of complementary feeding and risk of childhood obesity: a systematic review. *Int J Obes (Lond)* 2013; 37:1295–306.
75. Rasmussen KM, Geraghty SR. The quiet revolution: breastfeeding transformed with the use of breast pumps. *Am J Public Health* 2011; 101:1356–9.
76. World Health Organization. *Obesity: preventing and managing the global epidemic; report of a WHO consultation.* Geneva: World Health Organization; 2000.

Part Three

The role of eating patterns and other behavioural factors in obesity management

The role of dietary energy density in weight management

B. J. Rolls, R. A. Williams, K. L. Keller
The Pennsylvania State University, PA, USA

9.1 Introduction

Effective dietary therapy for weight management should include strategies that match energy intake to energy needs while providing optimal nutrition and controlling hunger. The ready availability of palatable, energy-dense foods makes it difficult to match energy intake and energy expenditure and is likely contributing to the prevalence of overweight and obesity. An evidence-based review by the 2010 US Dietary Guidelines Advisory Committee found 'a relationship between energy density and body weight in adults and in children and adolescents such that consuming diets lower in energy density may be an effective strategy for managing body weight'.[1] Although an understanding of the role that energy density (ED) plays in energy balance is quite recent, there have been a number of relevant laboratory-based studies, longitudinal population-based studies, and randomized controlled trials to inform this relationship.[2–4] These studies indicate that people eat a fairly consistent amount (weight or volume) of food on a day-to-day basis.[3,5,6] This holds true whether the amount of food eaten contains many or few calories. Therefore, the number of calories in a particular amount or weight of food, or the food's ED, has an impact on the total number of calories a person consumes. This review will summarize evidence related to the influence of ED on satiety, energy intake, and body weight and will provide practical approaches for using ED to manage obesity.

9.2 Energy density explained

Energy density is the amount of energy in a particular weight of food (calories per gram), and it ranges from 0 kcal/g to 9 kcal/g. The largest influence on ED is water, which contributes weight and volume to a food without supplying any energy (0 kcal/g). The macronutrient with the greatest influence on ED is fat, which is high in ED with around 9 kcal/g. Carbohydrate and protein are moderate in ED and each provides around 4 kcal/g. A food's ED depends upon its mix of macronutrients and water; the incorporation of water lowers ED, and removing water increases ED.

Modest changes in ED can have a significant impact on energy intake. For example, on a typical day an adult might consume 1,200 g of food with an average ED of 1.8 kcal/g, giving an energy intake of 2,160 kcal. If the average ED of the diet

Managing and Preventing Obesity. http://dx.doi.org/10.1533/9781782420996.3.137

Table 9.1 **Essential information for understanding why a diet low in energy density can be effective for enhancing satiety and facilitating weight management**

> • A high-energy-dense food has lots of calories in a small weight, while a low-energy-dense food has fewer calories for the same weight.
> • For the same number of calories, a larger portion of a low-energy-dense food can be eaten than of a food higher in energy density.
> • On a day-to-day basis, people tend to eat a similar amount of food by weight.
> • Choosing foods with a lower energy density allows individuals to eat their usual amount (weight) of food while reducing their energy intake.

was decreased by 0.1 kcal/g while the same weight of food was consumed, then the individual would ingest 2,040 kcal. Thus, a relatively small change in overall ED of the diet would reduce daily energy intake by 120 kcal. The fundamentals of using ED for weight management are summarized in Table 9.1.

9.3 Controlled studies demonstrate the influence of dietary energy density on satiety, satiation, and energy intake

Dietary ED has emerged in recent years as one of the most consistent influences on satiety and energy intake. A number of systematic studies show that when the macronutrient content of foods was varied, but the ED was kept constant, the effects of fat, carbohydrate, and protein on satiety were similar.[3–6] On the other hand, the ED of foods is a robust and significant determinant of satiety and energy intake regardless of macronutrient composition.[3, 7] Clearly the macronutrient composition of the diet is important for optimal nutrition and it can influence energy intake through effects on regulatory systems and on a food's sensory attributes; however, the ED of food has more robust effects on energy intake than the proportion of macronutrients.

Many of the studies on the effects of ED have been relatively short-term, examining individual meals or effects over several days. To show that ED affects satiety, a fixed amount of a defined food (a preload) is consumed and the effect of the preload on subsequent intake of a test meal is measured.[8] In one study, decreasing the ED of a milk-based preload by adding water, and thus increasing the volume, was shown to enhance satiety in that it led to a significant reduction in subsequent energy intake.[3] Other water-rich foods that are low in ED, such as soup, salad, or fruit, also significantly enhanced satiety and reduced energy intake at a meal when consumed as a preload.[9–12] Of particular interest is that drinking water as a beverage along with a food affected satiety less than incorporating the same amount of water into the food to lower the ED.[9]

ED can influence energy intake not only by enhancing satiety, but also through effects on *ad libitum* intake. *Ad libitum* intake is an indicator of satiation, or the processes leading to the termination of eating during a meal.[8] When the ED of meals was reduced by increasing the proportion of vegetables, it was found that adults who were offered *ad libitum* access ate a consistent weight of food.[3,5,6] This meant that energy intake varied directly with changes in ED. Participants reported similar ratings of hunger and fullness even when reductions in ED led to a decrease in energy intake of approximately 25% over two days.[6] Practical applications of this research that show how to use reductions in ED to prevent excess energy intake will be presented later.

9.4 Dietary energy density and weight management

The robust effects of ED on satiety, satiation, and energy intake indicate that ED could play a role in the control of body weight; however, until recently few studies have examined this relationship. Instead, much of the emphasis in the dietary management of obesity has been on how changing the proportion of macronutrients affects energy intake and body weight. Popular diets urge consumers to eat less fat or carbohydrates or to increase their protein intake. The results of randomized controlled trials aimed at determining whether such advice is effective have been mixed.[13–17] Even when a particular macronutrient was associated with the amount of weight lost during the active treatment phase, significant differences across diets were not sustained during the maintenance phase.[13,17] With similar results coming from several recent large trials, health policy recommendations for weight management have shifted away from macronutrient-based advice to a food-based approach emphasizing control of portion size, ED, and total energy intake.[18]

In the interest of identifying factors that contribute both to excess weight gain and to weight management, the 2010 Dietary Guidelines Advisory Committee conducted a systematic evidence-based review of the relationship between ED and body weight.[1] Their review included 17 studies (seven randomized controlled trials, one nonrandomized controlled trial, and nine cohort studies) in adults. The committee concluded 'that strong and consistent evidence in adults indicates that dietary patterns relatively low in energy density improve weight loss and weight maintenance'. In the rest of this review, rather than reiterating this evidence, we will provide a brief summary of the types of studies that have led to these recommendations and offer practical advice on applying these findings to weight management in clinical populations.

A number of studies in the US and Europe have examined the relationship between dietary ED and body weight.[1,19–22] Population-based studies have shown that normal-weight adults report consuming diets with a lower ED than obese individuals.[19,20] ED was also associated with the amount of weight gained over an eight-year period in a prospective study of over 50,000 middle-aged women in the US Nurses' Health Study.[21] While these data suggest that ED could be a determinant of weight status, results from epidemiologic studies have not been consistent, probably because of differences in dietary assessment methods. For example, some large population-based studies rely on food frequency questionnaires to determine intake,[21] and it is not clear that these adequately assess amounts of food consumed. Furthermore, the association between ED and weight status can be influenced by whether or not different types of beverages are included in the calculation of ED.[22–24] Beverages can have a disproportionate impact on ED because of their high water content. Agreement is needed upon the appropriate methods for calculating ED and assessing its relationship to energy intake and body weight.

Strong support for a relationship between the ED of the diet, excluding beverages, and body weight comes from several longitudinal studies that have tracked body weight and energy intake via dietary recalls which provide the best tool for capturing reports from free-living individuals.[1] In a six-year longitudinal study, it was observed that young women who reported a diet higher in ED gained two-and-a-half times as much weight as those reporting a lower-ED diet.[25] A secondary analysis of the results in the multi-center PREMIER trial that included three different lifestyle interventions found that changes in ED after six months were related to changes in body weight in 658 men and women. In addition to weight loss, reductions in ED were associated with improved diet quality.[26]

Several randomized controlled trials, the most rigorous test for dietary effects, confirm that consuming low-ED foods influences weight loss.[1,27–29] In one trial, daily incorporation of a low-ED food (soup) into a reduced-energy diet increased the magnitude of the weight loss and helped participants to maintain this loss.[28] In another trial, the effect of two strategies to reduce dietary ED on weight loss in obese women was tested.[29] One group was counseled to increase their intake of water-rich foods, such as fruits and vegetables, and to reduce dietary fat. A comparison group was counseled to restrict portions and to reduce dietary fat. Both groups reduced the ED of their diets, and both groups lost weight; however, after 12 months, the group counseled to eat more fruits and vegetables had a greater reduction in dietary ED and lost more weight (17.4 vs. 14.1 lb). Over the course of the year, participants who ate the lower-ED diet reported consuming 25% more food and reported less hunger than those in the comparison group.[29]

Additional clinical weight loss trials indicate that low-ED diets can also help patients maintain their weight loss. Greene and colleagues[30] examined dietary ED two years after participation in a hospital-based weight loss program that encouraged consumption of lower-ED foods. They found that weight loss maintainers reported eating a lower-ED diet than those who regained body weight. A secondary data analysis aimed at determining which dietary strategies were associated with weight loss maintenance found that consumption of a lower-ED diet, characterized by greater intake of vegetables and whole grains, was the most effective.[31] Several studies suggest that low-ED diets could be used to counsel patients attending outpatient clinics. One non-randomized intervention conducted without a control group in an outpatient clinic found that dietary counseling based primarily on food ED was associated with maintenance of weight lost after the treatment was terminated.[32] More recently Lowe and colleagues conducted a randomized controlled trial specifically to test the influence of an ED intervention on maintenance of weight loss.[33] Participants, who were recruited from a primary care clinic, lost weight over 12 weeks and were then randomized to one of four maintenance conditions: no intervention, meal replacements, instruction on lower-ED eating, or meal replacements and instruction on lower-ED eating. Instruction on how to lower dietary ED was the only condition associated with sustained weight loss 36 months after the start of the intervention.[33] Therefore, advising patients on how to lower the ED of their diet shows promise for weight-loss maintenance, and its utility to be widely disseminated in primary care settings should be explored further.

While data suggest that reducing dietary energy density can facilitate weight management, more long-term studies are needed to understand how to implement this approach and facilitate the maintenance of low-ED eating habits. If people were to adopt lower-ED eating patterns, they would be able to eat more satisfying amounts of food appropriate to meet both energy and nutrient needs.

9.5 Strategies to reduce dietary energy density

A goal for weight management is to provide dietary strategies that are sustainable and have moderate energy intake. Consuming a low-ED diet is one strategy that emphasizes intake of nutrient-dense foods like fruits and vegetables and allows individuals to control hunger, feel full, and eat a satisfying amount of food while lowering energy intake. A low-ED diet is versatile and does not restrict food groups; instead, its emphasis is on consuming larger portions of low-ED foods and controlling portions of higher-ED foods. Figure 9.1 shows how foods can be divided into four categories based on their ED, ranging from Category 1, very-low-ED foods, to Category 4, high-ED foods.[34] Foods in Category 1 can be eaten in satisfying portions, but as ED goes up in Categories 2, 3 and 4, the need to manage portions increases. Use of these categories can help with meal planning and provide ideas for simple swaps that can be made in order to choose lower-ED foods and decrease energy intake.[34] In addition to choosing foods that are lower in ED, individuals can use other strategies such as reducing the ED of mixed dishes[5,6] and strategically using low-ED foods as a first course at a meal.[9–12]

A number of well-controlled studies have investigated different methods for reducing ED, such as decreasing fat, increasing fruits and vegetables, adding water, and using fat or sugar substitutes.[3–6] Although the sensory and biological effects of these methods differ, they are all associated with decreased energy intake. In order to determine if there is an optimal way to reduce ED and influence energy intake, three methods of ED reduction (decreasing fat, increasing fruits and vegetables, and adding water) were compared.[7] Commonly consumed foods such as oatmeal, a pasta dish, and a chicken rice casserole were reduced in ED. Although there were some differences in energy intake across conditions, all three methods of ED reduction decreased daily energy intake relative to no ED reduction. This suggests that individuals can use a variety of methods to reduce ED, all of which can effectively decrease energy intake. Furthermore, a combination of methods can be used in order to modify foods for a more personalized and flexible dietary approach. Table 9.2 demonstrates how simple swaps can be made at meals in order to reduce ED using a combination of methods.

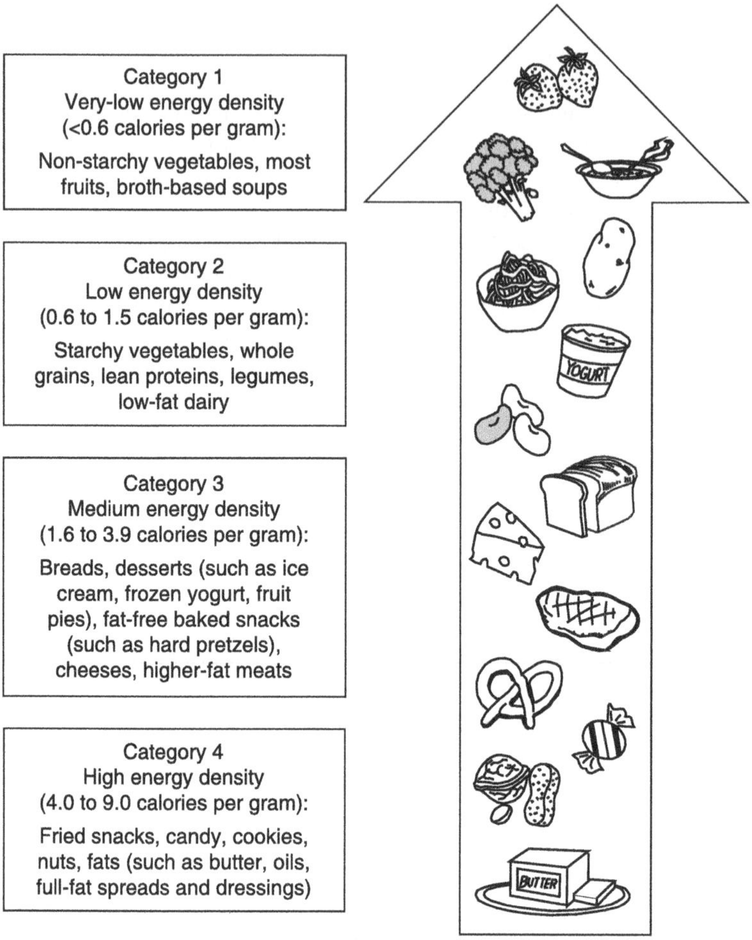

Figure 9.1 Four categories of energy density can be used to guide food choices and portion sizes:

Category 1: Satisfying portions can be consumed without many calories

Category 2: Start portion control at the upper end

Category 3: Manage portions as these foods can be easy to overeat

Category 4: Carefully manage portions and frequency of eating

Source: modified from Rolls (2012).[34]

While there continues to be debate about the optimal diet composition for weight management, there is agreement that most people should eat more vegetables. Recent research shows that some approaches to increasing vegetable intake to lower ED for weight management are likely to be more effective than others. Vegetables can be incorporated into meals in a variety of ways; for example, they can be served whole, chopped, shredded, or puréed, depending on whether they are provided as a side dish

Table 9.2 Sample menus varying in energy density

	Original version	Energy	Weight	Energy density	Lower-energy-dense version	Energy	Weight	Energy density
Breakfast	Oatmeal made with whole milk, dried cranberries	401	315	1.27	Oatmeal made with skim milk, blueberries	268	334	0.80
Lunch	Sandwich (roll, fried chicken, cheese, mayonnaise), cream soup	686	438	1.57	Sandwich (roll, grilled chicken, cheese, vegetables, mustard), minestrone soup	533	509	1.05
Snack	Celery with peanut butter	190	110	1.73	Celery with hummus	90	112	0.80
Dinner	Pasta dish (pasta, regular minced beef, parmesan cheese, Alfredo sauce), tossed salad, creamy Italian salad dressing, regular chocolate ice cream	790	481	1.64	Pasta dish (pasta, extra lean minced beef, parmesan cheese, tomato sauce), tossed salad with extra vegetables, Italian salad dressing, light chocolate ice cream	650	640	1.02
Total		2067	1344	1.54		1541	1595	0.97

Note: This table shows how lower-ED foods and ingredients can be exchanged for higher-ED foods and ingredients to achieve a reduction in total energy of nearly 500 calories over the day. The lower-ED menu on the right was developed with a combination of strategies, including decreasing fat (e.g. ice cream) and increasing water-rich foods including vegetables and broth-based soup. About 25% of the energy contained in the original version was eliminated, yet the amount of food consumed in the lower-ED version was increased.

or incorporated into a main dish. In order to reduce energy intake, however, vegetables should be substituted for higher-ED components of the meal. Previous research has shown that simply adding more vegetables to the meal while maintaining the portion of grain and meat did not reduce overall meal energy intake.[35] In contrast, increasing the portion of vegetables while decreasing the grain and meat components of the meal led to a reduction in meal energy intake. The substitution of vegetables for higher-ED meal components is critical for the reduction in energy intake but this strategy may not work if individuals dislike vegetables. One way to overcome this barrier is to incorporate puréed vegetables into mixed dishes to lower ED. The covert incorporation of puréed vegetables into the entrées served at all meals across a day significantly reduced daily energy intake, even in people who reported not liking vegetables.[36] Together, these findings indicate that substituting low-ED vegetables for either higher-ED meal components or higher-ED ingredients in mixed dishes can moderate energy intake.

Another approach to encouraging consumption of low-ED foods is to provide them at the start of a meal when hunger is elevated and there are no competing foods.[9–12] 'Filling up first' by consuming a large portion of a low-ED food such as salad with low-calorie dressing,[11] an apple,[12] or a broth-based soup[10] has been shown to reduce energy intake from the main course and over the entire meal compared to not consuming these foods as a first course. This strategy is most effective if the first course is a large portion of very-low-ED food that is less than 100 calories total. A recent study also emphasized that the utility of a low-ED first course to reduce meal energy intake depends upon what is served at the rest of the meal. For example, if a large, low-ED salad is followed by large portions of high-ED foods, people are still at risk of eating excess energy.[37] Although most studies that have shown the satiety enhancing effect of a low-ED first course have been short-term, a recent small study found that consuming a low-ED first course of salad and yogurt prior to the main course at both lunch and dinner reduced body weight over three months compared to consuming these foods with the main course.[38]

A low-ED diet is not restrictive and can be tailored to accommodate individual preferences. There are four ED categories, ranging from very-low-ED to high-ED; as the ED category increases, greater attention to portion control is needed (Figure 9.1). In order to lower dietary ED, meals should contain a larger proportion of very-low- and low-ED foods than of higher-ED foods. Decreases in energy intake can be achieved by swapping higher-ED foods for lower-ED foods, incorporating lower-ED ingredients into mixed dishes to reduce ED, and 'filling up first' with a low-ED first course. Since a range of eating patterns can be reduced in ED, this type of diet has wide applicability and thus can be a key component of a lifestyle that encourages a healthy well-balanced diet for weight management.

9.6 Future trends

Low-ED diets are now widely recognized as versatile, nutritious, and effective for managing energy intake and body weight. Nevertheless, greater understanding is needed on how consumers can lower ED affordably and sustainably without sacrificing palatability and enjoyment. The *optimal strategies* for lowering ED to promote satiety and persistently reduce energy intake are not known. For example, is it important to lower the ED of all foods or are there some foods, meals, or meal components that are particularly effective for satiety-enhancement and intake reduction? Does 'filling up first' with a low-ED food lower energy intake more than reducing the ED of the main course? Little research has been conducted to determine which ED reduction strategies are the most sustainable for weight loss and weight loss maintenance over the long-term. Such well-controlled longer-term studies could lead to the development of programs and products that will help consumers to maintain consumption of a lower-ED diet that meets their energy and nutrient requirements.[39]

If lower-ED foods become more widely available and are more frequently consumed than higher-ED foods, it will be important to determine whether this leads to the prevention of overweight and obesity. Over time people who are not actively trying to manage their weight may compensate for reductions in their energy intake associated with lower-ED foods. Biological regulatory systems may sense an accumulating energy deficit which leads to increased hunger and energy intake. Thus, well-controlled studies are needed to evaluate the persistence of the effects of ED reduction. In addition, innovative translational research should investigate the impact of lowering dietary ED in a person's everyday eating environment. Even small reductions in ED of frequently consumed foods could impact daily energy intake. A question of interest is whether such reductions will be most effective if done covertly or more overtly. Such research might identify new strategies that will help patients to more successfully navigate the current obesogenic environment and maintain healthy body weights.

9.7 Sources of further information and advice

A number of resources are available that enhance understanding of the science behind the impact of ED on satiety and weight management. The systematic evidence-based review from the 2010 Dietary Guidelines Advisory Committee summarizes the clinical trials and cohort studies published before May 2011.[1] Several other reviews provide an overview of the laboratory-based controlled studies that have been conducted on ED and energy intake[3,4] and describe mechanisms underlying the effects of ED.[2] Practical advice on to how to communicate ED to consumers is provided by health organizations.[40,41] A weight-loss program based on ED research is available for consumers.[34]

9.8 Acknowledgements

BJR is supported by National Institutes of Health grants RO1DK059853 and RO1DK082580.

References

1. Perez-Escamilla, R., Obbagy, J. E., Altman, J. M., *et al.* Dietary energy density and body weight in adults and children: a systematic review. *J Acad Nutr Diet*, 2012; **112**:671–84.
2. Keller, K. L., Kral, T. V. E. and Rolls, B. J. (2013), 'Impacts of energy density and portion size on satiation and satiety' in J. Blundell and F. Bellisle, *Satiation, Satiety and the Control of Food Intake: Theory and Practice.* Cambridge, Woodhead, 115–127.
3. Rolls, B. J. The relationship between dietary energy density and energy intake. *Physiol Behav*, 2009; **97**:609–615.
4. Rolls, B. J. Plenary Lecture 1: Dietary strategies for the prevention and treatment of obesity. *Proc Nutr Soc*, 2010; **69**:70–79.
5. Rolls, B. J., Bell, E. A., Castellanos, V. H., *et al.* Energy density but not fat content of foods affected energy intake in lean and obese women. *Am J Clin Nutr*, 1999; **69**:863–871.
6. Rolls, B. J., Roe, L. S. and Meengs, J. S. Reductions in portion size and energy density of foods are additive and lead to sustained decreases in energy intake. *Am J Clin Nutr.* 2006; **83**:11–17.
7. Williams, R. A., Roe, L. S. and Rolls, B. J. Comparison of three methods to reduce energy density. Effects on daily energy intake. *Appetite*, 2013; **66**:75–83.
8. Blundell, J., De Graaf, C., Hulshof, T., *et al.* Appetite control: methodological aspects of the evaluation of foods. *Obes Rev*, 2010; **11**:251–270.
9. Rolls, B. J., Bell, E. A. and Thorwart, M. L. Water incorporated into a food but not served with a food decreases energy intake in lean women. *Am J Clin Nutr*, 1999; **70**:448–455.
10. Flood, J. E. and Rolls, B. J. Soup preloads in a variety of forms reduce meal energy intake. *Appetite*, 2007; **49**:626–634.
11. Rolls, B. J., Roe, L. S. and Meengs, J. S. Salad and satiety: energy density and portion size of a first course salad affect energy intake at lunch. *J Am Diet Assoc*, 2004; **104**:1570–1576.
12. Flood-Obbagy, J. E. and Rolls, B. J. The effect of fruit in different forms on energy intake and satiety at a meal. *Appetite*, 2009; **52**:416–422.
13. Fogelholm, M., Anderssen, S., Gunnarsdottir, I., *et al.* Dietary macronutrients and food consumption as determinants of long-term weight change in adult populations: a systematic literature review. *Food Nutr Res*, 2012; **56**:doi: 10.3402/fnr.v56i0.
14. Foreyt, J., Salas-Salvado, J., Caballero, B., *et al.* Weight-reducing diets: Are there any differences? *Nutr Rev*, 2009; **67**:S99–101.
15. Hooper, L., Abdelhamid, A., Moore, H. J., *et al.* Effect of reducing total fat intake on body weight: systematic review and meta-analysis of randomised controlled trials and cohort studies. *BMJ*, 2012; **345**:e7666.
16. Vergnaud, A. C., Norat, T., Mouw, T., *et al.* Macronutrient composition of the diet and prospective weight change in participants of the EPIC-PANACEA study. *PLoS One*, 2013; **8**:e57300.
17. Sacks, F. M., Bray, G. A., Carey, V. J., *et al.* Comparison of weight-loss diets with different compositions of fat, protein, and carbohydrates. *N Engl J Med*, 2009; **360**:859–873.
18. *Dietary Guidelines for Americans, 7th edn* (2010). Washington, D.C. Government Printing Office.
19. Kant, A. K. and Graubard, B. I. Energy density of diets reported by American adults: association with food group intake, nutrient intake, and body weight. *Int J Obes (Lond)*, 2005; **29**:950–956.
20. Ledikwe, J. H., Blanck, H. M., Kettel-Khan, L., *et al.* Dietary energy density is associated with energy intake and weight status in US adults. *Am J Clin Nutr*, 2006; **83**:1362–1368.

21. Bes-Rastrollo, M., Van Dam, R. M., Martinez-Gonzalez, M. A., *et al.* Prospective study of dietary energy density and weight gain in women. *Am J Clin Nutr*, 2008; **88**:769–777.

22. Hartline-Grafton, H. L., Rose, D., Johnson, C. C., *et al.* Energy density of foods, but not beverages, is positively associated with body mass index in adult women. *Eur J Clin Nutr*, 2009; **63**:1411–1418.

23. Ledikwe, J. H., Blanck, H. M., Khan, L. K., *et al.* Dietary energy density determined by eight calculation methods in a nationally representative United States population. *J Nutr*, 2005; **135**:273–278.

24. Johnson, L., Wilks, D. C., Lindroos, A. K., *et al.* Reflections from a systematic review of dietary energy density and weight gain: is the inclusion of drinks valid? *Obes Rev*, 2009; **10**:681–92.

25. Savage, J. S., Marini, M. and Birch, L. L. Dietary energy density predicts women's weight change over 6 y. *Am J Clin Nutr*, 2008; **88**:677–684.

26. Ledikwe, J. H., Rolls, B. J., Smiciklas-Wright, H., *et al.* Reductions in dietary energy density are associated with weight loss in overweight and obese participants in the PREMIER trial. *Am J Clin Nutr*, 2007; **85**:1212–1221.

27. Raynor, H. A., Looney, S. M., Steeves, E. A., *et al.* The effects of an energy density prescription on diet quality and weight loss: a pilot randomized controlled trial. *J Acad Nutr Diet*, 2012; **112**:1397–1402.

28. Rolls, B. J., Roe, L. S., Beach, A. M., *et al.* Provision of foods differing in energy density affects long-term weight loss. *Obes Res*, 2005; **13**:1052–1060.

29. Ello-Martin, J. A., Roe, L. S., Ledikwe, J. H., *et al.* Dietary energy density in the treatment of obesity: a year-long trial comparing 2 weight-loss diets. *Am J Clin Nutr*, 2007; **85**:1465–1477.

30. Greene, L. F., Malpede, C. Z., Henson, C. S., *et al.* Weight maintenance 2 years after participation in a weight loss program promoting low-energy density foods. *Obesity*, 2006; **14**:1795–1801.

31. Raynor, H. A., Van Walleghen, E. L., Bachman, J. L., *et al.* Dietary energy density and successful weight loss maintenance. *Eat Behav*, 2011; **12**:119–25.

32. Schusdziarra, V., Hausmann, M., Wiedemann, C., *et al.* Successful weight loss and maintenance in everyday clinical practice with an individually tailored change of eating habits on the basis of food energy density. *Eur J Nutr*, 2011; **50**:351–361.

33. Lowe, M. R., Butryn, M. L., Thomas, J. G., *et al.* Meal replacements, reduced energy density eating and weight loss maintenance in primary care patients: A randomized controlled trial. *Obesity*, 2014; **22**:94–100.

34. Rolls, B. J. *The Ultimate Volumetrics Diet.* New York, New York. William Morrow, 2012.

35. Rolls, B. J., Roe, L. S. and Meengs, J. S. Portion size can be used strategically to increase vegetable consumption in adults. *Am J Clin Nutr*, 2010; **91**:913–922.

36. Blatt, A. D., Roe, L. S. and Rolls, B. J. Hidden vegetables: an effective strategy to reduce energy intake and increase vegetable intake in adults. *Am J Clin Nutr.* 2011; **93**:756–763.

37. Williams, R. A., Roe, L. S. and Rolls, B. J. Assessment of satiety depends on the energy density and portion size of the test meal. *Obesity*, 2014; **22**:318–324.

38. Azadbakht, L., Haghighatdoost, F., Karimi, G., *et al.* Effect of consuming salad and yogurt as preload on body weight management and cardiovascular risk factors: a randomized clinical trial. *Int J Food Sci Nutr*, 2013; **64**:392–9.

39. Institute of Medicine. 2011. *Leveraging Food Technology for Obesity Prevention and Reduction Efforts: Workshop Summary.* Washington, DC. The National Academies Press.

40. Centers for Disease Control and Prevention, Division of Nutrition, Physical Activity and Obesity. 2008. *Research to Practice Series, No. 5: Low-energy-dense foods and weight management: cutting calories while controlling hunger*. Atlanta, Centers for Disease Control and Prevention.
41. World Cancer Research Fund. 2012. Energy Density: finding the balance for cancer prevention. Available from: www.wcrf-uk.org/PDFs/EnergyDensity.pdf? [accessed 9/4/2014].

Controlling appetite and food intake by regulating eating frequency and timing

R. J. Stubbs
University of Derby, Derby, UK

10.1   Introduction

Eating is a behaviour influenced by numerous genetic, physiological, psychological, cultural, social and situational factors. This behaviour can be described or measured in terms of subjective motivation to eat (appetite, hunger, satiation and satiety), as amount and type of food and energy ingested, structure of dietary pattern, macronutrient profile and the frequency and timing of eating (Blundell and Stubbs, 2004; Stubbs and Blundell, 2011). The behaviours of interest in this current chapter are eating frequency (EF) and timing and how they may influence appetite and energy balance (EB). EF and timing are often tangled up with other issues such as type and composition of foods, how foods and beverages affect appetite, energy density (ED), portion size, environmental cues, cognitive processes, emotion regulation and circadian rhythms (de Castro, 2010; Stubbs *et al.*, 2012). Several of these issues are dealt with in other chapters, but in the real world these issues interact to determine patterns of eating behaviour and EB. Disentangling different sources of scientific evidence and their various limitations can be difficult.

10.2   The relationship between motivation to eat and eating behaviour

10.2.1 Patterns of intake

Mammalian (and human) feeding occurs regularly and intermittently and despite a general lack of conscious nutritional knowledge on the part of the animal, approximately matches energy intake (EI) and nutrient intakes with requirements (Stubbs and Blundell, 2011). This does not mean that we regulate our intake with great precision or accuracy in relation to energy requirements. Appetite regulation appears to be imprecise and numerous factors disrupt the relationship between eating behaviour and appetite (Mattes *et al.*, 2005). It is likely that our feeding behaviour is designed to protect us from deficiencies in energy and nutrients to ensure that physiological requirements are met (or at least deficiencies that produce functional impairments are avoided). It would appear that evolution has designed our behaviour and physiological systems to 'bank' surplus energy during times of abundance to protect us from times of uncertainty. Such a design would have a conveyed survival advantage in our ancient past because we frequently experienced seasonal food shortages and famines (Prentice, 2005; Prentice *et al.*, 2008).

Over the millennia we have become so successful at adapting to potential food shortages that in many parts of the world we now face unprecedented levels of disease associated with having too much food. Technological progress has shaped our environment faster than the environment can shape our genes, leaving humans with the biological design constraints of an optimal forager but an environment where food is ubiquitous (Stubbs and Tolkamp, 2006; Stubbs *et al.*, 2012). Many humans find it hard to resist weight gain when surrounded by an abundance of inexpensive, palatable and energy dense foods that can be obtained for minimal energy expenditure (Mattes *et al.*, 2005; Stubbs *et al.*, 2012). Being overweight has become a highly probable consequence of modern lifestyles. The characteristics of human feeding behaviour that were adaptive in resource-limiting environments appear to have become 'maladaptive' with reference to weight control and health in modern environments (Stubbs and Tolkamp, 2006).

Rather than being regulated, appetite and feeding behaviour might be said to be anticipatory or reactive since patterns of food intake (FI) are flexible and responsive to the state of the internal and external environment. Hunger and satiety have a large learned component rather than being the direct consequences of unconditioned physiological signals *per se*, such as reduced gastrointestinal content or circulating peptides. Such physiological events can act as important cues for feeding but they do not necessarily directly determine that behaviour (Stubbs and Blundell, 2011). Hence environmental factors can have a major impact on eating behaviour and EB (Mattes *et al.*, 2005; de Castro, 2010). The process of learning links feeding behaviour to physiological, sensory, nutritional, situational and other cues. This is important because meal timing and frequency for most individuals form part of patterns of learned behaviour. While there are considerable inter-individual differences in the timing and frequency of ingestive events, it is likely that intra-individual differences are somewhat less. In other words we are creatures of habit, although such habits are easier to demonstrate for patterns of mobility (Gonzalez *et al.*, 2008) than for patterns of EI (Blundell, 2000).

The relationship between a meal and a snack relates to timing and size of ingestive events in meal feeding animals and there is no universally accepted definition of either in the scientific literature. In non-human species (and indeed humans) that engage in numerous small feeding bouts throughout their diurnal cycle there is little if any distinction between a meal and a snack. Meal feeding animals are conditioned to ingest the majority of their EI in a few large ingestive events in their diurnal cycle, at approximately the same time points. Under these conditions, a snack can be defined as an energetically small, inter-meal ingestive event. To avoid confusion with a common use of the word to describe a certain type of commercially available food, it is useful to use the phrase 'commercially available snack foods' to describe those specific foods (Stubbs and Blundell, 2011).

10.2.2 Patterns of hunger, satiety and energy intake

Typically, hunger and appetite rise and fall in anticipation/response to FI. A scheme illustrating the relationship between hunger, appetite, satiation and satiety and FI is illustrated in Figure 10.1 (Blundell and Stubbs, 2004; Mattes *et al.*, 2005). It is important that we try to understand the impact of EF and timing on appetite, food and EI in the context of EB. In other words, we are subject to the laws of thermodynamics and if alterations in EF or timing have a significant impact on appetite control, they must influence EI or EE in a quantitatively significant manner.

Typically EI increases from earlier to later ingestive events across the day, such that EI at lunch exceeds that at breakfast and EI in the evening meal exceeds that at lunch (de Castro, 2004b; McCrory *et al.*, 2011). There appears to have been a secular trend of increased frequency of ingestive events over the last few decades. The more traditional 3–4 meals per day pattern has been replaced by one of an average of 5 ingestive events per day, in Americans at least (Leidy *et al.*, 2010).

10.2.3 How food composition impacts on satiety

The dietary macronutrients protein, carbohydrate, fat and alcohol together make up our total EI. ED is the energy per unit weight of a ready to eat food, and is usually expressed as kilocalories [kcal] per gram [kcal/g]. Macronutrients contribute 4, 4,

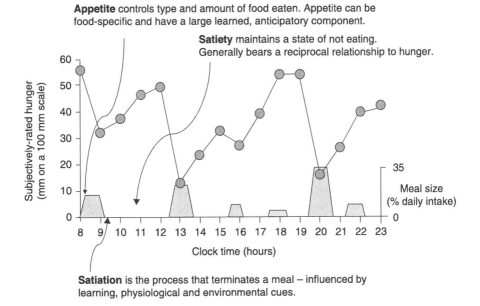

Figure 10.1 A schematic representation (not to scale) of the relationship between the subjectively expressed constructs of motivation in relation to feeding, and their relationship to quantitative and qualitative feeding behaviour.

7 and 9 kcal/g for carbohydrate, protein, alcohol and fat respectively, while water contains 0 kcal/g. Although the ED of foods can range from 0 [water] to 9 kcal/g [pure fat], for most of the frequently consumed individual foods it is around 0.5–2.4 kcal/g (Royal Society of Chemistry, 2002). Some foods are less energy dense, such as fruits and vegetables (0.25–0.5 kcal/g), and some considerably more so – savoury snack products are approximately 5.3 kcal/g (Royal Society of Chemistry, 2002).

Macronutrients are not all equal when it comes to how satisfied one feels after eating them. Protein has the greatest effect on satiety, followed by carbohydrate, followed by fat (Blundell and Stubbs, 2004; Stubbs et al., 2008). Thus while fat is the most energy dense food-based macronutrient it is also the least satisfying. Alcohol is the only macronutrient known to stimulate appetite (Caton et al., 2005; Yeomans, 2010a, 2010b). Because of the relative imprecision of appetite control, changes in dietary ED do not have a large effect on FI and so ED of foods has a leverage effect on EI such that high ED foods elevate EI (de Castro, 2004a) and low energy dense foods tend to lower EI (Ello-Martin et al., 2007; Ledikwe et al., 2007).

There is considerable confusion in both the scientific and popular literature about the role of EF and timing in appetite control and weight management (Mattson, 2005). The following sections consider current evidence on EF appetite regulation and weight control.

10.3   Eating frequency and energy balance – observational studies of free-living adults consuming self-selected diets

In 1997 Bellisle and Colleagues criticised early cross-sectional associations between meal frequency and adiposity with convincing arguments that (i) the inverse association between meal frequency and adiposity disappears when reported dietary intakes are adjusted for probable mis-reporting of EI and (ii) these associations are also likely to be affected by reverse causality, i.e. that more overweight people may omit more meals in an attempt to control their weight (Bellisle et al., 1997).

McCrory et al. (2011) have extensively reviewed evidence of EF and adiposity in free-living adults consuming self-selected diets in 19 cross-sectional studies (20 analyses). In 16 (10 significant) analyses, individuals who reported eating more frequently where leaner than those who reported eating less frequently. Four analyses (3 significant) showed the opposite effect. The different studies used different measures of EF and adiposity, and sample sizes ranged from 82 to 14,666. Taking up the arguments made by Bellisle et al. (1997), McCrory et al. (2011) examined data from the Continuing Survey of FIs by Individuals 1994–96 (n = 6,499). The relationship between self-reported EF and BMI was not significant. However, they then applied commonly used methods to estimate mis-reporting by comparing EI to estimated energy requirements to split the sample into those deemed to have plausible or implausible self-reported EIs (McCrory et al., 2002; Huang et al., 2004, 2005). Analysis of the 'plausible' sub-sample (n = 2,658) showed that the relationship

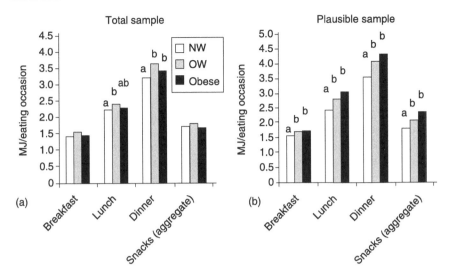

Figure 10.2 Energy intake from breakfast, lunch, dinner, and snacks (aggregate) in relation to weight status in 20–59 year olds from a total sample (n = 6499): (a) from Continuing Survey of Food Intake by Individuals 1994–96 (n = 6499); and (b) the 'plausible' sub-sample (n = 2685), i.e. having excluded those records deemed to exhibit implausibly low energy intakes relative to expected energy requirements. Within each eating occasion, labelled means without a common letter differ at P < 0.05 (McCrory *et al.*, 2011).

between reported EF and BMI changed from non-significant to significant and positive. Similar patterns were seen for the relationship between EI and BMI (Figure 10.2).

They confirmed these results by repeating the analysis in the Nationwide Food Consumption Survey 1977–78 (n = 13,750) and the Continuing Survey of FIs by Individuals 1989–91 (n = 2,474). These analyses suggest that in cross-sectional studies the relationship between EF, EI and adiposity is confounded by underreporting (McCrory *et al.*, 2011). Comparing results obtained in the total sample with plausible samples provided an indication that both breakfast and snacks may be selectively under-reported and that EF is associated with increased adiposity in cross-sectional studies when the effect of under-reporting has been corrected. Such corrections are based on a number of approximate assumptions (i.e. that subjects should be in EB, physical activity is a fixed multiple of basal metabolic rate and that basal metabolic rate can be predicted with linear regression equations) (Livingstone and Black, 2003).

10.4   Eating frequency and energy balance – intervention studies

Palmer (2009) identified (from 176 studies conducted between 1980 and 2009) 25 weight loss/maintenance interventions examining the impact of varying EF on weight outcomes in studies lasting between 2–8 weeks, with sample sizes between 5–38. For weight loss 1–9 eating occasions/day were studied and for weight maintenance 1–17 eating occasions/day. Palmer found no association between EF and weight status. A meta-analysis of the relationship between weight outcomes and EF was precluded by between-study differences in definitions of meals and snacks. Only two of the studies examined the impact of EF on hunger, one of which showed a transient effect over a single meal, but no differences over a whole day (Palmer, 2009).

McCrory et al. (2011) have also reviewed 5 studies in which high and low EF was prescribed. The studies lasted between 2–4 weeks per intervention in samples ranging between 10–19 adults. EF ranged from 3 to 9 ingestive events/day. Only one of the studies showed a significant change in body weight where participants lost slightly more weight when eating 6 versus 3 times/day. However, the difference in weight amounted to 0.3 kg over 4 weeks. In 5 studies EI increased (albeit slightly) with increased EF (McCrory et al., 2011).

10.5   Eating frequency and energy balance – controlled feeding studies

Leidy et al. (2010) reviewed current controlled feeding studies examining the effects of EF on appetite control and FI, whether increased EF improves appetite control, subsequently reduces EI or vice versa. They found minimal/no improvements in appetite control and regulation of FI with increased EF, beyond the typical 3 meals/day (Leidy et al., 2010). Reduced EF, i.e. less than 3 meals/day appeared to negatively affect appetite control (i.e. subjects felt hungrier, see for example Smeets and Westerterp-Plantenga (2008). As with the Palmer review, the limited number of studies, small sample sizes and short duration of studies constrained generalizability of conclusions (Leidy et al., 2010).

Parenthetically it is worth mentioning that controlled studies have also examined the effect of altered EF on energy expenditure and substrate utilisation. The studies have generally found little/no impact of altered EF per se on energy on nutrient metabolism beyond an increased periodicity of substrate utilisation and the thermic effect of food, which generally does not impact on 24-hour EB (Bellisle et al., 1997). Significant changes in EE may however affect eating frequency (Westerterp-Plantenga et al., 2003).

The effect of eating frequency (EF) on appetite and EB is still not entirely resolved. Evidence is indirect and fragmentary. Ostensibly cross-sectional studies tend to support no or a negative relationship between meal frequency and BMI (McCrory et al., 2011). Current evidence suggests that increased EF of modern foods is associated with greater adiposity once the effects of mis-reporting have been estimated (McCrory et al., 2011). However, the assumptions behind such estimates may in themselves create an artifact. These methods are essentially a means of verifying dietary intakes relative to an assumed habitual EB, rather than a direct means of measuring mis-reporting of food, energy or nutrient intakes. The definition of ingestive events in these studies is both arbitrary and variable between studies and measures of intake also vary between studies. It is therefore important to compare such analyses to controlled laboratory interventions over a number of weeks in humans, but there are not enough controlled studies to draw firm conclusions.

10.6   Small inter-meal ingestive events

Caloric beverages and commercial snack foods have the potential to be consumed with greater frequency than other foods at various points in the diurnal cycle. Calories contained in drinks appear to be poorly compensated for compared to the same calories contained in solid foods (McKiernan *et al.*, 2009; Cassady *et al.*, 2012; Mattes, 2010). Mattes has conducted an analysis of patterns of hunger and thirst and their relationships to eating and drinking in a convenience sample of 53 healthy adults (Mattes, 2010). He has considered the results in the context of evidence regarding beverages, satiety and weight control (McKiernan *et al.*, 2009; Mattes, 2010, Cassady *et al.*, 2012). Mattes suggested:

(i)   thirst sensations are higher than hunger and more stable over the day;
(ii)   the health consequence of drinking in excess of needs are minimal;
(iii) there are strong environmental influences on drinking;
(iv)   beverages are highly palatable inexpensive and convenient;
(v)   it is socially acceptable to drink in many social and professional settings;
(vi)   beverages have minimal impact on satiety and inasmuch are an ideal vehicle the delivery of nutrients (Mattes, 2010).

Commercially available snack foods tend to differ from the rest of the diet as they are more energy dense, high in fat and carbohydrate, low in protein and usually contain a large fraction of their edible mass as dry matter. They are by no means the only food eaten as a snack by many people at large. Like soft drinks, commercial snack foods are also attractively packaged, producing strong environmental influences on consuming them. They are highly palatable, inexpensive and convenient, and it is socially acceptable to consume them in many social and professional settings. Also they have minimal impact on satiety and inasmuch are also an ideal vehicle for the delivery of energy outside of a clear temporal pattern, or even perhaps below the threshold for strong detection by satiety mechanisms. Energy dense, high-carbohydrate and high-fat snacks have similar effects in increasing EI, under laboratory (Mazlan *et al.*, 2006) and free-living conditions (Whybrow *et al.*, 2007; Tey *et al.*, 2012), but not when of identical ED and composition to the rest of an *ad libitum* diet (Johnstone *et al.*, 2000). These effects are most pronounced in subjects who do not habitually eat snack foods between meals and least pronounced in subjects who incorporate such foods in their learned (habitual) patterns of behaviour (Westerterp-Plantenga *et al.*, 2002; Whybrow *et al.*, 2007).

While there is considerable research (albeit methodologically limited) on EF and indices of EB, there is less published research on the role of altering the timing of eating *per se* on these outcomes.

10.7   Timing of eating within a habitual diurnal rhythm

10.7.1 Observational studies

De Castro and colleagues have examined a number of correlates of self-reported FI in free-living humans ingesting their usual diets, using 7-day food diaries and concomitant measures of motivation to eat, mood and environmental circumstances (de Castro, 2004b). They found that meal sizes increase, whereas the after-meal intervals and satiety ratios decrease over the day. They then hypothesised that the time of day of FI would be related to total EI such that intake early in the day would tend to reduce overall EI, whereas intake later in the day would tend to increase EI over the entire day. This hypothesis was tested in a reanalysis of 7-day food diaries in 375 male and 492 female free-living individuals. The amounts of the macronutrients ingested and the density of intake occurring during five 4-h periods (0600–0959, 1000–1359, 1400–1759, 1800–2159 and 2200–0159 h) were identified and related to overall daily EI and meal intakes during the entire day. The proportion of intake in the morning was negatively correlated with daily EI ($r=-0.13$, $P<0.01$), whereas the proportion ingested late in the evening was positively correlated with daily EI ($r=0.14$, $P<0.01$) (de Castro, 2004b) (Figure 10.3).

EIs were then analysed by splitting days for each participant into those where intake during the morning, afternoon or evening were above or below each

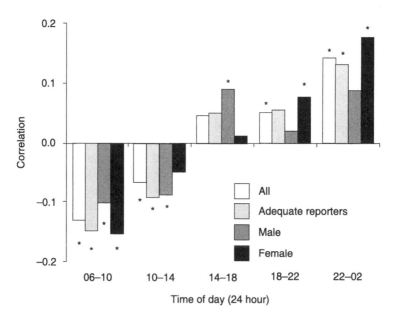

Figure 10.3 Correlations between the proportions of food energy ingested by humans self-reported in 7-day diet diaries during each of the five time periods and the total amount of energy ingested during the day for all subjects, for subjects identified as adequate reporters, for men only and for women only. *Different from zero, $P<0.01$ (de Castro, 2004b).

individual's mean daily intake for those periods and then relating proportionate intake in the morning, afternoon or evening to total daily EI. Correlation analysis suggested that high proportional intake during the morning was associated with low overall daily EI and high proportional intake during the evening was associated with high overall daily EI. The energy densities of intake during all periods of the day were positively related to overall intake (range, $r = 0.13$–0.23, $P < 0.01$). De Castro suggested that circadian and diurnal rhythms affect FI such that eating more earlier in the day can help limit EI and eating more late in the day may predispose people to overconsumption (de Castro, 2004b). Subsequent analysis suggested there was a macronutrient specificity to these effects. When a higher proportion of carbohydrate was ingested in the morning, less total energy and carbohydrate was ingested over the whole day. When the proportion of daily fat ingested in the morning was high, less energy, carbohydrate and fat were ingested over the whole day. When the proportion of protein intake was high in the morning protein intake was lower over the whole day. The opposite effects were also seen. When the proportionate intakes of carbohydrate, fat or energy were higher in the evening total daily EIs tended to be higher (de Castro, 2007).

De Castro argued that the problem of mis-reporting (under-reporting) of EI was corrected for by:

(i)   analysing absolute values and also the proportions of intake that are magnitude independent;
(ii) using within-subject comparisons;
(iii) examining data reported above and below a cut-off of $1.1 \times BMR$;
(iv) acknowledging that unsystematic, random, errors of measurement likely remain 'which should obfuscate relationships rather than produce them' (de Castro, 2004b, 2007).

There are potential limitations to this research:

(i)   relationships are correlational, cause and effect are hard to distentangle;
(ii) these are real world effects and relationships could be due to other (unmeasured) phenomena;
(iii) the cut-off of $1.1 \times BMR$ for estimated mis-reporting is low;
(iv) it is possible that misreporting could be selective, the McCrory analysis of EF suggests breakfasts are specifically under-reported (McCrory et al., 2011), which if present in the de Castro analysis would create an artefact;
(v)   the correlations were relatively small producing effect sizes on total EI of ~0.5 MJ/d;
(vi) these effects have not been replicated in other independent data-sets, which should be a research priority.

10.7.2 Intervention studies of free-living adults consuming self-selected diets

Recently, a prospective longitudinal study examining how timing of FI relates to weight loss effectiveness in humans has been reported in individuals following a 20 week diet and lifestyle weight loss treatment (49.5% female; mean age 42; mean BMI 31.4). Those who tended to eat lunch later lost less weight (7.7 versus 9.9 kg) and had a slower rate of weight loss, than those who tended to eat lunch earlier.

Those who ate lunch later tended to be more evening types, consumed less energy at breakfast and skipped breakfast more frequently than those who tended to eat lunch earlier (Garaulet *et al.*, 2013). This study did not detect any differences in EI, diet composition, estimated EE, appetite hormones or sleep patterns between the two groups, which is not surprising given the magnitude of weight differences observed over 20 weeks.

In the context of weight management it is interesting that in addition to current interest in the timing of eating behaviour *per se* as a factor that can affect appetite and weight control, the regularity and stability of eating behaviour may also be important. Eating patterns are a form of learned behaviour and evidence suggests that more chaotic, impulsive and unpredictable patterns in the frequency and timing of ingestive events are associated with less control over EI and body weight (Stubbs *et al.*, 2011, Stubbs and Lavin, 2013).

10.7.3 Intermittent fasting, appetite and weight control

The timing of eating is also altered during intermittent fasting, the most extensively studied example of which is Ramadan. A recent meta-analysis of self-controlled cohort studies comparing body weights, blood levels of lipids and fasting blood glucose levels before and after Ramadan showed that after Ramadan fasting, low-density lipoprotein and fasting blood glucose levels were decreased. In women weight remained unchanged and men lost a small amount of weight (Kul *et al.*, 2014). Haljek and Co-workers noted that 202 observers of Ramadan lost on average about a kilogram of weight over four weeks, and the lost weight was quickly regained (Hajek *et al.*, 2012). Roky *et al.* (2004) reviewed the effects of Ramadan fasting on physiological and behavioural variables in healthy subjects. They found that Ramadan fasting did not dramatically affect the metabolism of lipids, carbohydrates and proteins, or the daily mean of hormonal serum levels. Some beneficial changes (increased HDL, apoprotein A1, decreased LDL) were noted along with changes in the circadian distribution of body temperature, cortisol, melatonin and glycemia. Nocturnal sleep, daytime alertness and psychomotor performance were decreased (Roky *et al.*, 2004). Finch *et al.* (1998) studied hourly ratings of hunger (Figure 10.4), mood and thirst, food and drink intake on specified days before, during and after Ramadan in 15 men and 26 women.

Hunger increased substantially during the daily fast and was higher for the women than the men during the earlier days of Ramadan. On average, fasting levels of hunger were similar for both sexes as Ramadan progressed. Despite these marked changes, there were no significant changes in body weight over Ramadan (Finch *et al.*, 1998). What is most remarkable about the complete fast during the hours of sunrise to sunset during Ramadan is that it has minimal effect on body weight in a population who are not fasting for the purpose of losing weight. It is worth noting that intermittent fasting (i.e. between days) is becoming increasingly popular as a means of weight management. A recent review (Varady, 2011) found intermittent fasting in seven studies had a similar impact to caloric restriction (11 studies) on weight loss and fat loss.

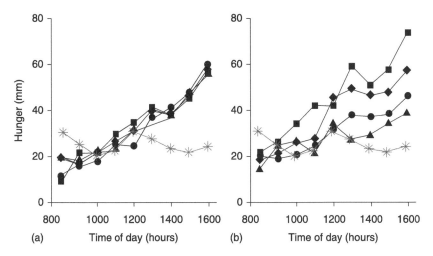

Figure 10.4 Mean hourly hunger ratings (100 mm line scale) during Ramadan for males (a), and females (b) for day 3 (squares), day 10 (diamonds), day 17 (circles) and day 24 (triangles), and mean hourly hunger ratings for the period after Ramadan (*). (Reprinted from Finch *et al.*, 1998, copyright © 1998, with permission from Elsevier.)

10.8   Timing of eating and disruption of diurnal rhythms

It is possible that an altered eating pattern, shorter sleep duration, international travel across time-zones, exposure to bright lights at night or shift work could impact on metabolic outcomes, health (de Castro, 2007, 2009; Garaulet *et al.*, 2010, 2013), and (in animal models at least), lifespans (Froy, 2010). The role of chrono-disruption in health and well-being is an emerging area with relevance for modern lifestyles although evidence in relation to appetite control humans is currently limited. There is a growing literature relating circadian disruption to the development of certain diseases or the impairment of existing pathologies including premature aging, cancer, cardiovascular diseases, cognitive impairment, mood disorders, obesity and metabolic syndrome (Garaulet *et al.*, 2010; Froy, 2010). On the other hand there is considerable plasticity in feeding behaviour. Despite large changes in the pattern of feeding, EI can potentially be adjusted to satisfy requirements (see below). But appetite and feeding behaviour are biased towards over-rather than under-consumption, which suggests circadian disruption could potentially uncouple the normal phase relationships between internal circadian rhythms (i.e. appetite and satiety signals) and 24-hour environmental cycles (feeding and activity schedules) (Froy, 2010; Garaulet *et al.*, 2010).

To date very few controlled studies in humans have examined how chrono-disruption *per se* influence appetite control when EI is controlled, or under *ad libitum* conditions. It is therefore useful to examine this issue in the context of rodent models. Fonken *et al.* (2010) have conducted a series of studies in rodents showing that night time light exposure increases body mass, body fatness and reduces glucose tolerance over 8 weeks compared with mice living under a standard light/dark cycle. Their results suggested that low levels of light at night disrupted the timing of Fl and other metabolic signals leading to excess weight gain. Similarly, Arble *et al.* (2009) showed that nocturnal mice fed a high-fat diet only during the 12 hour light phase gained significantly more weight than mice fed only during the 12 hour dark phase. In these studies there were no statistically significant differences in caloric intake and locomotor activity between groups. However, in the study by Arble and colleagues the light fed group were consistently less active and ate slightly more than the dark fed group–effects which might summate to influence EB. Subsequent studies have begun to characterize the molecular mechanisms by which shifts in light/dark patterns disrupt molecular clocks in rodent models e.g. (Fonken *et al.*, 2013a, 2013b, 2013c). It is not yet clear if disruptions of light/dark cycles have equally pronounced effects in humans.

The neurophysiology of eating behaviour and sleep/activity profiles are inter-connected and co-ordinated in that hunger and vigilance are paired during daylight hours and sleep/satiety are paired during the hours of darkness (Vanitallie, 2006). The interconnected nature of chronobiology, eating behaviour, EB and obesity illustrates the complexity of mechanisms at play (Froy, 2010; Garaulet *et al.*, 2010; Fonken and Nelson, 2011). Chrono-disruption may influence health and well-being but it is not clear if this operates through any changes in meal timing or frequency. Perhaps the real life intervention in humans that is closest to switching the light/dark cycle of rodents is shift work. Zhao *et al.* (2012) found that night-only shift work was associated with obesity in 2,086 nurses and midwives, but the relative risk was slight (1.02). A study by Itani *et al.* (2011) suggested that the relationship between shift work and obesity may be mediated through sleep-loss in 21,693 Japanese men and 2,109 women. Analysis using both engagement in shift work and sleep duration as dependent variables showed that the relative risks of new-onset obesity for those with a sleep duration of less than 5 h were 1.20 (95% Cl, 1.09–1.32) for men and 1.7 (95% Cl, 1.11–2.87) for women (Itani *et al.*, 2011). A systematic review by Antunes *et al.* (2010) suggested that shift workers seem to gain weight more often than those workers submitted to a usual work day and that shift work is associated with increased risk for obesity, diabetes and CVD. In a systematic review of 10 articles (Canuto *et al.* 2013), 8 found a positive association between shift work and the meta-bolic syndrome after controlling for socio-demographic and behavioural factors, although only 3 studies included sleep duration as a confounder (Canuto *et al.*, 2013). Vyas *et al.* (2012) conducted a systematic review and meta-analysis of 34 studies in 2,011,935 people. They found that: 'On the basis of the Canadian prevalence of shift work of 32.8%, the population attributable risks related to shift work were 7.0% for myocardial infarction, 7.3% for all coronary events, and 1.6% for ischaemic stroke' (Vyas *et al.*, 2012). Van Drongelen *et al.* (2011) conducted a systematic review of 8 articles examining the longitudinal effects of shift work on body weight change and found strong evidence for a crude relationship between shift work and body weight increase.

Appetite control is far less clearly studied in relation to shift work. Crispim *et al.* (2011) found that shift workers on an early morning shift had lower appetites and concentrations of leptin and nonacylated and acylated ghrelin than the workers on other shifts in very small samples of 6-9 subjects.

The balance of evidence suggests some association between shift work, weight gain, the metabolic syndrome and cardiovascular risk, which may be mediated by lack of sleep, associated circadian disturbances, psychosocial stress or other factors. Evidence relating shift work patterns to appetite control and eating behaviour barely exists. There is much work yet to be done in understanding how the timing of eating associated with altered diurnal patterns affects human appetite and energy balance.

10.9   Summary and future trends

Eating frequency and timing can be interrelated both with each other and a range of other variables that can impact on appetite and EB. This suggests that EF and timing operate in a complex matrix of influences and the studies reviewed here may often be affected by unmeasured variables. The definitions of EF and timing differ between studies as do measures of EF, timing and indices of EB. It is important to understand the limitations to current data and heterogeneity in the relationship between eating patterns, appetite and EB control. Current evidence suggests EF is associated with higher EIs and a positive EB. Foods eaten as small inter-meal ingestive events often tend to be different in ED and composition to foods eaten at main meals, which raises issues of the impact of food composition, ED and pre-packaged foods on EI and EB. There is very little evidence that eating less frequently promotes a positive or negative EB. The size and composition of meals eaten appears to change across the day. These findings take into account mis-reporting of EI and current corrections for this phenomenon make approximate assumptions that may create artefacts. There is little evidence that EF affects appetite except that decreasing eating frequency below three meals/day elevates hunger (Leidy et al., 2010). Gross changes in the timing of eating appears to have little impact on body weight with the possible exception of shift work, where evidence indicates some risk of weight gain although mechanisms are far from clear. EF and timing in relation to shift work are largely unstudied. Examinations of appetite control during shift work appear limited to pilot work. The relationship between EF and timing, appetite and EB requires a consideration of nutritional and non-nutritional properties of foods, the social and environmental context and that human eating behaviour is biased toward over- rather than under-consumption.

Future work should address the current lack of controlled studies on EF and timing, move towards standardising definitions of ingestive events and measures of food intake and reduce the considerable heterogeneity in measures made. Mis-reporting of food intake is an area that requires urgent attention for EF and timing, and relationships between diet and health in general. Many authors state the need for reliable biomarkers of energy and nutrient intake, but there is little sign that such techniques will be developed for large-scale or individual level assessments in the near future. Attempting to replicate the real-world correlates of EF and timing produced by de

Castro (2004a, 2004b, 2007, 2009, 2010) should also be a research priority, using more incisive measures of EB and mis-reporting, as the findings of this work are tantalising. The area of chrono-disruption requires structured investigation in terms of the mechanisms by which specific components of altered diurnal rhythms impact on overall patterns of eating behaviour, EB, health and well-being.

References

Antunes, L. C., Levandovski, R., Dantas, G., Caumo, W. and Hidalgo, M. P. (2010). Obesity and shift work: chronobiological aspects. *Nutr Res Rev*, 23, 155–68.

Arble, D. M., Bass, J., Laposky, A. D., Vitaterna, M. H. and Turek, F. W. (2009). Circadian timing of food intake contributes to weight gain. *Obesity (Silver Spring)*, 17, 2100–2.

Bellisle, F., McDevitt, R. and Prentice, A. M. (1997). Meal frequency and energy balance. *Br J Nutr*, 77 Suppl 1, S57–70.

Blundell, J. (2000). What foods do people habitually eat? A dilemma for nutrition, an enigma for psychology 1, 2. *American Journal of Clinical Nutrition*, 71, 3–5.

Blundell, J. E. and Stubbs, R. J. (2004). Diet and food intake in humans. *In:* Bray, G. A., Bouchard, C. and James, W. P. T. (eds) *Handbook of Obesity (2nd Edition)*. New York: Marcel Dekker Inc.

Canuto, R., Garcez, A. S. and Olinto, M. T. (2013). Metabolic syndrome and shift work: a systematic review. *Sleep Med Rev*, 17(6), 395–7.

Cassady, B. A., Considine, R. V. and Mattes, R. D. (2012). Beverage consumption, appetite, and energy intake: what did you expect? *Am J Clin Nutr*, 95, 587–93.

Caton, S. J., Marks, J. E. and Hetherington, M. M. (2005). Pleasure and alcohol: manipulating pleasantness and the acute effects of alcohol on food intake. *Physiol Behav*, 84, 371–7.

Crispim, C. A., Waterhouse, J., Damaso, A. R., Zimberg, I. Z., Padilha, H. G., *et al.* (2011). Hormonal appetite control is altered by shift work: a preliminary study. *Metabolism*, 60, 1726–35.

de Castro, J. M. (2004a). Dietary energy density is associated with increased intake in free-living humans. *J Nutr*, 134, 335–41.

de Castro, J. M. (2004b). The time of day of food intake influences overall intake in humans. *J Nutr*, 134, 104–11.

de Castro, J. M. (2007). The time of day and the proportions of macronutrients eaten are related to total daily food intake. *Br J Nutr*, 98, 1077–83.

de Castro, J. M. (2009). When, how much and what foods are eaten are related to total daily food intake. *Br J Nutr*, 102, 1228–37.

de Castro, J. M. (2010). The control of food intake of free-living humans: putting the pieces back together. *Physiol Behav*, 100, 446–53.

Ello-Martin, J. A., Roe, L. S., Ledikwe, J. H., Beach, A. M. and Rolls, B. J. (2007). Dietary energy density in the treatment of obesity: a year-long trial comparing 2 weight-loss diets. *Am J Clin Nutr*, 85, 1465–77.

Finch, G. M., Day, J. E., Razak, Welch, D. A. and Rogers, P. J. (1998). Appetite changes under free-living conditions during Ramadan fasting. *Appetite*, 31, 159–70.

Fonken, L. K., Aubrecht, T. G., Melendez-Fernandez, O. H., Weil, Z. M. and Nelson, R. J. (2013a). Dim light at night disrupts molecular circadian rhythms and increases body weight. *J Biol Rhythms*, 28, 262–71.

Fonken, L. K., Lieberman, R. A., Weil, Z. M. and Nelson, R. J. (2013b). Dim light at night exaggerates weight gain and inflammation associated with a high-fat diet in male mice. *Endocrinology*, 154(10), 3817–25.

Fonken, L. K. and Nelson, R. J. (2011). Illuminating the deleterious effects of light at night. *F1000 Med Rep*, 3, 18.

Fonken, L. K., Weil, Z. M. and Nelson, R. J. (2013c). Dark nights reverse metabolic disruption caused by dim light at night. *Obesity (Silver Spring)*, 21, 1159–64.

Fonken, L. K., Workman, J. L., Walton, J. C., Weil, Z. M., Morris, J. S., *et al.* (2010). Light at night increases body mass by shifting the time of food intake. *Proc Natl Acad Sci USA*, 107, 18664–9.

Froy, O. (2010). Metabolism and circadian rhythms – implications for obesity. *Endocr Rev*, 31, 1–24.

Garaulet, M., Gomez-Abellan, P., Alburquerque-Bejar, J. J., Lee, Y. C., Ordovas, J. M. and Scheer, F. A. (2013). Timing of food intake predicts weight loss effectiveness. *Int J Obes (Lond)*, 37, 604–11.

Garaulet, M., Ordovas, J. M. and Madrid, J. A. (2010). The chronobiology, etiology and pathophysiology of obesity. *Int J Obes (Lond)*, 34, 1667–83.

Gonzalez, M. C., Hidalgo, C. A. and Barabasi, A. L. (2008). Understanding individual human mobility patterns. *Nature*, 453, 779–82.

Hajek, P., Myers, K., Dhanji, A. R., West, O. and McRobbie, H. (2012). Weight change during and after Ramadan fasting. *J Public Health (Oxf)*, 34, 377–81.

Huang, T. T., Howarth, N. C., Lin, B. H., Roberts, S. B. and McCrory, M. A. (2004). Energy intake and meal portions: associations with BMI percentile in U.S. children. *Obes Res*, 12, 1875–85.

Huang, T. T., Roberts, S. B., Howarth, N. C. and McCrory, M. A. (2005). Effect of screening out implausible energy intake reports on relationships between diet and BMI. *Obes Res*, 13, 1205–17.

Itani, O., Kaneita, Y., Murata, A., Yokoyama, E. and Ohida, T. (2011). Association of onset of obesity with sleep duration and shift work among Japanese adults. *Sleep Med*, 12, 341–5.

Johnstone, A. M., Shannon, E., Whybrow, S., Reid, C. A. and Stubbs, R. J. (2000). Altering the temporal distribution of energy intake with isoenergetically dense foods given as snacks does not affect total daily energy intake in normal-weight men. *Br J Nutr*, 83, 7–14.

Kul, S., Savas, E., Ozturk, Z. A. and Karadag, G. (2014). Does Ramadan fasting alter body weight and blood lipids and fasting blood glucose in a healthy population? A meta-analysis. *J Relig Health*, 53, 929–42.

Ledikwe, J. H., Rolls, B. J., Smiciklas-Wright, H., Mitchell, D. C., Ard, J. D., *et al.* (2007). Reductions in dietary energy density are associated with weight loss in overweight and obese participants in the PREMIER trial. *Am J Clin Nutr*, 85, 1212–21.

Leidy H. J., Harris C. T. and Campbell W. W. (2010). Eating frequency and energy regulation in controlled feeding studies. *J Nutr*, 141, 154–7.

Livingstone, M. B. and Black, A. E. (2003). Markers of the validity of reported energy intake. *J Nutr*, 133 Suppl 3, S895–920.

Mattes, R. D. (2010). Hunger and thirst: issues in measurement and prediction of eating and drinking. *Physiol Behav*, 100, 22–32.

Mattes, R. D., Hollis, J., Hayes, D. and Stunkard, A. J. (2005). Appetite: measurement and manipulation misgivings. *J Am Diet Assoc*, 105, S87–97.

Mattson, M. P. (2005). The need for controlled studies of the effects of meal frequency on health. *Lancet*, 365, 1978–80.

Mazlan, N., Horgan, G., Whybrow, S. and Stubbs, J. (2006). Effects of increasing increments of fat- and sugar-rich snacks in the diet on energy and macronutrient intake in lean and overweight men. *Br J Nutr*, 96, 596–606.

McCrory, M. A., Howarth, N. C., Roberts, S. B. and Huang, T. T. (2011). Eating frequency and energy regulation in free-living adults consuming self-selected diets. *J Nutr*, 141, 148–53.

McCrory, M. A., Hajduk, C. L. and Roberts, S. B. (2002). Procedures for screening out inaccurate reports of dietary energy intake. *Public Health Nutr*, 5, 873–82.

McKiernan, F., Hollis, J. H., McCabe, G. P. and Mattes, R. D. (2009). Thirst-drinking, hunger-eating; tight coupling? *J Am Diet Assoc*, 109, 486–90.

Palmer, M. A. (2009). Association between eating frequency, weight, and health. *Nutrition Reviews*, 67, 379–90.

Prentice, A. M. (2005). Starvation in humans: evolutionary background and contemporary implications. *Mech Ageing Dev*, 126, 976–81.

Prentice, A. M., Hennig, B. J. and Fulford, A. J. (2008). Evolutionary origins of the obesity epidemic: natural selection of thrifty genes or genetic drift following predation release? *Int J Obes (Lond)*, 32, 1607–10.

Roky, R., Houti, I., Moussamih, S., Qotbi, S. and Aadil, N. (2004). Physiological and chronobiological changes during Ramadan intermittent fasting. *Ann Nutr Metab*, 48, 296–303.

Royal Society of Chemistry (2002). *The Composition of Foods*, London.

Smeets, A. J. and Westerterp-Plantenga, M. S. (2008). Acute effects on metabolism and appetite profile of one meal difference in the lower range of meal frequency. *Br J Nutr*, 99, 1316–21.

Stubbs, J., Whybrow, S., Teixeira, P., Blundell, J., Lawton, C., et al. (2011). Problems in identifying predictors and correlates of weight loss and maintenance: implications for weight control therapies based on behaviour change. *Obes Rev*, 12, 688–708.

Stubbs, R. and Blundell, J. (2011). Appetite: psychobiological and behavioural aspects. *The Enclyclopedia of Human Nutrition 3rd Edition*. London.

Stubbs R. J. and Lavin, J. H. (2013). The challenges of implementing behaviour changes that lead to sustained weight management. *Nutrition Bulletin*, 38, 5–22.

Stubbs, R. J., Gail, C., Whybrow, S. and Gilbert, P. (2012). The evolutionary inevitability of obesity in modern society: implications for behavioral solutions to weight control in the general population. *In:* Martinez, M. P. and Robinson, H. (eds.) *Obesity and Weight Management: Challenges, Practices and Health Implications*. Novo Publishing.

Stubbs, R. J. and Tolkamp, B. J. (2006). Control of energy balance in relation to energy intake and energy expenditure in animals and man: an ecological perspective. *Br J Nutr*, 95, 657–76.

Stubbs, R. J., Whybrow, S. and N., M. (2008). Macronutrients, feeding behavior, and weight control in humans. *In:* Harris, R. B. S. and Mattes, R. D. (eds.) *Appetite and Food Intake: Behavioral and Physiological Considerations*. Boca Ranton: Taylor and Francis Group.

Tey, S. L., Brown, R. C., Gray, A. R., Chisholm, A. W. and Delahunty, C. M. (2012). Long-term consumption of high energy-dense snack foods on sensory-specific satiety and intake. *Am J Clin Nutr*, 95, 1038–47.

van Drongelen, A., Boot, C. R., Merkus, S. L., Smid, T. and van der Beek, A. J. (2011). The effects of shift work on body weight change – a systematic review of longitudinal studies. *Scand J Work Environ Health*, 37, 263–75.

Vanitallie, T. B. (2006). Sleep and energy balance: interactive homeostatic systems. *Metabolism*, 55, S30–5.

Varady, K. A. (2011). Intermittent versus daily calorie restriction: which diet regimen is more effective for weight loss? *Obes Rev*, 12, e593–601.

Vyas, M. V., Garg, A. X., Iansavichus, A. V., Costella, J., Donner, A., *et al.* (2012). Shift work and vascular events: systematic review and meta-analysis. *BMJ*, 345, e4800.

Westerterp-Plantenga M.S., Kovacs E.M.R. and Melanson K.J. (2002). Habitual meal frequency and EI regulation in partially temporally isolated men. *Int J Obes Rel Metab Dis*, 26, 102–10.

Westerterp-Plantenga, M. S., Goris, A. H., Meijer, E. P. and Westerterp, K. R. (2003). Habitual meal frequency in relation to resting and activity-induced energy expenditure in human subjects: the role of fat-free mass. *Br J Nutr*, 90, 643–9.

Whybrow, S., Mayer, C., Kirk, T. R., Mazlan, N. and Stubbs, R. J. (2007). Effects of two weeks' mandatory snack consumption on energy intake and energy balance. *Obesity (Silver Spring)*, 15, 673–85.

Yeomans, M. R. (2010a). Alcohol, appetite and energy balance: is alcohol intake a risk factor for obesity? *Physiol Behav*, 100, 82–9.

Yeomans, M. R. (2010b). Short term effects of alcohol on appetite in humans. Effects of context and restrained eating. *Appetite*, 55, 565–73.

Zhao, I., Bogossian, F. and Turner, C. (2012). A cross-sectional analysis of the association between night-only or rotating shift work and overweight/obesity among female nurses and midwives. *J Occup Environ Med*, 54, 834–40.

Managing food portion size and its effect on weight control

I. H. M. Steenhuis, M. P. Poelman[1], W. M. Vermeer[2]
[1]VU University, Amsterdam, The Netherlands; [2]Leiden University Medical Center, Leiden, The Netherlands

11.1 Introduction: trends in food portion sizes

Research shows that food portion sizes have increased during the past decades. Studies have been conducted in the USA (Nielsen and Popkin, 2003; Smiciklas-Wright *et al.*, 2003; Young and Nestle, 2002, 2007, 2012), the UK (Wrieden *et al.*, 2008; Benson, 2009), Denmark (Matthiessen *et al.*, 2003) and the Netherlands (Steenhuis *et al.*, 2010). Young and Nestle (2002) showed that the portion sizes of numerous foods offered in the USA have increased, and that current sizes of, for example, French fries, hamburgers or soda are two to five times larger than the original sizes (Young and Nestle, 2002). They also illustrated that since the 1970s, there has been a tremendous increase in the number of available 'large' and 'super' sizes. This trend has continued during the first decade of this century (Young and Nestle, 2012). Although food portions in the USA tend to be larger than in Europe, portion sizes have also increased in Europe. A study conducted in Denmark showed that portion sizes of particularly high-energy dense foods and beverages such as chocolate bars, ice creams, and sugar-sweetened beverages have increased during the past decades (Matthiessen *et al.*, 2003). A study conducted in the UK confirmed the increased availability of king and giant sizes, and increasing portion sizes, especially in fast-food chains (Wrieden *et al.*, 2008). The increase in portion sizes in the UK was also demonstrated by Benson and colleagues (2009) who concluded that the most significant increases in portion sizes in Britain occurred during the last two decades (Benson, 2009). Research conducted in the Netherlands demonstrated also a trend of increased portion sizes. Three major trends were identified (Steenhuis *et al.*, 2010). First, original sizes of products have enlarged, with the smaller original size being no longer available on the market; second, larger sizes have been added to the portion size portfolio; and third, multi-packages have been introduced, with an increased number of sub items within a multi-package since their introduction.

Portion sizes as well as the portion size portfolio are changing continuously. The reason why portion sizes keep changing is that they form an important marketing tool to increase market share. Larger portion sizes can be offered by food companies at a relatively low cost, since the costs of the food are relatively cheap compared to other

Managing and Preventing Obesity. http://dx.doi.org/10.1533/9781782420996.3.167

costs such as labor (Young and Nestle, 2012). Besides the above mentioned studies conducted in the USA, UK, Denmark and the Netherlands, virtually no data on changing portion size are available. In order to be able to monitor the changes in portion sizes systematically, it is advisable to set up a consistent monitoring system across countries. A first step to provide insight in such changes over time is already being undertaken as in 2011 the Global Food Monitoring Group was established. This initiative currently exists in 31 countries and seeks to monitor and report the nutritional composition of processed foods available in different countries, including data on the packages and portion sizes (Dunford et al., 2012).

11.2   Effects of food portion size on energy intake

Numerous studies have proved that a person's energy intake increases when being offered a larger portion (Zlatevska et al., 2014). This also accounts for food with a perceived unfavorable taste, e.g. stale popcorn (Wansink and Kim, 2005). The effects have been shown for a variety of foods, such as macaroni (Rolls et al., 2002), pre-packaged snacks (Rolls et al., 2004), and beverages (Flood et al., 2006). Effects of at least 30% higher consumption levels due to portion size are frequently reported (e.g. Diliberti et al., 2004; Raynor and Wing, 2007; Rolls et al., 2002, 2004; Wansink and Park, 2001; Wansink and Kim, 2005; Wansink et al., 2005), with larger effects for larger portion sizes. In a meta-analytic review, Zlatevska and colleagues showed that doubling a portion led on average to an increase in consumption of 35% (Zlatevska et al., 2014). Furthermore, research has shown that the effects of portion size can persist at least over several days, with no indication of meal to meal compensation (Rolls et al., 2006, 2007). Rolls and co-workers showed that the average increase in caloric intake, owing to 50% larger portions, did not decline over a period of eleven days. This resulted in a cumulative increase of, on average, more than 4600 kcal during the research period (Rolls et al., 2007).

11.3   Explanations for the effects of portion size on energy intake

Important factors found in the literature, explaining why people buy and eat larger portion sizes than they actually need, are the notions of 'value for money' and 'portion distortion'. Larger portions are made attractive by offering more value for money, i.e. having a lower price per unit. Lower unit costs also explain why larger package or portion sizes lead to a higher user volume (French, 2005; Swinburn et al., 2004; Wansink, 1996). Based on focus group interviews, it seems that consumers experience the lower price per unit in the case of larger portions as a natural pattern that they are used to and expect to occur (Vermeer et al., 2010b).

Next, continuous exposure to larger food portion sizes contributes to 'portion distortion' among consumers (Matthiessen et al., 2013; Penisten and Litchfield,

2004). People experiencing portion distortion perceive larger portion sizes than recommended by nutritional guidelines as an appropriate amount to consume at a single occasion (Schwartz and Byrd-Bredbenner, 2006). It also refers to the fact that individuals do not realize that their portion size commonly exceeds the serving size (Bryant and Dundes, 2005). With respect to portion distortion, a number of aspects are relevant. First, larger portions have become standard and, as a consequence, consumers have difficulty selecting amounts of food that are appropriate for their weight and activity levels (Young and Nestle, 2003). Second, market-place portions differ increasingly from recommended standard portion sizes defined by federal agencies (Young and Nestle, 2003). In fact, market-place portions are often three to four times larger than the recommended portion size, while consumers perceive market-place portions as standard portions (Hogbin and Hess, 1999). Several studies have shown that people tend to select substantially larger portions than the recommended portion sizes (Bryant and Dundes, 2005; Burger *et al.*, 2007; Condrasky *et al.*, 2007; Schwartz and Byrd-Bredbenner, 2006). Third, labels on food packaging are not always clear with respect to the serving size. Sometimes, unrealistic small serving sizes are used on food packages in order to give consumers a positive impression about the number of servings in one package and the caloric content (Bryant and Dundes, 2005). Similarly, using the terms 'small', 'medium' and 'large' also creates confusion, as people's interpretation of these terms differs (Young and Nestle, 1998). Moreover, the absolute amounts for a 'small', 'medium' or 'large' also vary greatly and may also create confusion (unpublished data). A fourth factor relevant in portion distortion is the 'unit bias' people might experience. Geier *et al.* (2006) define unit bias as 'a sense that a single entity is the appropriate amount to engage, consume or consider'. The size of the unit or package sets a consumption norm for consumers, which might not be an appropriate norm in accordance with food recommendations (Geier *et al.*, 2006; Wansink, 2004). Many people interpret package size as a single serving size and are unaware of the fact that a package contains multiple servings (Pelletier *et al.*, 2004). Fifth, tableware also contributes to portion distortion. It seems that people serve themselves more food if using a larger dinnerware such as a bowl, glass, plate or spoon (Pelletier *et al.*, 2004; Ittersum and Wansink, 2012; Wansink and Cheney, 2005; Wansink *et al.*, 2006). Sixth, and finally, the extended portion size portfolio (see section 11.2) leads to a shift in the perception of what the 'normal' size is. The larger the portion sizes available in the portion size portfolio, the larger the selected portion (Vermeer *et al.*, 2010a). This might be caused by people's so-called 'preference for the middle'; when adding larger sizes to the portion size portfolio consumers will shift up their choice to select a portion size more in the middle (Sharpe *et al.*, 2008).

Once larger portions have been selected because of the value for money and portion distortion principle, passive over-consumption is likely to occur. In particular, people tend to overeat palatable, high energy-dense (e.g. high in fat) foods, without deliberate intention (Blundell and MacDiarmid, 1997). This mindless eating occurs especially in situations in which individuals are distracted during eating and when they are not focused on the food they are consuming. When eating mindlessly, individuals are at risk of consuming surplus amounts when enough food is available (Stroebele and de Castro, 2004). Watching television, playing a computer game, listening to the radio and dining with others are factors that typically lead to mindlessly eating larger amounts than intended (Bellisle *et al.*, 2004; Blass *et al.*, 2006; Hetherington *et al.*, 2006; Higgs and Woodward, 2009; Oldham-Cooper *et al.*, 2011). Mindless eating might also reduce individuals' sensory-specific satiety, meaning that perceived pleasantness from the food declines less gradually and therefore postpones meal termination. When eating mindlessly, people have difficulty memorizing the amount of food consumed recently. These consequences of mindless eating result in an increase in the quantity consumed (Bellisle *et al.*, 2004; Blass *et al.*, 2006; (Hetherington *et al.*, 2006), and also the amount of food consumed later that day (Higgs and Woodward, 2009; Oldham-Cooper *et al.*, 2011).

11.4 Environmental strategies influencing portion control behaviors

Since increased portion sizes are part of a changed food environment, it is a challenge to change this into an environment that makes it easier to not overeat. Physical, economic, political and socio-cultural aspects of the environment can be distinguished according to the ANGELO-grid (ANalysis Grid for Environments Linked to Obesity) (Swinburn *et al.*, 1999). The physical environment refers to available options to make a healthy choice; the economic environment refers to the cost of healthy choices; the political environment refers to rules and regulations that may influence healthy choices; and the socio-cultural environment refers to social and cultural norms influencing healthy choices (Swinburn *et al.*, 1999). Interventions aimed at portion size can be put in place in all four types of environment. In the following, intervention opportunities within the physical, economic and political environment will be identified.

Physical environment. Decreasing portion sizes, or the option to order half a portion, are examples of interventions aimed at the physical environment (Schwartz *et al.*, 2012; Steenhuis and Vermeer, 2009; Wansink and Huckabee, 2005). An experiment conducted in 26 worksite cafeterias showed that around 10% of customers who normally ordered a standard sized hot meal switched to a smaller size (which was about two-thirds of the original standard available size) when made available (Vermeer *et al.*, 2011b). Schwartz *et al.* (2012) demonstrated that this percentage can be increased to a third, if consumers are actively offered to downsize their order. After offering a smaller snack, people did not report more feelings of hunger and craving compared to a larger snack (van Kleef *et al.*, 2013). Visual segmentation cues in packages appears to promote a reduction in consumption as well (Geier *et al.*, 2012; Wansink and Huckabee, 2005). Segmentation cues enhance monitoring of consumption, can set a consumption norm, and can interrupt automatic eating (Geier *et al.*, 2012). Smaller servings in multi-packs, for example mini candy bars, can also be regarded as a segmentation cue. However, it is also recognized that these smaller servings might undermine self-control mechanisms (Vale *et al.*, 2008). As the number of sub items in multi-packages has increased (see before), offering smaller servings in larger multi-packages might not be the solution to control energy intake adequately. More research is needed into the optimum size of products, when people are still satisfied with the product and do not opt for more than one unit as a serving size.

Economic environment. Since the value for money principle is a quite strong mechanism, and price remains an important determinant in food choice, pricing strategies to make smaller portions more attractive can be put in place (Steenhuis *et al.*, 2011; Steenhuis and Vermeer, 2009; Young and Nestle, 2012. Only very few experiments have been conducted with respect to removing the value size pricing and using proportional pricing instead. Harnack *et al.* (2008) and Vermeer *et al.* (2011a) applied value size pricing for fast food meal choices in a research setting and hot meal choices in worksite cafeterias respectively (Harnack *et al.*, 2008; Vermeer *et al.*, 2011b). They found no effects of proportional pricing, possibly due to a minimal exposure to the intervention (Harnack *et al.*, 2008) or the relatively small differences in absolute price between the different portion sizes (Harnack *et al.*, 2008; Vermeer *et al.*, 2011b). More studies into attractive pricing strategies for smaller portions are needed, since intervention effects of pricing strategies in general are promising (Epstein *et al.*, 2012).

Political environment. It might be somewhat unrealistic to expect the food industry to voluntarily reduce portion sizes. There are some good starting points for policy measures with respect to portion sizes (Steenhuis and Vermeer, 2009; Young and Nestle, 2012). Clear and realistic serving size standards should be defined. The same accounts for the expressions 'small', 'medium', 'large' et cetera (Just and Wansink, 2014). Package labels should be in accordance with the defined standards. Although portion size labeling has not convincingly proven to be effective in changing consumers' behavior (e.g. Vermeer *et al.*, 2011a), portion size information should be clear and consistent which is not the case right now (see before). Other potential policy measures include actual limitations on the amount of food marketed or sold as single servings (Young and Nestle, 2012). This might be easier to accomplish in, for example, a school setting (Hartstein *et al.*, 2008), but should be studied further on feasibility and effectiveness for all different kinds of point of purchase settings.

11.5   Self-regulation strategies to control portion sizes

Environmental interventions in the physical, economic and political environment as described above are necessary in order to help consumers to control their portion sizes. However, the environment with respect to portion sizes will not change back to the sixties of the last century. For example, the attempt of New York's former major Bloomberg to ban the sale of single-serve sugar-sweetened beverages larger than 16 oz in New York restaurants, movie theaters and mobile food vendors was stopped by the New York Country Supreme Court shortly before the regulation would be implemented (March 2013) because the regulation was judged to be 'arbitrary and capricious because it applies to some but not all food establishments in the city'

Therefore, complementary to the environmental interventions, consumers need to learn to cope with an obesogenic environment with food in large amounts and portion sizes available. Educational interventions should address awareness to decrease portion distortion and teach behavioral strategies for portion control. Self-regulation might be helpful in this. Self-regulation refers to all efforts to steer attention, emotions and behaviors to reach beneficial long-term goals (i.e. weight loss), even when there are short-term temptations (i.e. a tasty cookie) or conflicting long-term goals (de Ridder and de Wit, 2006). In the context of controlling portion sizes, self-regulation refers to efforts to control and maintain adequate selection and intake of the amount of food, thereby resisting or adapting temptations and situations by which one is triggered to overeat (Poelman et al., 2014).

To support self-regulation to resisting large portion sizes, educational interventions might offer so-called 'portion control strategies'. These are simple behavioral strategies to eliminate the risk of *selecting* large food portions or *consuming* surplus servings/portions/amounts The strategies are derived from studies explaining why larger portions lead to an increased energy intake (see also section 11.3). Portion control strategies can help individuals decrease their energy intake. Moreover, a higher usage of such strategies are associated with a healthy body weight, indicating the efficacy of such strategies in weight-management (Poelman et al., 2014). Table 11.1 provides some examples of portion control strategies.

11.5.1 Integrated interventions aimed at portion control behavior

To encourage the use of portion control behavior among individuals, comprehensive interventions are needed. Interventions need to focus on the awareness about appropriate normal-size portions and the use of behavioral strategies. Because eating behavior is such a strong habitual process, educational interventions need to incorporate several general self-regulatory strategies aimed at applying the portion control behavior (Verplanken, 2006). Goal setting, action planning, coping planning and self-monitoring are general self-regulation strategies that have been found effective in archiving health behavioral changes (Sniehotta et al., 2005).

11.6   Summary and conclusions

In general, portion sizes have (been) increased over the past decades, extra portion sizes have (been) added to the portion size portfolio, super- and jumbo-size portions and multi-packs have become available. From a public health perspective this is unfavorable as larger portions lead to an increased energy intake. Explanations for increased energy intake levels due to portion sizes are the value for money principle and the portion distortion phenomenon. In order to reverse the trend of large portions,

Table 11.1 **Examples of drivers of portion size selection and consumption and portion control strategies to eliminate these factors**

Examples of drivers of portion size selection and intake	Examples of portion control strategies
Purchase behaviour during grocery shopping	
Increased purchases might be driven by several price marketing strategies that stimulate individuals to increase the amount of food purchased. Relevant price marketing strategies used to persuade consumers to buy larger amounts and more products are value size pricing (Wansink, 1996), bundle promoting (Foubert and Gijsbrechts, 2007) and free sampling (Heilman *et al.* 2011), as consumers will select a larger package or quantity that maximizes utility (Wansink, 1996).	*When grocery shopping, make a list in advance and do not deviate from it when you are in the supermarket. Do not be tempted by special deals and offers (bundle promotions such as buy-two-get-$1-off or buy-one-get-one-free).* *Do not taste free samples at shops.* *Don't buy jumbo-sized packages (e.g. 30% extra or the largest package) and do not buy large quantities at once.*
Food exposure and stockpiling	
Individuals' desire to consume larger amounts and also the actual portion size that they consume is actual intake evoked by food exposure (Fedoroff *et al.*, 1997; Ferriday and Brunstrom, 2008; Marcelino *et al.*, 2001). When exposed to easily accessible foods (e.g. snacks within reach), individuals perceive that obtaining these foods requires less effort to consume (Wansink *et al.*, 2006). Moreover, easily accessible foods are perceived as more difficult to resist and are more attention-grabbing (Engell *et al.*, 1996; Maas *et al.*, 2012; Wansink *et al.*, 2006). An important factor that can contribute to in-home food exposure is the quantity and manner of stockpiling. The incidence of the consumption of high-convenience foods increases when the foods are stockpiled more visibly. For both high- and low-convenience foods, large amounts of stockpiled foods also induce increased usage, the intake of larger amounts (Chandon and Wansink, 2002) and thus greater energy intake (Raynor and Wing, 2007).	*Store tempting foods (such as sweets and candies) well packaged, out of sight and out of reach.* *When at a party put yourself out of reach of tempting foods.* *Don't store (tempting) foods in several places such as in the glove compartment of the car or the desk drawer at work. Keep these places snack-free!*

Package size

People consume more from large packages than out of small packages (Flood *et al.*, 2006; Rolls *et al.*, 2004). This phenomenon arises for packages of high-convenience foods (e.g. chips) (Rolls *et al.*, 2004), as well as for packages of low-convenience food that requires preparation before consumption (e.g. spaghetti strings) (Wansink, 1996). Moreover, large packages influences food intake for high-energy food even when the portion size is the same but served in a smaller package (Machiori *et al.*, 2012).

When eating palatable and tempting foods, determine a normal serving in advance and store the rest of the package out of sight and reach.

When preparing a meal, decide what a normal serving size of the ingredients per person is beforehand. Do not use the whole package automatically, but take the number of people who will be eating into account.

Food establishments and takeaway food

Participants are driven by several aspects to select larger portions when eating out. In addition to 'standard' restaurants or fast-food outlets, most buffet-style restaurants offer an 'all-you-can-eat' system where visitors are responsible for the amount they serve to themselves. Because such restaurants offer of a great variety of food, people might experience more hedonic properties of the foods offered and consequently are prompted to serve themselves with surplus amounts (Rolls *et al.*, 1981). Moreover, since most buffet-style restaurants have fixed-price offers, most visitors are motivated by the desire to get their money's worth and consume as much as possible. Consequently, the more people pay for their all-you-can-eat deal, the more they consume (Just, 2008).

When eating out, only order a maximum of two dishes or share one or more dishes with someone else.

When there is a choice of portion size, pick the smallest one.

When going to a buffet, serve yourself small amounts of the dishes. Take into account that the total amount you are taking should fit on one plate.

Mindless eating

This mindless eating occurs especially in situations in which individuals are distracted during eating and when they are not focused on the food they are consuming. When eating mindlessly, individuals are at risk of consuming surplus amounts when enough food is available (Stroebele and de Castro, 2004). Individuals should avoid eat mindlessly to eliminate the influence of this phenomenon on overconsumption.

Avoid other activities such as watching television, reading or driving a car when eating.

Avoid eating during work-related activities such as meetings, working at your desk or making telephone calls.

the physical, economic as well as the political environment should be changed with respect to portion sizes. Nevertheless, it is unrealistic to expect the desired change to come from self-regulatory efforts from the food industry only and governmental action should also be considered to realize change. At the same time, consumers need to be educated how they can apply portion control strategies, in order to deal adequately with an obesogenic environment filled with supersized food.

11.7 Acknowledgement

This chapter is partly based on:

Steenhuis, I. H. M., Leeuwis, F. H. and Vermeer, W. M. (2010) Small, medium, large or supersize: trends in food portion sizes in the Netherlands. *Public Health Nutrition*, 13(6): 852–7.

Steenhuis, I. H. M. and Vermeer, W. M. (2009) Portion size: review and framework for interventions. *International Journal of Behavioural Nutrition and Physical Activity*, 6: 58.

Poelman, M. P., de Vet, E., Velema, E., Seidell, J. C. and Steenhuis, I. H. (2014) Behavioural strategies to control the amount of food selected and consumed. *Appetite*, 72: 156–65.

References

Bellisle, F., Dalix, A. M. and Slama, G. (2004). Non food-related environmental stimuli induce increased meal intake in healthy women: comparison of television viewing versus listening to a recorded story in laboratory settings. *Appetite*, 43, 175–80.

Benson, C. (2009). Increasing portion size in Britain. *Society, Biology and Human Affairs.*, 74, 4–20.

Blass, E. M., Anderson, D. R., Kirkorian, H. L., Pempek, T. A., Price, I. and Koleini, M. F. (2006). On the road to obesity: television viewing increases intake of high-density foods. *Physiol Behav*, 88, 597–604.

Blundell, J. E. and MacDiarmid, J. I. (1997). Fat as a risk factor for overconsumption: satiation, satiety, and patterns of eating. *J Am Diet Assoc*, 97, S63–9.

Bryant, R. and Dundes, L. (2005). Portion distortion: a study of college students. *J Cons Aff*, 39, 399–408.

Burger, K. S., Kern, M. and Coleman, K. J. (2007). Characteristics of self-selected portion size in young adults. *J Am Diet Assoc*, 107, 611–18.

Chandon, P. and Wansink, B. (2002). When are stockpiled products consumed faster? A convenience-salience framework of postpurchase consumption incidence and quantity. *J Mar Res*, 39, 321–35.

Condrasky, M., Ledikwe, J. H., Flood, J. E. and Rolls, B. J. (2007). Chefs' opinions of restaurant portion sizes. *Obesity (Silver Spring)*, 15, 2086–94.

de Ridder and de Wit, J. (2006). *Self-regulation in Health Behaviour*. Sussex, UK: John Wiley.

Diliberti, N., Bordi, P. L., Conklin, M. T., Roe, L. S. and Rolls, B. J. (2004). Increased portion size leads to increased energy intake in a restaurant meal. *Obes Res*, 12, 562–8.

Dunford, E., Webster, J., Metzler, A. B., Czernichow, S., NI Mhurchu, C., *et al.*, (2012). International collaborative project to compare and monitor the nutritional composition of processed foods. *Eur J Prev Cardiol*, 19, 1326–32.

Engell, D., Kramer, M., Malafi, T., Salomon, M. and Lesher, L. (1996). Effects of effort and social modeling on drinking in humans. *Appetite*, 26, 129–38.

Epstein, L. H., Jankowiak, N., Nederkoorn, C., Raynor, H. A., French, S. A. and Finkelstein, E. (2012). Experimental research on the relation between food price changes and food-purchasing patterns: a targeted review. *Am J Clin Nutr*, 95, 789–809.

Fedoroff, I. C., Polivy, J. and Herman, C. P. (1997). The effect of pre-exposure to food cues on the eating behavior of restrained and unrestrained eaters. *Appetite*, 28, 33–47.

Ferriday, D. and Brunstrom, J. M. (2008). How does food-cue exposure lead to larger meal sizes? *Br J Nutr*, 100, 1325–1332.

Flood, J. E., Roe, L. S. and Rolls, B. J. (2006). The effect of increased beverage portion size on energy intake at a meal. *J Am Diet Assoc*, 106, 1984–90; discussion 1990–1.

Foubert, B. and Gijsbrechts, E. (2007). Shopper response to bundle promotions for packaged goods. *J Mar Res*, 44, 647–62.

French, S. A. (2005). Public health strategies for dietary change: schools and workplaces. *J Nutr*, 135, 910–12.

Geier, A., Wansink, B. and Rozin, P. (2012). Red potato chips: segmentation cues can substantially decrease food intake. *Health Psychology*, 31, 398–401.

Geier, A. B., Rozin, P. and Doros, G. (2006). Unit bias. A new heuristic that helps explain the effect of portion size on food intake. *Psychol Sci*, 17, 521–5.

Harnack, L. J., French, S. A., Oakes, J. M., Story, M. T., Jeffery, R. W. and Rydell, S. A. (2008). Effects of calorie labeling and value size pricing on fast food meal choices: results from an experimental trial. *Int J Behav Nutr Phys Act*, 5, 63.

Hartstein, J., Cullen, K. W., Reynolds, K. D., Harrell, J., Resnicow, K., *et al.* (2008). Impact of portion-size control for school a la carte items: changes in kilocalories and macronutrients purchased by middle school students. *J Am Diet Assoc*, 108, 140–4.

Heilman, C., Lokishyk, K. and Radas, S. (2011). An empirical investigation of in-store sampling promotions. *Br Food J*, 113, 1252–66.

Hetherington, M. M., Anderson, A. S., Norton, G. N. and Newson, L. (2006). Situational effects on meal intake: a comparison of eating alone and eating with others. *Physiol Behav*, 88, 498–505.

Higgs, S. and Woodward, M. (2009). Television watching during lunch increases afternoon snack intake of young women. *Appetite*, 52, 39–43.

Hogbin, M. B. and Hess, M. A. (1999). Public confusion over food portions and servings. *J Am Diet Assoc*, 99, 1209–11.

Ittersum, K. V. and Wansink, B. (2012). Plate size and color suggestibility: the Delboeuf Illusion's bias on serving and eating behaviour. *J Con Res*, 39, 215–28.

Just D. R. (2008). Personal communication. The Fixed Price Paradox: conflicting effects of 'All-You-Can-Eat' pricing. Cornell University: http://www.agecon.purdue.edu/news/seminarfiles/MS12118.pdf.

Just, D. R. and Wansink, B. (2014). One man's tall is another man's small: how the framing of portion size influences food choice. *Health Econ*, 23(7), 776–91.

Maas, J., de Ridder, D. T., de Vet, E. and de Wit, J. B. (2012). Do distant foods decrease intake? The effect of food accessibility on consumption. *Psychology and Health*, 59–73.

Marcelino, A. S., Adam, A. S., Couronne, T., Koster, E. P. and Sieffermann, J. M. (2001). Internal and external determinants of eating initiation in humans. *Appetite*, 36, 9–14.

Marchiori, D., Corneille, O. and Klein, O. (2012). Container size influences snack food intake independently of portion size. *Appetite*, 58, 814–17.

Matthiessen, J., Biltoft-Jensen, A., Fagt, S., Knudsen, V. K., Tetens, I. and Groth, M. V. (2013). Misperception of body weight among overweight Danish adults: trends from 1995 to 2008. *Public Health Nutr*, 1–8.

Matthiessen, J., Fagt, S., Biltoft-Jensen, A., Beck, A. M. and Ovesen, L. (2003). Size makes a difference. *Public Health Nutr*, 6, 65–72.

Nielsen, S. J. and Popkin, B. M. (2003). Patterns and trends in food portion sizes, 1977–1998. *JAMA*, 289, 450–3.

Oldham-Cooper, R. E., Hardman, C. A., Nicoll, C. E., Rogers, P. J. and Brunstrom, J. M. (2011). Playing a computer game during lunch affects fullness, memory for lunch, and later snack intake. *Am J Clin Nutr*, 93, 308–13.

Pelletier, A. L., Chang, W. W., Delzell, J. E., Jr. and McCall, J. W. (2004). Patients' understanding and use of snack food package nutrition labels. *J Am Board Fam Pract*, 17, 319–23.

Penisten, M. B. and Litchfield, R. E. (2004). Nutrition education delivered at the state fair: are your portions in proportion? *J Nutr Educ Behav*, 36, 275–7.

Poelman, M. P., De Vet, E., Velema, E., Seidell, J. C. and Steenhuis, I. H. (2014). Behavioural strategies to control the amount of food selected and consumed. *Appetite*, 72, 156–65.

Raynor, H. A. and Wing, R. R. (2007). Package unit size and amount of food: do both influence intake? *Obesity (Silver Spring)*, 15, 2311–19.

Rolls, B. J., Morris, E. L. and Roe, L. S. (2002). Portion size of food affects energy intake in normal-weight and overweight men and women. *Am J Clin Nutr*, 76, 1207–13.

Rolls, B. J., Roe, L. S. and Meengs, J. S. (2006). Larger portion sizes lead to a sustained increase in energy intake over 2 days. *J Am Diet Assoc*, 106, 543–9.

Rolls, B. J., Roe, L. S. and Meengs, J. S. (2007). The effect of large portion sizes on energy intake is sustained for 11 days. *Obesity (Silver Spring)*, 15, 1535–43.

Rolls, B. J., Roe, L. S., Meengs, J. S. and Wall, D. E. (2004). Increasing the portion size of a sandwich increases energy intake. *J Am Diet Assoc*, 104, 367–72.

Rolls, B. J., Roe, L. S., Kral, T. V., Meengs, J. S. and Wall, D. E. (2004). Increasing the portion size of a packaged snack increases energy intake in men and women. *Appetite*, 42, 63–9.

Rolls, B. J., Rowe, E. A., Rolls, E. T., Kingston, B., Megson, A. and Gunary, R. (1981). Variety in a meal enhances food intake in man. *Physiol Behav*, 26, 215–21.

Schwartz, J. and Byrd-Bredbenner, C. (2006). Portion distortion: typical portion sizes selected by young adults. *J Am Diet Assoc*, 106, 1412–18.

Schwartz, J., Riis, J., Elbel, B. and Ariely, D. (2012). Inviting consumers to downsize fast-food portions significantly reduces calorie consumption. *Health Affairs*, 31, 399–407.

Sharpe, K. M., Staelin, R. and Huber, J. (2008). Using extremeness aversion to fight obesity: policy implications of context dependent demand. *J Con Res*, 35, 406–22.

Smiciklas-Wright, H., Mitchell, D. C., Mickle, S. J., Goldman, J. D. and Cook, A. (2003). Foods commonly eaten in the United States, 1989–1991 and 1994–1996: are portion sizes changing? *J Am Diet Assoc*, 103, 41–7.

Sniehotta, F. F., Scholz, U., Schwarzer, R., Fuhrmann, B., Kiwus, U. and Voller, H. (2005). Long-term effects of two psychological interventions on physical exercise and self-regulation following coronary rehabilitation. *Int J Behav Med*, 12, 244–55.

Steenhuis, I. H., Leeuwis, F. H. and Vermeer, W. M. (2010). Small, medium, large or supersize: trends in food portion sizes in The Netherlands. *Public Health Nutr*, 13, 852–7.

Steenhuis, I. H. and Vermeer, W. M. (2009). Portion size: review and framework for interventions. *Int J Behav Nutr Phys Act*, 6, 58.

Steenhuis, I. H., Waterlander, W. E. and de Mul, A. (2011). Consumer food choices: the role of price and pricing strategies. *Public Health Nutr*, 14, 2220–6.

Stroebele, N. and de Castro, J. M. (2004). Effect of ambience on food intake and food choice. *Nutrition*, 20, 821–38.

Swinburn, B., Egger, G. and Raza, F. (1999). Dissecting obesogenic environments: the development and application of a framework for identifying and prioritizing environmental interventions for obesity. *Prev Med*, 29, 563–70.

Swinburn, B. A., Caterson, I., Seidell, J. C. and James, W. P. (2004). Diet, nutrition and the prevention of excess weight gain and obesity. *Public Health Nutr*, 7, 123–46.

Vale, R. C. D., Rik Pieters, R. and Zeelenberg, M. (2008). Flying under the radar: perverse package size effects on consumption self-regulation. *J Con Res*, 35, 380–90.

van Kleef, E., Shimizu, M. and Wansink, B. (2013). Just a bite: considerably smaller snack portions satisfy delayed hunger and craving. *Food Quality and Preference*, 27, 96–100.

Vermeer, W. M., Steenhuis, I. H., Leeuwis, F. H., Bos, A. E., De Boer, M. and Seidell, J. C. (2010a). Portion size labeling and intended soft drink consumption: the impact of labeling format and size portfolio. *J Nutr Educ Behav*, 42, 422–6.

Vermeer, W. M., Steenhuis, I. H., Leeuwis, F. H., Bos, A. E., De Boer, M. and Seidell, J. C. (2011a). View the label before you view the movie: a field experiment into the impact of portion size and Guideline Daily Amounts labelling on soft drinks in cinemas. *BMC Public Health*, 11, 438.

Vermeer, W. M., Steenhuis, I. H., Leeuwis, F. H., Heymans, M. W. and Seidell, J. C. (2011b). Small portion sizes in worksite cafeterias: do they help consumers to reduce their food intake? *Int J Obes (Lond)*, 35, 1200–7.

Vermeer, W. M., Steenhuis, I. H. and Seidell, J. C. (2010b). Portion size: a qualitative study of consumers' attitudes toward point-of-purchase interventions aimed at portion size. *Health Educ Res*, 25, 109–20.

Verplanken, B. (2006). Beyond frequency: habit as mental construct. *Br J Soc Psychol*, 45, 639–56.

Wansink, B. (1996). Can package size accelerate usage volume? *Journal of Marketing*, 60, 1–14.

Wansink, B. (2004). Environmental factors that increase the food intake and consumption volume of unknowing consumers. *Annu Rev Nutr*, 24, 455–79.

Wansink, B. and Cheney, M. M. (2005). Super Bowls: serving bowl size and food consumption. *JAMA*, 293, 1727–8.

Wansink, B. and Huckabee, M. (2005). De-marketing obesity. *California Management Review*, 47, 6–18.

Wansink, B. and Kim, J. (2005). Bad popcorn in big buckets: portion size can influence intake as much as taste. *J Nutr Educ Behav*, 37, 242–5.

Wansink, B., Painter, J. E. and Lee, Y. K. (2006). The office candy dish: proximity's influence on estimated and actual consumption. *Int J Obes*, 30(5), 871–5.

Wansink, B., Painter, J. E. and North, J. (2005). Bottomless bowls: why visual cues of portion size may influence intake. *Obes Res*, 13, 93–100.

Wansink, B. and Park, S. B. (2001). At the movies: how external cues and perceived taste impact consumption volume. *Food Quality and Preference*, 12, 69–74.

Wansink, B., Van Ittersum, K. and Painter, J. E. (2006). Ice cream illusions bowls, spoons, and self-served portion sizes. *Am J Prev Med*, 31, 240–3.

Wrieden, W. L., Longbottom, P. J., Adamson, A. J., Ogston, S. A., Payne, A., *et al.* (2008). Estimation of typical food portion sizes for children of different ages in Great Britain. *Br J Nutr*, 99, 1344–53.

Young, L. R. and Nestle, M. (1998). Variation in perceptions of a medium' food portion: implications for dietary guidance. *J Am Diet Assoc*, 98, 458–9.

Young, L. R. and Nestle, M. (2002). The contribution of expanding portion sizes to the US obesity epidemic. *Am J Public Health*, 92, 246–9.

Young, L. R. and Nestle, M. (2003). Expanding portion sizes in the US marketplace: implications for nutrition counseling. *J Am Diet Assoc*, 103, 231–4.

Young, L. R. and Nestle, M. (2007). Portion sizes and obesity: responses of fast-food companies. *J Public Health Policy*, 28, 238–48.

Young, L. R. and Nestle, M. (2012). Reducing portion sizes to prevent obesity: a call to action. *Am J Prev Med*, 43, 565–8.

Zlatevska, N., Dubelaar, C. and Holden, S. S. (2014). Sizing up the effect of portion size on consumption: a meta-analytic review. *Journal of Marketing*, 78(3), 140–54.

Eating in response to external cues

12

J. Polivy, C. P. Herman
University of Toronto, Toronto, ON, Canada

12.1 Introduction

There is currently a paradox in Western societies: the thin ideal for body shape that dominates our culture makes dieting normative, but at the same time, obesity has become 'epidemic'. Given the extent of dieting to lose weight, supporting a multi-billion-dollar diet industry, with millions of participants in diet programs, not to mention the never-ending stream of best-selling diet books – many of them repeat best-sellers, as new generations discover them – given the myriad of pills, devices, fitness regimes and medical 'breakthroughs' offered in the last 45 years, North Americans should be the thinnest, most physically fit humans on the planet! But we all know that that is not the case. We have managed to produce record numbers of eating disorders, including several whole new categories, while obesity is more prevalent than it has ever been.

Several relatively recent societal developments have been identified as contributors to the increased prevalence of obesity, as was discussed earlier in this volume. To recap briefly, portion sizes have grown inordinately large (e.g., Nielsen and Popkin, 2003), food cues have generally proliferated, and there appears to be generally greater access to appealing, high calorie foods (Brownell and Horgen, 2003; Polivy *et al.*, 2008). Brownell describes this constant exposure to food cues as a 'toxic food environment' that contributes to the prevalence of overweight (Brownell, 2002).

12.2 Effects of food cues

Evolutionarily, food cues are useful, indicating when, where, and what food is available for us to eat. Thus, food cues should trigger appetite and eating behavior. Exposure to attractive food cues has been shown to elicit the urge to eat (Loxton *et al.*, 2011), and merely reading a list of foods and rating their nutritional values caused students to report increases in hunger, desire to eat, and number of foods currently hungry for, as well as reduced fullness (Oakes and Slotterback, 2000). The sight and smell of salient food cues do seem to increase food intake (Coelho *et al.*, 2009a), as do the smell and thought of food (Fedoroff *et al.*, 1997; Jansen and Van den Hout, 1991). In fact, such cues can operate in a highly specific manner, such that after exposure to food cues for one particular food (such as cookies, or pizza),

Managing and Preventing Obesity. http://dx.doi.org/10.1533/9781782420996.3.181

people craved and ate more of only the food that they had been exposed to (i.e., those exposed to pizza craved and ate pizza more whereas those exposed to cookies craved and ate cookies more) (Fedoroff *et al.*, 2003). One might even argue that the well-documented increased eating in response to larger portion sizes (e.g., Rolls *et al.*, 2002) reflects an effect of exposure to increased food cues.

Large-scale correlational studies also indicate that exposure to food cues through television viewing is associated with increased food intake and weight in children (Crespo *et al.*, 2001; Halford and Boyland, 2013; Wiecha *et al.*, 2006) and even predicts adult obesity (Viner and Cole, 2005). Moreover, girls who viewed more television each day also ate more energy dense snacks (Francis *et al.*, 2003). A laboratory test of these findings showed that children exposed to the sorts of food advertisements seen on television ate more than did children shown non-food-related ads (Halford *et al.*, 2004), demonstrating that these food cues do promote eating in children. Similarly, Folkvord *et al.*, (2013) had children play food- or non-food-related advergames (free online games that integrate advertising messages and logos) and found that they ate more after playing an advergame containing food cues regardless of what brand or product type (energy-dense snacks or fruit) was displayed. Moreover, such games promoted increased eating of energy-dense snack foods, even when fruits were the food depicted in the game (fruit consumption did not increase).

12.3   Potential moderators influencing responding to food cues

Studies on the effects of food cues often find that everyone responds to the cues by eating more, but this is not always the case. Ever since Stanley Schachter pointed out that obese people are hyper-responsive to external cues, particularly food cues (Schachter, 1971), research has focused first on differences between obese and normal people in their responses to food, and then between those who are concerned about their weight (restrained eaters) and those who are not (e.g., Herman and Polivy, 1988; Polivy and Herman, 1987). Our research on chronic dieting, or as we somewhat ironically called it, restrained eating, over the past three decades has demonstrated that such dieting is common among young women, and has what appear to be para-doxical effects. Nondieters (or unrestrained eaters) often eat a lot when they are given nothing to eat initially, but they eat very little if you 'preload' them with 16 ounces of rich chocolate milkshake. Chronic on-again off-again dieters, or restrained eaters, on the other hand, eat somewhat less in laboratory situations under 'normal' (i.e., no preload) circumstances, maintaining their diets, but after a fattening milkshake or other food, they tend to eat more. We (and others) have found over the years that a disturbingly large variety of manipulations results in restrained eaters eating signi-ficantly more than do either their nonmanipulated restrained eater peers, or than do unrestrained eaters in a similar situation. In other words, in almost any situation other than a calm, neutral environment, restrained eaters are more likely to 'break' their diets than to stick to them. It is thus not surprising that restrained eaters also have been found not to lose weight over six months or a year, and in the short term, their weight fluctuates significantly more than does that of unrestrained eaters (Heatherton *et al.*, 1991).

12.4   How plentiful food cues affect dieters/ overweight individuals

So how do obese people and restrained eaters respond to food cues? Apparently quite strongly. Overweight children responded more strongly than did normal weight children to food words on a Stroop test (Braet and Crombez, 2003). More importantly, overweight children overate after being exposed to the smell and taste of palatable food, whereas normal weight children ate less after such exposure (Jansen *et al.*, 2003). Halford and colleagues (Halford *et al.*, 2008) showed that although all children ate more after viewing food advertisements than after viewing non-food ads, the increase was significantly greater in obese children and the amount eaten after the food ads was significantly correlated with degree of fatness.

Similarly, overweight adults respond more strongly to food cues by ordering cued desserts in restaurants (Herman *et al.*, 1983). Overweight adults also report increased urges to eat and increases in desired portion size of a cued food (Tetley *et al.*, 2009), as well as increased salivation (Ferriday and Brunstrom, 2011). Tetley and colleagues concluded that such elevated reactivity to food cues could signal a risk for overeating and becoming overweight, and/or maintaining an overweight status. These authors replicated this work in female participants who differed with respect to deprivation level (hungry vs non-hungry), impulsivity, and sensitivity to reward, finding results similar to those found with overweight versus normal participants (Tetley *et al.*, 2010). The women with higher levels of trait impulsivity experienced greater changes in appetite ratings in response to exposure to food cues whether food-deprived or not. Moreover, these individuals reported wanting larger portions of a cued food when food deprived. The participants with a high sensitivity to reward also desired larger portions of the cued food, but only when they were not food-deprived. The authors interpreted these results as indicating that individual differences in food-cue reactivity could be related to an inability to exercise sufficient self-control in the presence of tempting environmental stimuli in general, suggesting that overweight individuals should show greater impulsivity than normal.

Talmi *et al.* (2013) found that hungry individuals had a differential bias toward recall of food-related words, not evident in sated individuals. Looking at attentional focus measures as well as food intake, Nijs *et al.* (2010) found an attentional bias towards food pictures in all participants, hungry, sated, obese, and normal weight. Hungry people, however, showed greater automatic attention to food cues than did satiated individuals, as did overweight/obese as compared to normal-weight individuals. Other measures of attentional bias toward food pictures were less clear and consistent, but what was clear was that it was the hungry overweight participants who ate the most food in a taste test. The authors concluded that 'overweight/obese individuals appear to automatically direct their attention to food-related stimuli, to a greater extent than normal-weight individuals, particularly when food-deprived' (p. 243).

Tetley *et al.* (2009) included the DEBQ measure of restrained eating (van Strien *et al.*, 1986) in their examination of responses to food cues and found no effects of restraint on responses to food cues, but Ouwehand and Papies (2010) found that exposure to attractive food cues differentially affected restrained eaters (measured with the Herman – Polivy Restraint Scale, 1980), and did so in conjunction with obesity. They found a decrease in desire for high-calorie food in normal-weight restrained eaters who were primed with attractive food cues, but increased desire for the food in overweight restrained eaters. Unrestrained eaters all responded to the priming manipulation regardless of weight. The measure of restraint used does seem to matter; heightened responding to food cues by restrained eaters seems to be found primarily in studies using the Herman – Polivy Restraint Scale, rather than the DEBQ or TFEQ (Stunkard and Messick, 1985). As has been discussed previously (Heatherton *et al.*, 1988; van Strein, 1999), the RS measure of restrained eating seems to identify a population different from that identified by the DEBQ and TFEQ. Thus it is the reaction to food cues of RS restrained eaters that we will be discussing in this chapter, as they are the restrained eaters who seem to behave like overweight and obese individuals, despite being of normal weight (Heatherton *et al.*, 1988).

For some time, it has been noted that restrained eaters respond more strongly to food cues than do unrestrained eaters. Rogers and Hill (1989) found that restrained eaters exposed to attractive photographs of food and the actual food itself ('to study' rather than to eat) report more hunger and desire to eat, and do indeed eat more than do unrestrained eaters or restrained eaters exposed to neutral cues. Fedoroff *et al.* (1997, 2003) showed that restrained eaters report more craving and desire to eat, and also eat more than do unrestrained eaters in response to olfactory and cognitive food cues.

Cognitive responses to food cues show similar results. Restrained eaters were found to respond faster than unrestrained eaters in a visual search task, when asked to detect a food word within a neutral group of words or when asked to detect a neutral word in a group of food words compared to a group of neutral words (Hollit *et al.*, 2010). Using a go/no-go task, Meule *et al.*, (2011) found restrained eaters to be generally better at the task, but significantly slowed by food words, indicating an attentional bias to food words. Finally, restrained eaters perceived attractive foods as larger after priming with tempting food cues (van Koningsbruggen *et al.*, 2011).

An innovative study of responses to food cues manipulated food cue exposure and then measured handgrip force (which presumably would allow participants to acquire the object depicted) while presenting participants with pictures of healthy food objects (van Koningsbruggen *et al.*, 2012). Exposure to tempting food cues led restrained eaters, but not unrestrained eaters, to exert less forceful grip strength in response to (and as an attempt to acquire) healthy food objects. The authors point out that this sort of finding adds to our understanding of why restrained eaters are so susceptible to the temptations of food-rich environments.

12.5   Factors influencing overweight/obese people and restrained eaters to respond more to salient food cues

Not every study shows hyper-reactivity to food cues by either overweight (e.g., Legoff and Spigelman, 1987) or restrained individuals (e.g., Coelho *et al.*, 2009b; Oakes and Slotterback, 2001). This failure to over-react might indicate a weakness of the tendency, or it might suggest something about when such hyper-responsiveness is more likely to occur. As Coelho *et al.* (2009b) point out, highly salient food cues may overwhelm attempts to diet and resist temptation, but less obtrusive, less salient food cues might serve to trigger or bolster dietary restraint. Coelho *et al.* (2009a) tested this possibility directly by exposing weight concerned and non-concerned participants to salient food cues to which they were forced to attend, or to less salient incidental food cues, or to no food cues. Only the highly weight concerned participants ate more after exposure to the salient cues, and those exposed to the incidental food cues did not differ from controls exposed to no food cues. The salience or potency of the food cues present thus seems to determine whether they will elicit more eating from overweight or restrained individuals.

With the increased availability of fMRI equipment, the brains of restrained eaters have been scrutinized to see if their fMRI responses to food cues differ from those of unrestrained eaters. The short answer is that they do. The longer answer is that different studies find activation in different brain regions, but there is agreement on the fact that restrained eaters' brains light up more reliably in response to food intake (Burger and Stice, 2011) and food cues than do the brains of unrestrained eaters (e.g., Shur *et al.*, 2012). Shur and colleagues conclude that deciding to restrain one's eating behavior alters the brain's response to food cues, which may be what makes restrained eaters more susceptible to salient, tempting food cues.

Another source of enhanced response to food cues is craving, which might also be related to restraining one's food intake, specifically restraining one's intake of highly palatable but high calorie preferred foods. Fedoroff *et al.* (1997, 2003) found that restrained eaters reported more cravings for cued foods, and that the cravings (like the increased consumption) were specific to the food cues presented. Restrained eaters deprived of chocolate (Polivy *et al.*, 2005) or carbohydrates more generally (Coelho *et al.*, 2006) reported increased craving for the missing food, and when confronted with it, ate more than did equally deprived unrestrained eaters or non-deprived restrained eaters. Even if one simply eats less of a favorite food rather than avoiding it altogether, one may feel subjectively deprived, which may contribute to experiencing cravings, or strong desires, for the avoided food (Herman *et al.*, 2005). The enhanced craving stimulated by food cues experienced by people restraining their intake of attractive foods may make it harder to resist the temptation to eat larger amounts of those foods when they become available.

12.6   Psychological processes governing eating behavior

We need to fully understand the psychological processes that govern eating behavior in general if we want to learn to control the excess eating induced by environmental food cues in overweight and restrained individuals. Eating behavior is influenced by aspects of both individual differences among people, as we have seen in the discussion of restrained eating and overweight/obesity (but which also include other personality traits such as impulsivity, memory, degree of deprivation, and beliefs about food), and the situation. Food cues are one aspect of the situation, but other factors such as social influence (the behavior of other people present), portion size, the palatability of the food, and the variety of foods available all affect eating behavior (e.g., Herman *et al.*, 2005). We cannot review all of these literatures here, but will give a brief summary of the salient findings.

12.6.1 The psychology of the person

We have seen that obese and overweight people seem to respond more strongly to food cues, as do restrained eaters. There is also evidence that trait impulsivity is similarly predictive of a cognitive bias toward food cues (Hou *et al.*, 2011), is associated with increases in appetite ratings and desired portion sizes after food-cue exposure (Tetley *et al.*, 2010), and is associated with weight gain over a 10-year period and with a tendency to give in to temptation (Sutin *et al.*, 2013).

Other aspects of the person, such as memory about recent eating and beliefs about the food that one has eaten or is about to eat, have also been shown to influence food intake (Higgs, 2008). Moreover, lesions to the hippocampus, which is the area of the brain thought to be responsible for learning and memory, produce excessive eating in the lesioned animals (Higgs, 2008).

It is clear that visceral factors such as hunger due to food deprivation affect people's behaviors, and as such factors become more intense or increase, they focus behavior more and more toward the relief of visceral discomfort (Loewenstein, 1996). Thus, food deprivation has been shown to affect the reinforcing value of food and to influence intake (Epstein and Leddy, 2006), as well as to shift people's food choices from preferred, palatable foods to anything that is immediately available to be eaten (Hoefling and Strack, 2010). Simply anticipating being food deprived by having to go on a diet later produces overeating in restrained eaters (Urbszat *et al.*, 2002). Mere perceived deprivation, or the feeling that one has been deprived or cannot eat as much as one would like, seems to be as influential as actual food deprivation. This perception correlates strongly with restrained eating and susceptibility to weight gain (Markowitz *et al.*, 2008).

12.6.2 The psychology of the situation

As we have seen, food cues in the environment affect eating in everyone, but especially in overweight and restrained eaters. Other aspects of the situation exert strong influences on food intake. Social influences (i.e., responses to the presence and/or behavior of other people) are particularly potent; for example, modeling of another person's intake (or even just a piece of paper indicating how much other people in the situation have eaten) produces matching in people exposed to the model (Herman *et al.*, 2003). The presence of others also affects how much people eat; social facilitation makes us eat more the more people present at the meal (Herman *et al.*, 2003). Both modeling and social facilitation may operate by setting social norms for what is appropriate in a given eating situation. A different social factor is impression management; people eat different foods or different amounts of food in order to project a particular image of themselves (Herman *et al.*, 2003). For example, when trying to impress an attractive male, females will eat less or will eat a salad rather than something more 'masculine' such as a burger and French fries. The presence of other people thus exerts powerful effects on eating by those with them.

Other situational factors can be equally powerful. The amount of food presented as a portion dictates how much people eat; those served large portions eat more than do those served small portions (e.g., Rolls *et al.*, 2002). Similarly, palatability is a powerful determinant of intake; not surprisingly, people eat more good-tasting food than bad-tasting food, and the better the food tastes, the more people eat (Pliner *et al.*, 1990). Other aspects of the environment such as the variety of foods available, plate or package size, and even lighting have much greater influences on how much individuals eat than most people realize (Wansink, 2004). As Wansink points out, these sorts of environmental elements interfere with people's attempts to monitor their intake and also set social norms that dictate how much to eat.

12.6.3 The interaction between person and situation

It should be clear by this point that eating and overeating are not simply responses to hunger or even the simple presence of food cues. Both person variables and aspects of the situation have strong effects on eating behavior. The next question is how these two sorts of influences interact with each other. We have proposed that different people respond to the same food-related environmental cues in different but predictable ways (Herman and Polivy, 2008). Some cues are sensory in nature; these cues relate to sensory aspects of the food such as appearance, smell, taste, or even texture/feeling. Even thinking about food can be sensory-based if the thoughts are about how good the food tastes, smells, looks or feels. Other environmental cues are not directly connected to the food itself, but provide information about norms concerning food intake, such as how much one should eat, or when and where it is appropriate to eat the food (e.g., breakfast foods vs dinner foods). Reviewing the research on responses to such cues, we found that normative food cues seem to have a universal effect, influencing everyone exposed to them. If the norm set is a low one, people generally do not violate the norm and eat a lot; but if the norm is high then everyone eats more heartily. Sensory food cues, however, are the cues to which overweight/obese people and restrained eaters respond more strongly than do their normal-weight or unrestrained counterparts (Herman and Polivy, 2008). So it follows that an increase in sensory food cues in the environment (such as smells of attractive cinnamon rolls, pictures of fattening foods in advertisements on television or billboards, etc.) will have a stronger effect on overweight and restrained eaters than on normal weight, non-diet-conscious people.

12.7   Implications for obesity management

If people who are overweight, obese, or weight-conscious restrained eaters are more susceptible to the abundant food cues characterizing Western society, then perhaps controlling their exposure to such cues or even teaching them to react less to the cues might help curb their overeating (Jansen, 1998). Fifteen years ago, Jansen reviewed several promising pilot studies using cue exposure and response prevention to get binge eaters to stop bingeing. Unfortunately, this treatment does not seem to have been effective, and there are no recent reports (in the last decade) of its successful use to control eating behavior and reduce weight.

Another possible intervention might be making people aware of the factors that influence their eating, as Wansink (2004) suggests. We tried something along these lines, informing participants about the impact of portion sizes on intake, or giving them a series of mindfulness exercises designed to make them aware of how portion size influences their eating (Cavanagh et al., in press). Neither of these interventions was successful at preventing participants from eating more when given larger portions, however. Similarly, awareness interventions that entail making people aware of the calories in the food they are about to order at fast-food restaurants have also failed to reduce the amount of food ordered, and in one study, made restrained eaters switch from ordering salads more often to ordering pasta, when they are told that the actual calorie counts in the two dishes are comparable (Girz et al., 2012).

Thus an intervention aimed at sensory food cues (exposure to them combined with response prevention so that people cannot eat after exposure) and others aimed at normative cues (portion size) have both failed to change people's responses to food cues. Chronic on-again-off-again dieting such as that practiced by restrained eaters has also been shown over the last 30 plus years to be a fruitless endeavor—the 'obesity epidemic' that purportedly began around 1980 (Brownell and Horgen, 2003) coincided with an upsurge in dieting that began in the 1970s (Polivy and Herman, 1987). Some might see this correlation as indicating that dieting increased as a means of dealing with the increased overweight in the population, but we suggest that the correlation reflects the reverse process; dieting is not only not a solution to the problem of overeating and overweight, but in many cases it makes the problem worse (Polivy and Herman, 1987, 2002). As we have just shown, restrained eaters are the ones who resemble the obese in their heightened response to external, sensory food cues. It seems that if we want to change people's eating behavior in response to environmental food cues, whether sensory or normative, we must recognize the complexity of the endeavor. Ideally, we might recommend a reduction in the prevalence of attractive food cues and normative messages promoting inflated intake. Given the power of the food industry, however, it seems unlikely that the ubiquity of food cues is going to decrease anytime soon. Telling people to disregard food cues and/or to eat less regardless of the presence of food cues seems likewise to be a strategy doomed to failure. Removing food and eating cues from the environment and/or getting vulnerable people to ignore them might be helpful, but the odds against successfully implementing such strategies are steep. Obesity is a complicated phenomenon; eliminating it will not be easily accomplished in the current food-abundant environment.

References

Braet, C. and Crombez, G. (2003). Cognitive interference due to food cues in childhood obesity. *Journal of Clinical Child and Adolescent Psychology*, *32*, 32–39.

Brownell, K.D. (2002). The environment and obesity. In C.G. Fairburn and K.D. Brownell (eds). *Eating Disorders and Obesity: A Comprehensive Handbook*. New York: Guilford, pp. 433–438.

Brownell, K.D. and K.B. Horgen (2003). *Food Fight: The inside story of the food industry, America's obesity crisis, and what we can do about it*. New York: McGraw-Hill.

Burger, K.S. and Stice, E. (2011). Relation of dietary restraint scores to activation of reward-related brain regions in response to food intake, anticipated intake, and food pictures. *Neuroimage*, *55*, 233–239.

Cavanagh, K., Vartanian, L. R., Herman, C. P. and Polivy, J. (in press). The effect of portion size on food intake is robust to brief education and mindfulness exercises. *Journal of Health Psychology*.

Coelho, J., Polivy, J., and Herman, C.P. (2006). Selective carbohydrate or protein restriction: effects on subsequent food intake and cravings. *Appetite*, *47*, 352–360.

Coelho, J.S., Jansen, A., Roefs, A. and Nederkoorn, C. (2009a). Eating behavior in response to food-cue exposure: examining the cue-reactivity and counteractive-control models. *Psychology of Addictive Behaviors*, *23*, 131–139.

Coelho, J., Polivy, J., Herman, C.P. and Pliner, P. (2009b). Wake up and smell the cookies: the effects of olfactory food cue exposure in restrained and unrestrained eaters. *Appetite*, *52*, 517–520.

Crespo, C.J., Smit, E., Troiano, R.P., Bartlett, S.J., Macera, C.A., and Andersen, R.E. (2001). Television watching, energy intake and obesity in US children, *Archives of Pediatrics and Adolescent Medicine*, 360–365.

Epstein, L. and Leddy, J.J. (2006). Food reinforcement. *Appetite*, *46*, 22–25.

Fedoroff, I., Polivy, J. and Herman, C.P. (1997). The effect of pre-exposure to food cues on the eating behavior of restrained and unrestrained eaters. *Appetite*, *28*, 33–47.

Fedoroff, I., Polivy, J. and Herman, C.P. (2003). The specificity of restrained versus unrestrained eaters' responses to food cues: general desire to eat, or craving for the cued food? *Appetite*, *41*, 7–13.

Ferriday, D. and Brunstrom, J. (2011). 'I just can't help myself': effects of food-cue exposure in overweight and lean individuals. *International Journal of Obesity*, *35*, 142–149.

Folkvord, F., Anschutz, D.J., Buijzen, M. and Valkenburg, P.M. (2013). The effect of playing advergames that promote energy-dense snacks or fruit on actual food intake among children. *American Journal of Clinical Nutrition*, *97*, 239–245.

Francis, L.A., Lee, Y. and Birch, L.L. (2003). Parental weight status and girls' television viewing, snacking, and body mass indexes. *Obesity Research*, *11*, 143–51.

Girz, L., Polivy, J., Herman, C.P. and Lee, H.H. (2012). The effects of calorie information on food selection and intake. *International Journal of Obesity*, *36*, 1340–1345.

Halford, J.C.G., Boyland, E.J., Hughes, G.M., Stacey, L., McKean, S. and Dovey, T.M. (2008). Beyond-brand effect of television food advertisements on food choice in children: The effects of weight status. *Public Health Nutrition, 11*, 897–904.

Halford, J.S.C., Gillespie, J., Brown, V., Pontin, E.E. and Dovey, T.M. (2004). Effect of television advertisements for foods on food consumption in children. *Appetite, 42*, 221–225.

Halford, J.C.G. and Boyland, E.J. (2013). Television advertising and branding. Effects on eating behaviour and food preferences in children. *Appetite, 62*, 236–241.

Heatherton, T., Herman, C.P., Polivy, J., King, G.A. and McGree, T. (1988). The (mis)measurement of restraint: an analysis of conceptual and psychometric issues. *Journal of Abnormal Psychology, 97*, 19–28.

Heatherton, T.F., Polivy, J. and Herman, C.P. (1991). Restraint, weight loss, and variability of body weight. *Journal of Abnormal Psychology, 100*, 78–83.

Herman, C.P., Olmsted, M.P. and Polivy, J. (1983). Obesity, externality, and susceptibility to social influence: an integrated analysis. *Journal of Personality & Social Psychology, 45*, 926–934.

Herman, C.P. and Polivy, J. (1980). Experimental and clinical aspects of restrained eating. In A. Stunkard (ed.), *Obesity: Basic mechanisms and treatment*. Philadelphia: W.B. Saunders, pp. 208–225.

Herman, C.P. and Polivy, J. (1988). Studies of eating in normal dieters. In B.T. Walsh (ed.), *Eating Behavior in Eating Disorders*. Washington, D.C.: American Psychiatric Association Press, pp. 95–112.

Herman, C.P. and Polivy, J. (2008). External cues in the control of food intake in humans: the sensory-normative distinction. *Physiology & Behavior, 94*, 722–728.

Herman, C.P., Polivy, J. and Leone, T. (2005). The psychology of overeating. In D. Mela (ed.). *Food, Diet, and Obesity*, pp. 115–136, Cambridge, UK: Woodhead Publishing.

Herman, C.P., Roth, D. and Polivy, J. (2003). Effects of the presence of others on food intake: a normative interpretation. *Psychological Bulletin, 129*, 873–886.

Higgs, S. (2008). Cognitive influences on food intake: the effects of manipulating memory for recent eating. *Physiology & Behavior, 94*, 734–739.

Hoefling, A. and Strack, F. (2010). Hunger induced changes in food choice. When beggars cannot be choosers even if they are allowed to choose. *Appetite, 54*, 603–606.

Hollitt, S., Kemps, E., Tiggemann, M., Smeets, E. and Mills, J.S. (2010). Components of attentional bias for food cues among restrained eaters. *Appetite, 54*, 309–313.

Hou, R., Mogg, K., Bradley, B.P., Moss-Morris, R., Peveler, R. and Roefs, A. (2011). External eating, impulsivity and attentional bias to food cues. *Appetite, 57*, 424–427.

Jansen, A. (1998). A learning model of binge eating: cue reactivity and cue exposure. *Behaviour Research and Therapy, 36*, 257–272.

Jansen, A. and Van den Hout, M. (1991). On being led into temptation: 'Counterregulation' of dieters after smelling a preload. *Addictive Behaviors, 16*, 247–253.

Jansen, A., Theunissen, N., Slechten, K., Nederkoorn, C., Boon, B., Mulkens, S. and Roefs, A. (2003). Overweight children overeat after exposure to food cues. *Eating Behaviors, 4*, 197–209.

Legoff, D.B. and Spigelman, M.N. (1987). Salivary response to olfactory food stimuli as a function of dietary restraint and body weight. *Appetite, 8*, 29–36.

Loewenstein, G. (1996). Out of control: visceral influences on behavior. *Organizational Behavior and Human Decision Processes, 65*, 272–292.

Loxton, N.J., Dawe, S. and Cahill, A. (2011). Does negative mood drive the urge to eat? The contribution of negative mood, exposure to food cues and eating style. *Appetite, 56*, 368–374.

Markowitz, J.T., Butryn, M.L. and Lowe, M. (2008). Perceived deprivation, restrained eating and susceptibility to weight gain. *Appetite*, *51*, 720–722.

Meule, A., Lukito, S., Vogele, C. and Kubler, A. (2011). Enhanced behavioral inhibition in restrained eaters. *Eating Behavior*, *12*, 152–155.

Nielsen, S.J. and Popkin, B.M. (2003). Patterns and trends in food portion sizes, 1977–1998. *Journal of the American Medical Association*, *289*, 450–453.

Nijs, I.M.T., Muris, P., Euser, A.S. and Franken, I.H.A. (2010). Differences in attention to food and food intake between overweight/obese and normal-weight females under conditions of hunger and satiety. *Appetite*, *54*, 243–254.

Oakes, M.E. and Slotterback, C.S. (2000). Self-reported measures of appetite in relation to verbal cues about many foods. *Current Psychology*, *19*, 137–142.

Oakes, M.E. and Slotterback, C.S. (2001). The effects of a list of food items on motivations to eat in dieters and nondieters. *Journal of Applied Social Psychology*, *31*, 1939–1950.

Ouwehand, C. and Papies, E.K. (2010). Eat it or beat it. The differential effects of food temptations on overweight and normal-weight restrained eaters. *Appetite*, *55*, 56–60.

Pliner, P., Herman, C.P. and Polivy, J. (1990). Palatability as a determinant of eating: Finickiness as a function of taste, hunger, and the prospect of good food. In E. Capaldi and T. Powley (eds.), *The Role of Experience in Modifying Taste and its Effects on Feeding*. American Psychological Association, Washington, D.C., pp. 210–226.

Polivy, J. and Herman, C.P. (1987). The diagnosis and treatment of normal eating. *Journal of Consulting and Clinical Psychology*, *55*, 635–644.

Polivy, J. and Herman, C.P. (2002). If at first you don't succeed: false hopes of self-change. *American Psychologist*, *57*, 677–689.

Polivy, J., Coleman, J. and Herman, C.P. (2005). The effect of deprivation on food cravings and eating behavior in restrained and unrestrained eaters. *International Journal of Eating Disorders*, *38*, 301–309.

Polivy, J., Herman, C.P. and Coelho, J. (2008). Caloric restriction in the presence of attractive food cues: external cues, eating, and weight. *Physiology & Behavior*, *94*, 729–733.

Rogers, P.J. and Hill, A. (1989). Breakdown of dietary restraint following mere exposure to food stimuli: interrelationships between restraint, hunger, salivation and food intake. *Addictive Behaviors*, *14*, 387–397.

Rolls, B.J., Morris, E.L. and Roe, L.S. (2002). Portion size of food affects energy intake in normal-weight and overweight men and women. *American Journal of Clinical Nutrition*, *76*, 1207–1213.

Schachter, S. (1971). Some extraordinary facts about obese humans and rats. *American Psychologist*, *26*, 129–144.

Shur, E A., Kleinhans, N.M., Goldberg, J., Buchwald, D.S., Polivy, J., *et al.* (2012). Acquired differences in brain responses among monozygotic twins discordant for restrained eating. *Physiology & Behavior*, *105*, 560–567.

Stunkard, A.J. and Messick, S. (1985). The Three-Factor Eating Questionnaire to measure restraint, disinhibition, and hunger. *Journal of Psychosomatic Research*, *29*, 71–83.

Sutin, A.R., Costa, P.T. Jr., Chan, W., Milaneschi, Y., Eaton, W.W., *et al.* (2013). I know not to, but I can't help it: weight gain and changes in impulsivity-related personality traits. *Psychological Science*, *24*, 1323–1328.

Talmi, D., Ziegler, M., Hawksworth, J., Lalani, S., Herman, C.P. and Moscovitch, M. (2013). Emotional stimuli exert parallel effects on attention and memory. *Cognition and Emotion*, *27*, 530–538.

Tetley, A.C., Brunstrom, J.M. and Griffiths, P. (2009). Individual differences in food-cue reactivity. The role of BMI and everyday portion-size selections. *Appetite*, *52*, 614–620.

Tetley, A.C., Brunstrom, J.M. and Griffiths, P. (2010). The role of sensitivity to reward and impulsivity in food-cue reactivity. *Eating Behaviors*, *11*, 138–143.

Urbszat, D., Herman, C.P. and Polivy, J. (2002). Eat, drink, and be merry, for tomorrow we diet: effects of anticipated deprivation on food intake in restrained and unrestrained eaters. *Journal of Abnormal Psychology*, *111*, 396–401.

van Koningsbruggen, G.M., Stroebe, W. and Aarts, H. (2011). Through the eyes of dieters: biased size perception of food following tempting food primes. *Journal of Experimental Social Psychology*, *47*, 293–299.

van Koningsbruggen, G.M., Stroebe, W. and Aarts, H. (2012). Mere exposure to palatable food cues reduces restrained eaters' physical effort to obtain healthy food. *Appetite*, *58*, 593–596.

van Strien, T. (1999). Success and failure in the measurement of restraint: Notes and data. *International Journal of Eating Disorders*, *25*, 441–449.

van Strien, T., Frijters, J.E., van Staveran, W.A., Defares, P.B. and Deurenberg, P. (1986). The predictive validity of the Dutch Restrained Eating Scale. *International Journal of Eating Disorders*, *5*, 747–755.

Viner, R.M. and Cole, T.J. (2005). Television viewing in early childhood predicts adult body mass index. *Journal of Pediatrics*, *147*, 429–435.

Wansink, B. (2004). Environmental factors that increase the food intake and consumption volume of unknowing consumers. *Annual Review of Nutrition*, *24*, 455–479.

Wiecha, J.L., Peterson, K.E., Ludwig, D.S., Kim, J., Sobol, A. and Gortmaker, S.L. (2006). When children eat what they watch. impact of television viewing on dietary intake in youth. *Archives of Pediatrics & Adolescent Medicine*, *160*, 436–442.

The interaction of diet and physical activity in managing obesity

13

M. Fogelholm
University of Helsinki, Helsinki, Finland

13.1   Introduction

Since managing and preventing obesity is related to energy balance, it is natural to consider both sides of the equation, that is, energy expenditure (physical activity) and energy intake (diet). But how do these two together affect or associate with obesity?

This chapter focuses on the potential interaction between diet and physical activity in preventing and managing obesity. Interaction exists when the effect of one modifiable factor (i.e. physical activity or diet) upon the outcome (e.g. obesity, weight change, obesity-related risk factors, etc.) is different at different levels of the other factor (i.e. diet or physical activity) (Woodward, 1999). The illustrative term 'effect modification' is also used instead of interaction.

Figure 13.1 illustrates the potential interactions relevant for this book. An arbitrary outcome is used to indicate the magnitude of change in, e.g., weight or risk-factors for chronic diseases. Both physical activity and the general diet are dichotomized in this illustration: people are thought to follow one of the two physical activity programmes (e.g. no activity vs. increase activity, or activity programme 1 vs. activity programme 2), and similarly for the diet programme. It should be noted that the examples are only illustrative and they are not based on actual research data.

In Figure 13.1(a), the effects of physical activity are similar for both diet groups, and vice versa. Although diet and physical activity have additive effects, they do not really interact. In Figure 13.1(b), the different physical activity programs have no additional effects if the participants are following one of the diets (e.g. a weight-reducing diet), whereas the effect is clear for those following the other diet (e.g. unrestricted energy intake). This is called unilateralism. Figure 13.1(c) shows the cases of synergism, when both diet and physical activity have a positive effect, but the effects of physical activity are stronger together with the other diet.

It is also important to consider the possibility of confounding effects, that is, whether physical activity and diet are simply confounders. A confounder is a factor that totally or partially accounts for the observed effects of another risk factor and disease (Woodward, 1999). If, for instance, dietary habits are related both to physical activity and obesity, diet may also be considered a confounder.

Managing and Preventing Obesity. http://dx.doi.org/10.1533/9781782420996.3.193

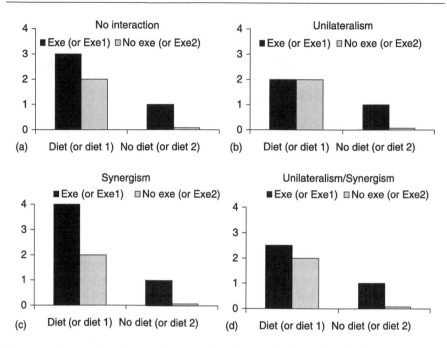

Figure 13.1 Examples of potential interactions of diet and physical activity in managing and preventing obesity. The scale on the Y-axis is arbitrary unit.

The aim of this chapter is to examine the possibility of real interaction between diet, physical activity and obesity. Moreover, the case of confounder effects is also discussed. One of the main objectives is to give 'food for thought' to researchers and to stimulate new study ideas and analytical designs.

The questions are approached from four different settings: (1) prevention of weight gain and/or obesity; (2) weight reduction intervention; (3) prevention of weight regain after weight reduction; (4) management of obesity-related diseases and risk-factors without change in weight. Contrary to the simple example in Figure 13.1, physical activity is much more than a dichotomous (yes/no) variable. In this chapter, the main views are on energy expenditure (quantity) and intensity (quality) of physical activity.

Diet is even more complicated than physical activity. In weight-reduction studies, the main factor is often energy intake or the level of reduction in energy intake. Recently there has been increasing interest in the effects of different types of diets during weight reduction, e.g., low-carbohydrate or high-protein diets (Brinkworth *et al.*, 2009; Josse *et al.*, 2011). Moreover, epidemiological studies have started to use foods, food-groups and total diets as the risk-factor (Fogelholm *et al.*, 2012) more often than earlier. Here 'total diets' may refer to scores given according to a theoretical premise (e.g. dietary recommendations) or to data-driven dietary analyses (e.g. principal component analysis) (Barbaresko *et al.*, 2013).

13.2   The independent and combined roles of physical activity and diet in prevention of weight gain

Primary prevention of weight gain is most often studied by using large popula-tion cohorts, with several years' follow-ups (Fogelholm *et al.*, 2012). Some studies (e.g. Nurse's Health Study) have repeated measurements (e.g. every 3 to 4 years) (Mozaffarian *et al.*, 2011), but most rely on baseline assessment as the sole predictor of weight change. Typically the behavioural components, including diet and phys-ical activity, are assessed at baseline. The change in weight or waist circumference is used as the main outcome; data on body composition are rare. The term 'weight gain' in this chapter includes also waist circumference and body fat, if not indicated otherwise.

Cohort studies on the association between physical activity and weight gain have been systematically reviewed by several authors during the last ten years (Fogelholm and Kukkonen-Harjula, 2000; Summerbell *et al.*, 2009; Wareham *et al.*, 2005). All of there three systematic reviews came to a similar conclusion: there is suggestive evid-ence that low levels of physical activity at baseline predict future weight gain, but the magnitude of effect is modest. There seems to be a trend that the most recent reports are more positive on physical activity as a preventive measure (Summerbell *et al.*, 2009), but whether this is due to improved methodology (e.g. larger datasets, more precise evaluation of physical activity) or to publication bias is uncertain.

There are several methodological challenges in studying the associations between physical activity and weight change in large cohorts. An apparent problem is what the precise exposure should be and how to measure it. Daily physical activity is a sum of several kinds of activities which take place in different settings (work, home, commuting) and have varying intensities and energy expenditures. Moreover, part of the time spent in low physical activity can be classified as totally sedentary (sitting or lying) and this component has also recently been associated with, e.g., obesity (Summerbell *et al.*, 2009; Wareham *et al.*, 2005) and mortality (Petersen *et al.*, 2014).

Since weight gain is a function of energy balance, it would be natural to try to assess total daily energy expenditure (Summerbell *et al.*, 2009). However, in past studies, this has not been possible, since most of the subjective measures only assess one or two components of physical activity. Hence, the data even today are restricted by incomplete description of total physical activity, and of inaccurate assessment of the component which was assessed. The recent increased used of accelerometers may provide new insights by giving simultaneously objective data for total activity and for different intensities, including time for total sedentariness (Rich *et al.*, 2012).

The above reviews also concluded that the associations between higher physical activity and less weight gain are stronger if physical activity is measured at the end of the follow-up, or if the change in physical activity from baseline is used as the exposure variable (Fogelholm and Kukkonen-Harjula, 2000; Summerbell *et al.*, 2009; Wareham *et al.*, 2005). However, these analytical designs are in fact cross-sectional (retrospective) in their design, not prospective. Therefore, reverse causality (weight gain and obesity leads to decreased physical activity) is at least partly a likely explanation for these stronger associations.

Numerous cohort studies have data with diet as the exposure and weight or waist circumference gain as the outcome (Fogelholm *et al.*, 2012; Summerbell *et al.*, 2009). In these studies, the choice of exposure variable could be considered even more difficult than for studies with physical activity. Namely, diet could be described by using, e.g., total energy intake, energy density (kJ/kg) proportion of macronutrients in total energy intake, dietary glycaemic index (GI), several food groups, the entire diet (Fogelholm *et al.*, 2012) or different dietary patters (Fuglestad *et al.*, 2012). Also the assessment of food consumption and dietary intake is demanding, and the results are often both biased (underestimated) and inaccurate.

In our systematic review on diet and weight gain (Fogelholm *et al.*, 2012), we found probable evidence for high intake of dietary fibre and nuts predicting less weight gain, and for high intake of meat in predicting more weight gain. Suggestive (weaker than 'probable') evidence was found for a protective role against increasing weight from whole grains, cereal fibre, high-fat dairy products and high scores in an index describing a prudent dietary pattern. Likewise, there was suggestive evidence for both fibre and fruit intake in protection against larger increases in waist circumference. Also suggestive evidence was found for high intake of refined grains, and sweets and desserts in predicting more weight gain, and for refined (white) bread and high energy density in predicting larger increases in waist circumference. The results suggested that the proportion of macronutrients in the diet was not important in predicting changes in weight or waist circumference.

In cohort studies predicting weight gain by using physical activity and/or diet as the exposure, age, socio-demographic status, baseline obesity, etc. are used as confounders. The important question for this chapter is if physical activity and diet are confounders for each other – or whether they interact? How should these two variables be used in the analyses?

A confounder should be related to both the other risk factor (exposure) and to the disease (obesity, in this case), but it should not be a caused by either of these (Woodward, 1999). A premise for the next discussion is that at least some components of diet and physical activity are associated with weight gain (Fogelholm *et al.*, 2012; Summerbell *et al.*, 2009). But are diet and physical activity associated with each other? Several studies have shown an association between lower physical activity and unhealthy eating behaviours (Mesas *et al.*, 2012), skipping breakfast (Corder *et al.*, 2014; Fuglestad *et al.*, 2012) and high meat consumption (Kappeler *et al.*, 2013). Moreover, watching TV was positively associated with an excessive urge to eat (Chapman *et al.*, 2012). Nevertheless, the associations between different components of diet, physical activity and health behaviour seem to be complex and very inconsistent (Leech *et al.*, 2014).

In a recent study, several food groups and a diet-quality score were associated with cardiorespiratory fitness, independent of physical activity levels (Shikany *et al.*, 2013). The result is interesting, although very difficult to explain, particularly since also some unhealthy dietary patterns (e.g. consumption of processed meat) were positively related to fitness.

The above data indicate that high physical activity and prudent diet go somewhat hand in hand and that by doing so they may support each other's effects on body weight and health. Unfortunately, it is not fully clear which components of activity and diet show the strongest correlations. Given this fact and the problems we face with assessment of both diet and physical activity accurately, it is very likely that the relationships between exposure (diet or physical activity) on the outcome (obesity or health/disease) are partly explained by residual confounding (Lawlor et al., 2004).

But the question of interaction exists – do physical activity and diet really interact? Are the associations between diet and weight change different for different physical activity levels and/or patterns? Data on insulin resistance as a modifier of the relationship between diet and weight gain (Mosca et al., 2004) could offer an explanation for the hypothesis of an interaction between diet and physical activity in predicting weight gain: by improving insulin sensitivity (Roberts et al., 2013), physical activity may make an individual less susceptible to the fattening effects of certain dietary components (e.g. fat or carbohydrates).

To the best of my knowledge, this question has only been assessed in papers from the European Prospective Investigation into Cancer and Nutrition (EPIC) cohort. A significant interaction between diet and physical activity was reported in one study (Vergnaud et al., 2010): the positive relationship between meat consumption and weight gain was stronger in individuals with high physical activity. The interaction between several other dietary factors (not meat), physical activity and weight gain was reported to be non-significant (Romaguera et al., 2010; Vergnaud et al., 2012).

The result on meat, physical activity and weight (Vergnaud et al., 2010) was surprising, since it could be hypothesized that the increased energy expenditure from physical activity would make it easier to control body weight, even when eating more foods which are associated with weight gain. However, since the relation between meat and weight gain was stronger in men than in women (Vergnaud et al., 2010), higher physical activity in men might explain the interaction between physical activity, meat consumption and weight change.

In conclusion, certain dietary components may have different associations with weight gain, depending on the amount of physical activity. Unfortunately, the data are far too inadequate to make any firm conclusions. Even less is known about different kinds of activities. It could be hypothesized that high-intensity training, with more emphasis on intramuscular energy sources compared to moderate-intensity activities, might have an interaction with, e.g., carbohydrate intake and/or dietary glycaemic index.

13.3 Physical activity and diet during weight reduction programmes

The data from weight reduction studies give more insight on the interaction of diet and exercise, compared to data from epidemiological designs. The literature allows

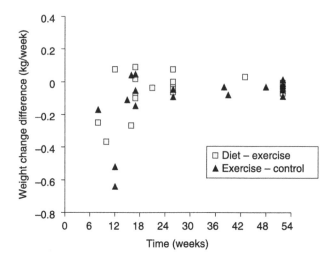

Figure 13.2 Difference in weight change (kg/week) between exercise/diet + exercise vs. control/diet only, as a function of duration of the intervention. Data from Wing (1999) and Ross and Janssen (2001).

assessment of the hypothesis that the effects of increased exercise are dependent on whether obese participants are following an energy-restricted diet or not.

Figure 13.2 combines the results from two earlier, comprehensive and systematic reviews on the effects of exercise in treatment of obesity. The figure shows the difference in weekly weight reduction as a function of study duration in two different designs: (1) an exercise group (mostly aerobic exercise) is compared to a control group (no exercise) (Ross and Janssen, 2001); (2) a combined exercise and diet group is compared against a diet only group (Wing, 1999). The figure suggests that there is apparently no interaction between exercise and diet: the additional effects of exercise on body weight reduction seem to be similar with or without an energy-restricted diet. It should be noted that the figure does not indicate that the prescribed dose of exercise was really high in two of the included studies (the two dots showing an approximately 600 g weekly weight reduction during a 12-week intervention) which is the likely explanation for the very good result in these studies.

A more recent Cochrane-review (Shaw et al., 2006) estimated that adding exercise to a weight-reducing diet lead to an increased average weight loss of 1.1 kg. Using the weighed mean difference of the studies comparing exercise alone against no treatment suggested a larger weight reduction as a result of exercise, namely 2.5 kg. However, because of great heterogeneity between the studies, the authors did not carry out an official meta-analysis. In the same review, high intensity exercise appeared to lead to an average of 1.5 kg greater weight reduction, compared to moderate or low-intensity aerobic exercise with similar estimated energy expenditure. This positive effect was observed only in trials without a simultaneous weight-reducing diet, which indicates an interaction with unilateralism (effects of exercise are only seen without a diet).

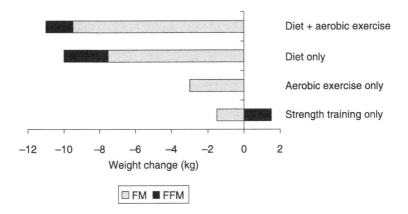

Figure 13.3 Change in body composition during weight reduction with or without physical exercise: meta-analytic findings. Data from Garrow and Summerbell (1995). FM = fat mass, FFM = fat-free mass.

There are rather few studies on the interaction between diet and physical activity on body composition changes during weight reduction. The key question from a health view-point is how to maximize body fat mass loss (FM) and simultaneously how to minimize loss of fat-free mass (FFM). An earlier review (Garrow and Summerbell, 1995) was able to give insight on these data (Figure 13.3). According to this review, adding exercise to diet improves weight loss and increases the proportion of FM loss, compared to diet only. However, the positive effects of exercise seemed to be slightly better when exercise without diet was compared to simply no exercise. This review therefore suggests that there is an interaction which is incompletely directed towards unilateralism. A more recent review (Weinheimer *et al.*, 2010) reached an approximately similar conclusion. However, this review was restricted to middle-aged and older individuals, and to changes in FFM.

In treatment of obesity, weight reduction should not be considered an end in itself; the main aim is to reduce risk-factors and to improve health prognosis. The independent and combined effects of diet and exercise in individuals with obesity have been systematically reviewed (Katzmarzyk and Lear, 2012; Shaw *et al.*, 2006). Both reviews concluded that adding exercise to a weight-reducing diet does not lead to clinically or statistically significant improvements in major risk-factors, such as systolic and diastolic blood pressure, fasting blood glucose, serum LDL- and HDL-cholesterol and serum triglycerides. The effects of exercise on risk-factors seem to be better observed when exercise alone is compared against a no treatment (Shaw *et al.*, 2006).

Again, the above results points towards unilateralism, that is, the effects of diet on body weight reduction and risk-factors are likely to be so marked that there simply is not 'space' for additional effects of physical activity. The effects may also be related to the outcome: Cox *et al.* (2004) did not find an additive effect of exercise on body composition changes, compared to diet only, but a positive effect on changes in insulin sensitivity. It is also possible that a higher exercise dose than used in studies is needed to overcome the effects of diet. Typically the exercise-induced energy expenditure has been 1000–1500 kcal (4.3 to 6.3 MJ) per week, that is, no more than 200 kcal (0.8 MJ) per day. In an interesting series of studies, Ross and colleagues used a very high amount of exercise (500–700 kcal or 2.1–2.9 MJ per day as energy expenditure) to induce a 6–7 kg weight reduction in men (Ross *et al.*, 2000) and women (Ross *et al.*, 2004). The results suggested that, compared to a similar magnitude of weight reduction achieved by diet without exercise, the high-volume exercise regimen lead to significantly better metabolic results (e.g. more reduction in fat and visceral fat mass, greater improvement in insulin sensitivity, etc.).

Earlier studies on diet and exercise in weight reduction were mostly interested in comparing exercise against no exercise and an energy-restricted diet against no diet. Typically diets were low in fat and high in carbohydrates. More recently, studies have started to compare different diets, and even leaving a no-diet group out of the study. For instance, the role of GI or glycaemic load in preventing obesity and treating Type 2 diabetes has been studied intensively during recent years (Thomas and Elliott, 2010). Varying protein levels are another point of interest. Data with obese individuals as participants suggest that, combined with exercise training, increasing dietary protein intake preserves FFM (Josse *et al.*, 2011) and that reducing dietary GI improves insulin sensitivity (Solomon *et al.*, 2010). However, since these studies have only one level of exercise, a true interaction cannot be examined.

There has been a great interest in the effects of low-carbohydrate, high-protein (LCHP) diets in treatment of obesity and obesity-related diseases (Hession *et al.*, 2009). It is interesting to note that, at least in the majority of weight reductions with LCHP diet, physical activity has not been included in the programme. Deduced from the findings of Josse *et al.* (2011), one could hypothesize that resistance training combined with LCHP might give an even better effect on the ratio between FM and FFM loss during weight reduction, compared to LCHP diet only. To really get more insight on the interactions, a comparison with increased aerobic exercise would also be interesting.

Limited data suggest that an energy-reduced diet may lead to decreased physical activity (Martin *et al.*, 2007). This effect could be exacerbated during a LCHP diet when reduced muscle glycogen stores might make physical activity even more difficult. Therefore, one unanswered question specifically related to the LCHP diet is whether the lack of carbohydrates has an effect on physical activity. One study has given indirect evidence on this issue (Brinkworth *et al.*, 2009). This study examined the effects of a low-carbohydrate diet on maximal oxygen uptake capacity (VO_2max). In contrast to the hypothesis, the study did not reveal any differences in change of VO_2max in low-carbohydrate vs. low-fat diet groups. Since weight reduction improves VO_2max, when expressed as ml/kg per min, this outcome may not be the best to study if carbohydrate restriction has a long-term effect on physical activity.

13.4 The roles of physical activity and diet in maintenance of reduced body weight

The real challenge in treating obesity with a lifestyle approach is not weight reduction *per se*, but long-term maintenance of reduced body weight (Turk *et al.*, 2009). The National Weight Control Registry (NWCR) gives an interesting possibility to observe determinants of successful weight loss in formerly obese individuals in the United States (Phelan *et al.*, 2006; Thomas *et al.*, 2014). The NWCR is a registry of participants who have lost at least 13.6 kg and maintained the loss for at least one year. The cross-sectional comparisons of individuals entering the study between years 1995 and 2003 show that the proportion of dietary carbohydrates was relatively high initially, but that the proportion has been gradually decreasing: in 1995, the proportion of carbohydrates in total energy intake was 56.0%, whereas the respective intake in 2003 was 49.3% (Phelan *et al.*, 2006). This might be connected with the increasing popularity of low-carbohydrate diet even among individuals in the NWCR. The proportion of protein intake has remained stable, around 19% in total energy intake.

Physical activity in individuals of the NWCR was high (mean physical activity corresponds to >2300 kcal or about 10 MJ per week) and quite stable throughout the years (Phelan *et al.*, 2006). In a recent study, the determinants of long-term weight change in 2880 NWCR participants (Thomas *et al.*, 2014) was studied. About half of the participants were followed for ten years. A decrease in physical activity, dietary restraint and weighing and an increase in the proportion of dietary fat were determinants of higher weight gain. In this study, it appeared that physical activity and following a prudent diet have additive effects (or associations, strictly speaking). A real interaction was not studied.

Several weight-reduction interventions have included a follow-up of at least six months' duration. These studies give additional observational evidence on the associations between physical activity and maintenance of reduced body weight. As concluded already for primary prevention of weight gain, the strongest and most consistent evidence for beneficial associations are from studies measuring physical activity in the end of the study, or as a change from baseline (immediately after weight reduction) to follow-up (Donnelly *et al.*, 2009; Fogelholm and Kukkonen-Harjula, 2000). In these designs, it is not possible to exclude reverse causation. That is, maintenance of body weight by, for example, prudent diet might make higher levels of physical activity easier.

Only very few studies have used a randomized design to test the hypothesis that prescribed physical activity after weight reduction improves weight maintenance, and the results are inconclusive (Curioni and Lourenço, 2005; Fogelholm and Kukkonen-Harjula, 2000). We have published two earlier studies with a similar design: weight loss by a very-low energy diet (3 months), followed by a group-guided weight maintenance intervention (6–9 months) and a 2-yr follow-up. All participants received dietary guidance and some were also randomized to increased physical activity groups during the weight maintenance intervention. The first study suggested that a moderate amount (1000 kcal or 4.2 MJ weekly) of increased physical activity reduced, but did not prevent, body weight regain in obese women (Fogelholm *et al.*, 2000). A higher exercise prescription (2000 kcal or 8.4 MJ weekly) did not improve weight maintenance, compared to dietary counselling only. The other study did not find an additional effect of adding aerobic or strength training to dietary counselling after weight reduction in obese men (Kukkonen-Harjula *et al.*, 2005). Higher prescribed physical activity levels do not necessarily help in maintaining reduced body weight due to poor compliance with high physical activity (Fogelholm *et al.*, 2000; Tate *et al.*, 2007).

Our studies used counselling for a healthy diet in all participants. Therefore, a true interaction with varying dietary exposure could not be examined. An observational analysis showed that control of overeating, as indicated by a lower disinhibition factor of the TFEQ, and daily physical activity, as indicated by a higher number of daily steps, were positive and independent predictors of weight maintenance (Fogelholm *et al.*, 1999). The results are similar to those observed recently in the NWCR (Thomas *et al.*, 2014).

There are only a few randomized studies on the effects of different dietary macronutrient composition on maintenance of body weight after weight reduction. In our systematic review (Fogelholm *et al.*, 2012), we did not find enough evidence to conclude that a certain macronutrient composition would be superior in preventing weight regain after prior weight reduction. However, one reason may be that the number of studies using comparable comparisons is too limited (typically no more than two studies for a given design and diet comparison) to reach any firm conclusions.

Nevertheless, one large dietary intervention on weight maintenance deserves mentioning (Larsen *et al.*, 2010). Using a large, international, multi-centre design, the DioGenes study examined the effects of four different intervention diets on weight maintenance after a 2-month weight-reduction with a low-energy diet. In this study, the only diet with almost complete 6-month weight maintenance had lowered GI and increased protein content. As already mentioned for the weight-reduction interventions, it would be really important to combine at least two different diets and at least two physical activity programmes in a large weight-maintenance intervention, in order to study if the effects of diet on body weight maintenance are modified by physical activity.

13.5 Conclusions

An interaction between diet and exercise in preventing and managing obesity means that the effects of diet are dependent on the chosen physical activity regimen, or vice-versa. In theory, the potential interactions may be outlined as shown in Figure 13.4.

To study an interaction, at least two levels for both diet and physical activity are needed. The simplest approach is to have a 'no diet, no exercise' group in the design. However, it has become evident that there are many potential interactions related to the macronutrient composition of the diet or to choice of food items. Particularly the interactions between dietary composition of carbohydrates and proteins have

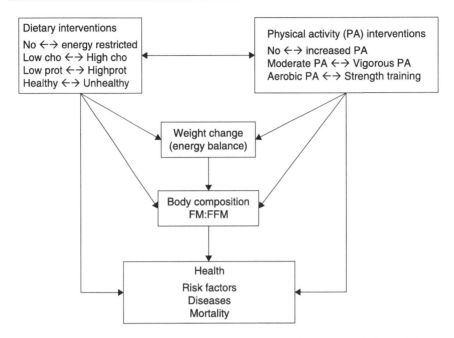

Figure 13.4 An outline of possible mechanisms for potential interactions of diet and physical activity in managing and preventing obesity. Cho = carbohydrates; Prot = proteins; PA = physical activity, FM = fat mass, FFM = fat-free mass.

theoretically important interactions with both the intensity (moderate vs. vigorous) and type (aerobic vs. strength) of physical activity.

Weight as an outcome is simple and often used, but it tells obviously very little about the real health-related effects and interactions of physical activity and diet in preventing and managing obesity. Intervention studies suggest that adding exercise to a weight-reducing diet improves weight reduction, but that the additive (positive) effects of exercise are less than without diet (Shaw *et al.*, 2006). It is hard to find a physiological explanation for this finding, but one explanation could be that the compliance to an exercise programme is worse during a simultaneous energy-restricted diet. Hence, in this case the effects of diet on physical activity may cause a true interaction.

Body weight changes are related to changes in body composition, but the effects are modified by physical activity (Garrow and Summerbell, 1995; Weinheimer *et al.*, 2010). Similar to what was already concluded for weight change, it seems that the additive effects of aerobic exercise on the proportions of FM and FFM losses in total weight reduction are more positive (meaning proportionally more FM and less FFM lost) without a concomitant energy-restricted diet. Apparently some of the metabolic effects of an energy-reduced diet on body composition changes are too strong to be overcome by added exercise. It would be important to study the interactions between different dietary macronutrients and different types of exercise programmes on body composition.

The general conclusion when using metabolic-risk factors as outcomes is directed towards unilateralism: examining the interaction shows that in most cases adding exercise to a weight-reducing diet has no additional effects on the outcome (Shaw *et al.*, 2006). While the randomized interventions give some, albeit limited, insight on the interaction between diet and physical activity in managing obesity, hardly anything is known about this in connection to primary prevention of weight gain. As pointed out earlier in this chapter, most population studies have only used physical activity and diet as confounder variables. Studies show independent, reverse associations between physical activity and weight gain. The evidence is not very strong, however, and the magnitude of the potential effect is modest (Summerbell *et al.*, 2009). Similarly, independent from physical activity levels, some dietary components and patterns (e.g. high consumption of meat, refined grains and sugary products) are positively related to weight gain, while some others (e.g. fibre-rich foods) have a reverse association (Fogelholm *et al.*, 2012). How physical activity and diet interact is not known.

It would be very important to understand how different diets and physical activity programmes really interact in preventing and managing obesity. For instance, if we recommend a low-carbohydrate diet for weight loss, should we include a physical activity programme or not? If yes, what kind of activity? Are people with healthier diets less dependent on physical activity levels for prevention of weight gain, compared to individuals with less prudent diets? New designs are needed to tackle these kinds of questions.

References

Barbaresko, J., Koch, M., Schulze, M.B. and Nöthlings, U. (2013). Dietary pattern analysis and biomarkers of low-grade inflammation: a systematic literature review. *Nutr. Rev.* 71, 511–527.

Brinkworth, G.D., Noakes, M., Clifton, P.M. and Buckley, J.D. (2009). Effects of a low carbohydrate weight loss diet on exercise capacity and tolerance in obese subjects. *Obes. Silver Spring Md* 17, 1916–1923.

Chapman, C.D., Benedict, C., Brooks, S.J. and Schiöth, H.B. (2012). Lifestyle determinants of the drive to eat: a meta-analysis. *Am. J. Clin. Nutr.* 96, 492–497.

Corder, K., van Sluijs, E.M., Ridgway, C.L., Steele, R.M., Prynne, C.J., *et al.* (2014). Breakfast consumption and physical activity in adolescents: daily associations and hourly patterns. *Am. J. Clin. Nutr.* 99, 361–368.

Cox, K.L., Burke, V., Morton, A.R., Beilin, L.J. and Puddey, I.B. (2004). Independent and additive effects of energy restriction and exercise on glucose and insulin concentrations in sedentary overweight men. *Am. J. Clin. Nutr.* 80, 308–316.

Curioni, C.C. and Lourenço, P.M. (2005). Long-term weight loss after diet and exercise: a systematic review. *Int. J. Obes.* 29, 1168–1174.

Donnelly, J.E., Blair, S.N., Jakicic, J.M., Manore, M.M., Rankin, J.W. and Smith, B.K. for the American College of Sports Medicine (2009). American College of Sports Medicine Position Stand. Appropriate physical activity intervention strategies for weight loss and prevention of weight regain for adults. *Med. Sci. Sports Exerc.* 41, 459–471.

Fogelholm, M., Anderssen, S., Gunnarsdottir, I. and Lahti-Koski, M. (2012). Dietary macro-nutrients and food consumption as determinants of long-term weight change in adult populations: a systematic literature review. *Food Nutr. Res.* 56, 19103.

Fogelholm, M. and Kukkonen-Harjula, K. (2000). Does physical activity prevent weight gain – a systematic review. *Obes. Rev. Off. J. Int. Assoc. Study Obes.* 1, 95–111.

Fogelholm, M., Kukkonen-Harjula, K., Nenonen, A. and Pasanen, M. (2000). Effects of walking training on weight maintenance after a very-low-energy diet in premenopausal obese women: a randomized controlled trial. *Arch. Intern. Med.* 160, 2177–2184.

Fogelholm, M., Kukkonen-Harjula, K. and Oja, P. (1999). Eating control and physical activity as determinants of short-term weight maintenance after a very-low-calorie diet among obese women. *Int. J. Obes. Relat. Metab. Disord. J. Int. Assoc. Study Obes.* 23, 203–210.

Fuglestad, P.T., Jeffery, R.W. and Sherwood, N.E. (2012). Lifestyle patterns associated with diet, physical activity, body mass index and amount of recent weight loss in a sample of successful weight losers. *Int. J. Behav. Nutr. Phys. Act.* 9, 79.

Garrow, J.S. and Summerbell, C.D. (1995). Meta-analysis: effect of exercise, with or without dieting, on the body composition of overweight subjects. *Eur. J. Clin. Nutr.* 49, 1–10.

Hession, M., Rolland, C., Kulkarni, U., Wise, A. and Broom, J. (2009). Systematic review of randomized controlled trials of low-carbohydrate vs. low-fat/low-calorie diets in the management of obesity and its comorbidities. *Obes. Rev. Off. J. Int. Assoc. Study Obes.* 10, 36–50.

Josse, A.R., Atkinson, S.A., Tarnopolsky, M.A. and Phillips, S.M. (2011). Increased consumption of dairy foods and protein during diet- and exercise-induced weight loss promotes fat mass loss and lean mass gain in overweight and obese premenopausal women. *J. Nutr.* 141, 1626–1634.

Kappeler, R., Eichholzer, M. and Rohrmann, S. (2013). Meat consumption and diet quality and mortality in NHANES III. *Eur. J. Clin. Nutr.* 67(6), 598–606.

Katzmarzyk, P.T. and Lear, S.A. (2012). Physical activity for obese individuals: a systematic review of effects on chronic disease risk factors. *Obes. Rev. Off. J. Int. Assoc. Study Obes.* 13, 95–105.

Kukkonen-Harjula, K.T., Borg, P.T., Nenonen, A.M. and Fogelholm, M.G. (2005). Effects of a weight maintenance program with or without exercise on the metabolic syndrome: a randomized trial in obese men. *Prev. Med.* 41, 784–790.

Larsen, T.M., Dalskov, S.-M., van Baak, M., Jebb, S.A., Papadaki, A., *et al.*, (Diet, Obesity, and Genes (Diogenes) Project) (2010). Diets with high or low protein content and glycemic index for weight-loss maintenance. *N. Engl. J. Med.* 363, 2102–2113.

Lawlor, D.A., Davey Smith, G., Kundu, D., Bruckdorfer, K.R. and Ebrahim, S. (2004). Those confounded vitamins: what can we learn from the differences between observational versus randomised trial evidence? *Lancet* 363, 1724–1727.

Leech, R.M., McNaughton, S.A. and Timperio, A. (2014). The clustering of diet, physical activity and sedentary behavior in children and adolescents: a review. *Int. J. Behav. Nutr. Phys. Act.* 11, 4.

Martin, C.K., Heilbronn, L.K., de Jonge, L., DeLany, J.P., Volaufova, J., *et al.* (2007). Effect of calorie restriction on resting metabolic rate and spontaneous physical activity. *Obes. Silver Spring Md* 15, 2964–2973.

Mosca, C.L., Marshall, J.A., Grunwald, G.K., Cornier, M.A. and Baxter, J. (2004). Insulin resistance as a modifier of the relationship between dietary fat intake and weight gain. *Int. J. Obes. Relat. Metab. Disord. J. Int. Assoc. Study Obes.* 28, 803–812.

Mozaffarian, D., Hao, T., Rimm, E.B., Willett, W.C. and Hu, F.B. (2011). Changes in diet and lifestyle and long-term weight gain in women and men. *N. Engl. J. Med.* 364, 2392–2404.

Petersen, C.B., Bauman, A., Grønbæk, M., Helge, J.W., Thygesen, L.C. and Tolstrup, J.S. (2014). Total sitting time and risk of myocardial infarction, coronary heart disease and all-cause mortality in a prospective cohort of Danish adults. *Int. J. Behav. Nutr. Phys. Act.* 11, 13.

Phelan, S., Wyatt, H.R., Hill, J.O. and Wing, R.R. (2006). Are the eating and exercise habits of successful weight losers changing? *Obes. Silver Spring Md* 14, 710–716.

Rich, C., Griffiths, L.J. and Dezateux, C. (2012). Seasonal variation in accelerometer-determined sedentary behaviour and physical activity in children: a review. *Int. J. Behav. Nutr. Phys. Act.* 9, 49.

Roberts, C.K., Little, J.P. and Thyfault, J.P. (2013). Modification of insulin sensitivity and glycemic control by activity and exercise. *Med. Sci. Sports Exerc.* 45, 1868–1877.

Romaguera, D., Angquist, L., Du, H., Jakobsen, M.U., Forouhi, N.G., *et al.* (2010). Dietary determinants of changes in waist circumference adjusted for body mass index – a proxy measure of visceral adiposity. *PloS One* 5, e11588.

Ross, R., Dagnone, D., Jones, P.J., Smith, H., Paddags, A., *et al.* (2000). Reduction in obesity and related comorbid conditions after diet-induced weight loss or exercise-induced weight loss in men. A randomized, controlled trial. *Ann. Intern. Med.* 133, 92–103.

Ross, R. and Janssen, I. (2001). Physical activity, total and regional obesity: dose-response considerations. *Med. Sci. Sports Exerc.* 33, S521–527; discussion S528–529.

Ross, R., Janssen, I., Dawson, J., Kungl, A.-M., Kuk, J.L., *et al.* (2004). Exercise-induced reduction in obesity and insulin resistance in women: a randomized controlled trial. *Obes. Res.* 12, 789–798.

Shaw, K., Gennat, H., O'Rourke, P. and Del Mar, C. (2006). Exercise for overweight or obesity. *Cochrane Database Syst. Rev.* CD003817.

Shikany, J.M., Jacobs, D.R., Jr, Lewis, C.E., Steffen, L.M., Sternfeld, B., *et al.* (2013). Associations between food groups, dietary patterns, and cardiorespiratory fitness in the Coronary Artery Risk Development in Young Adults study. *Am. J. Clin. Nutr.* 98, 1402–1409.

Solomon, T.P., Haus, J.M., Kelly, K.R., Cook, M.D., Filion, J., *et al.* (2010). A low-glycemic index diet combined with exercise reduces insulin resistance, postprandial hyper-insulinemia, and glucose-dependent insulinotropic polypeptide responses in obese, prediabetic humans. *Am. J. Clin. Nutr.* 92, 1359–1368.

Summerbell, C.D., Douthwaite, W., Whittaker, V., Ells, L.J., Hillier, F., *et al.* (2009). The association between diet and physical activity and subsequent excess weight gain and obesity assessed at 5 years of age or older: a systematic review of the epidemiological evidence. *Int. J. Obes.* 33 (Suppl 3), S1–92.

Tate, D.F., Jeffery, R.W., Sherwood, N.E. and Wing, R.R. (2007). Long-term weight losses associated with prescription of higher physical activity goals. Are higher levels of physical activity protective against weight regain? *Am. J. Clin. Nutr.* 85, 954–959.

Thomas, D.E. and Elliott, E.J. (2010). The use of low-glycaemic index diets in diabetes control. *Br. J. Nutr.* 104, 797–802.

Thomas, J.G., Bond, D.S., Phelan, S., Hill, J.O. and Wing, R.R. (2014). Weight-loss maintenance for 10 years in the National Weight Control Registry. *Am. J. Prev. Med.* 46, 17–23.

Turk, M.W., Yang, K., Hravnak, M., Sereika, S.M., Ewing, L.J. and Burke, L.E. (2009). Randomized clinical trials of weight loss maintenance: a review. *J. Cardiovasc. Nurs.* 24, 58–80.

Vergnaud, A.-C., Norat, T., Romaguera, D., Mouw, T., May, A.M., *et al.* (2012). Fruit and vegetable consumption and prospective weight change in participants of the European Prospective Investigation into Cancer and Nutrition-Physical Activity, Nutrition, Alcohol,

Cessation of Smoking, Eating Out of Home, and Obesity study. *Am. J. Clin. Nutr.* 95, 184–193.

Vergnaud, A.-C., Norat, T., Romaguera, D., Mouw, T., May, A.M., *et al.* (2010). Meat consumption and prospective weight change in participants of the EPIC-PANACEA study. *Am. J. Clin. Nutr.* 92, 398–407.

Wareham, N.J., van Sluijs, E.M.F. and Ekelund, U. (2005). Physical activity and obesity prevention: a review of the current evidence. *Proc. Nutr. Soc.* 64, 229–247.

Weinheimer, E.M., Sands, L.P. and Campbell, W.W. (2010). A systematic review of the separate and combined effects of energy restriction and exercise on fat-free mass in middle-aged and older adults: implications for sarcopenic obesity. *Nutr. Rev.* 68, 375–388.

Wing, R.R. (1999). Physical activity in the treatment of the adulthood overweight and obesity: current evidence and research issues. *Med. Sci. Sports Exerc.* 31, S547–552.

Woodward, M. (1999). *Epidemiology. Study Design and Data Analysis.* Chapman & Hall/CRC Press, Boca Raton, Florida.

Part Four

Structured dietary interventions in the treatment of obesity

Defined energy deficit diets for the treatment of obesity

C. Grace
King's College Hospital, London, UK

14.1   Introduction

Defined energy prescriptions are an evidence-based dietary treatment option which can be used to guide individuals towards an improved understanding of their likely energy needs for weight loss, and importantly what this means in terms of food choices and portion sizes. They are not, as is sometimes suggested, a precise individual prescription for weight loss due to the limitations in predicting resting metabolism and physical activity energy expenditure in the clinical setting. Nevertheless they provide a useful starting point for the patient and practitioner to explore possible dietary changes and clinical trials support their value in achieving meaningful clinical outcomes in the short to medium term. There are a number of interesting questions and challenges which arise in their clinical use including the choice of regression equation for predicting resting metabolism, the advised energy deficit and the best estimate of physical activity level. This chapter defines energy prescription approaches, considers their practical application, outlines the evidence for their effectiveness and considers some of the common challenges faced by practitioners in clinical practice.

14.2   History of defined energy prescriptions

Traditionally dietary advice was formulated following a diet history in which the patient would recall their usual food intake and the practitioner would aim to support the patient in identifying areas amenable to subsequent modification. However, this proved an unhelpful approach given the substantial under-reporting of energy intake by many obese individuals [1]. Frequently practitioners would be left in the predicament of how best to guide individuals struggling to lose weight while reporting an energy intake well below their estimated energy requirement. This led to the recommendation to base advised dietary changes on an estimate of the individual's energy requirements for weight loss and the subsequent development of defined energy prescriptions for the treatment of obesity.

Managing and Preventing Obesity. http://dx.doi.org/10.1533/9781782420996.4.211

14.3   Terminology and definitions

Defined energy prescriptions for weight loss can be broadly divided into two categories.

14.3.1 Fixed energy prescriptions

For many years fixed energy prescriptions, often 1500 kcal for women and 1800 kcal for men, were advised regardless of an individual's starting weight. Although this may be helpful for some individuals, for the heavier patient this may pose a potentially greater challenge as the magnitude of the advised energy deficit is higher given greater levels of energy expenditure. This led to the development of tailored energy prescriptions.

14.3.2 Tailored energy prescriptions

Limited evidence suggests this approach may be easier to adhere to compared to fixed energy diets [2] although more research is required to clarify this issue. Tailored energy prescriptions are often used by dietitians as a foundation for dietary plans and as a starting point for discussions on energy requirements and food choices. This approach calculates an individual's energy requirements for weight loss by first estimating resting metabolism using prediction equations and multiplying this result by a factor that accounts for physical activity. A daily number of calories, which often equates to a theoretical weekly loss of 0.5–1 kg, can then be subtracted. Subsequent dietary plans will be based on this energy prescription with the aim of achieving dietary guidelines for macronutrient composition.

14.4   Estimating total energy requirements

14.4.1 Predicting resting metabolic rate

Measuring resting metabolic rate using indirect calorimetry is the gold standard in determining energy requirements in obese individuals in clinical settings [3]. However in most clinical situations particularly outpatient settings, this is not feasible and using predictive equations is a practical alternative. Resting metabolic rate generally accounts for ~70% of total daily energy expenditure, particularly in sedentary individuals [4] and given it is such a major contributor making an accurate estimation is important. Predictive equations are developed from a reference population and are based on a regression analysis of weight, height, gender and age as independent variables and RMR measured by indirect calorimetry as the dependant variable.

14.4.1.1 Derivation of prediction equations

There are a number of different prediction equations available and variability is known to exist in the choice of equation used by practitioners [5]. Many studies on energy requirements in the obese have come from critically ill obese patients rather than those attending outpatients for support with weight management. Determining energy requirements in the acute setting is beyond the scope of this chapter, however comprehensive reviews have been published which summarize current knowledge [6] with consideration given to the consequences of under and overfeeding.

For practitioners to be confident in the use of predictive equations a low margin of error is needed to reduce the potential effects on treatment outcomes. Although this is particularly important in critical care patients it is also relevant to those individuals in weight management programmes where the energy prescription forms the basis of their dietary plan.

Understanding the derivation of the predication equations is important as it highlights potential differences between the reference population from which the equation has been developed and the individual/population in which energy requirement is being predicted. Some equations have been derived from predominantly white populations and it is uncertain how accurate these will be when used in other ethnic groups where variation in body composition is known to exist. For example, studies have found altered body composition and lower resting metabolism, of up to 15% (~274 kcal/day) in African American women [7]. Little is also known about the prediction accuracy of commonly used equations in older age groups [8]. Likewise although overweight and obese individuals have been included in some reference populations it is unclear how much of a contribution their data has made to the final equation. These limitations have important implications for the use of equations, particularly with individuals, and highlight the importance of using clinical judgement as well as appropriate monitoring and response to treatment.

14.4.1.2 Choosing a prediction equation

Predictive equations are less accurate when used to estimate resting metabolism in obese compared to non obese individuals and this may be even greater in those with severe obesity. One validation study found 70% of obese individuals had metabolic rates accurately predicted compared to 82% in non-obese individuals, when accuracy was defined as the predicted value within 10% of the measured [9]. Part of the difficulty in accurately predicting resting metabolism in obese individuals relates to changing body composition with weight gain. As obesity develops, fat tissue increases disproportionally and what is unclear is the extent to which this excess weight is metabolically active. Debate continues on the appropriateness of using adjusted versus actual weight to modulate for these body composition changes [10].

Although there is undoubtedly variation in the accuracy of prediction equations in the obese, a systematic review and recent report by the Academy of Nutrition and Dietetics concluded that the Mifflin-St Jeor equation [11] (Table 14.1) was the most accurate in determining RMR for US individuals when compared against three other common equations (Harris Benedict, Owen and Schofield equations) [12–14]. A validation study in Belgian comparing normal weight to obese women

Table 14.1 **Mifflin-St Jeor Equations**

Men: RMR = (9.99 × weight) + (6.25 × height) − (4.92 × age) + 5
Women: RMR = (9.99 × weight) + (6.25 × height) − (4.92 × age) − 161
Equations use weight in kilograms (kg), height in centimeters (cm).

also found the Mifflin equation to be one of the most accurate in the overweight group although in severe obesity the Siervo equation performed best [15]. The American Dietetic Association has recommended the Mifflin-St Jeor equation as the most suitable for use with obese individuals and this has been adopted by their Nutrition Care Manual [12]. A recent review by the British Dietetic Association also suggested the Mifflin equation predicted resting metabolic rate more accurately in more obese individuals than other equations (Madden *et al.*, personal communication).

The Mifflin-St Jeor equation was derived from a population that included healthy weight, overweight and obese individuals although there was limited representation from older age groups and ethnicity was not reported [11]. It produced fewer inaccurate predictions in obese individuals compared to other equations although there are likely to be limitations associated with its use in older individuals and certain ethnic groups [13].

The equation produces more underestimates of RMR than overestimates, with a maximum underestimate of 20% and maximum overestimate of 15% of measured RMR [9]. It is important to consider the impact this may have on treatment outcomes although given its tendency to under rather than overestimate energy requirements this lessens concerns about advising an energy prescription above energy needs.

It is important to recognize that, even using the most accurate prediction equation, approximately 20% of patients are likely to have a predicted RMR below the accepted level of accuracy [13] and therefore monitoring treatment response and adjusting dietary plans accordingly will be critical. In evaluating treatment response consideration should also be given to the range and complexity of factors which influence an individual's ability to change their eating behaviour of which knowledge and understanding of energy requirements for weight loss and associated food changes is only one aspect.

14.4.2 *Determining physical activity level [PAL]*

The term physical activity describes a complex set of behaviours which encompass routine lifestyle activities as well as structured exercise [16]. Measuring such complex behaviours in a research setting is challenging and estimating in clinical practice is even more difficult. Given there are currently no precise measures of activity energy expenditure which can be used in the outpatient setting this represents a substantial source of error in estimating energy needs for some obese individuals.

Table 14.2 Distribution of Physical Activity Level [21]

Typical activity (median) = 1.63
Less active (25th centile) = 1.49
More active (75th centile) = 1.78

Physical activity is the most variable component of total energy expenditure with estimates in the free living population suggesting contributions ranging from 20–50% [17]. Some of this variability may be accounted for by factors such as body weight and fitness levels with obese individuals generally having a higher energy cost for a given activity [18]. A comprehensive summary of the energy costs of individual activities have been previously published [19].

The Physical Activity Level or PAL ascribes a numerical value to activity which represents multiples of BMR such that PAL=TEE/RMR. These values have been formulated from studies where measures of resting metabolism using indirect calorimetry are combined with total energy expenditure from doubly labelled water. The range of PAL values for the general population ranges from 1.38 in the most sedentary (immobile) groups to 2.5 in the very active groups [20]. Recent evidence from a contemporary US population, which included 60% of subjects defined as overweight or obese, found a median PAL value of 1.63 and probably represents a light activity population. The group with below-average activity had a PAL value of 1.49 and those with above average activity a PAL of 1.78 [21–23] (Table 14.2). Interestingly, mean PAL values in different BMI categories have not been found to differ significantly and BMI was not a significant explanatory factor in the variation of PAL [21]. It is important to remember these are population-derived PAL values and although these represent the best current estimate, using with individuals will inevitably introduce errors of unknown magnitude.

Increasing activity in line with recent recommendations for health improvement would increase PAL by 0.15 if 30 minutes of moderate intensity activity on 5 or more days a week was undertaken and by 0.3 with 60 minutes of active sport [24].

14.5   Magnitude of energy deficit

Various factors may influence the level of energy deficit chosen including starting BMI, co-morbidities and risk factors, previous dieting experience, patient preference and perceived capacity to implement various changes. One of the key factors influencing the chosen energy deficit is the target weight loss outcome. In those with a BMI below 35 kg/m2, where associated co-morbidities are less likely, and a 5–10% weight loss target is appropriate, a modest energy deficit of 500–600 kcal/day may be sufficient. However for those with severe and complex obesity a greater energy deficit of 600–1000 kcal/day may be more appropriate given the likelihood of associated co-morbidities and the need to reduce weight beyond 10% to see improvement in associated disease or dysfunction.

14.6 Practical worked example of prescribed energy calculations

Table 14.3 shows a practical worked example of how to calculate energy requirements for weight loss in a theorectical case. It is assumed that reducing daily calorie intake by 500–600 kcal below estimated energy requirement will equate to a 3500 kcal deficit over 7 days equivalent to a theoretical 0.5 kg/1 lb weekly weight loss [36]. Although there are clearly limitations to this assumption due to the metabolic adaption associated with weight loss it does provide a baseline energy prescription from which adjustments can be made depending on treatment response.

Sharing information with patients on their calculated energy prescription may be helpful in improving their understanding of daily energy needs for weight loss and putting food choices and portion size changes into perspective. The skill of the practitioner is critical in collaboratively conveying this information in a helpful and practical way which the patient can understand and which takes account of their preferences and needs. It is common for this energy prescription to be divided into allowances/portions/points from various food groups so a detailed food plan can be developed between the patient and practitioner. This can form the basis of discussions regarding portion sizes and their contribution to energy intake and with the aid of food photographs can help patients visualise the limitations needed to the daily energy intake.

Table 14.4 converts the calorie prescription into food portions from the six food groups (sometimes referred to as exchanges/points/units/servings). Using the previous worked example a dietary plan of 2400 kcal would translate into

   10 starch
    9 fruit and vegetables
    3 meat or other protein foods
    4 milk and dairy
    4 fats
  260 kcal/day allowance for high fat and/or high sugar foods or alcoholic drinks

Lists are then provided which describe what one serving/unit/point from each food group consists of and ideally food photographs are incorporated to provide a visual

Table 14.3 Worked example

Male aged 45, BMI=42, weight=135 kg, height=1.8 m. Presents with severe osteoarthritis with poor mobility

1. Predict RMR [Mifflin-St Jeor equation used]
   RMR=(1349)+(1125)−(221)+5=2258 kcal/day
2. Calculate total daily energy needs
   TEE=RMR × PAL
   TEE=2258 × 1.49=3364 kcal/day
3. Minus energy deficit ~ 600–1000 kcal/day

Energy prescription for weight loss ~ 2400 kcal/day

Table 14.4 **Food group allocation based on daily energy prescription**

Daily energy prescription	Starch (80 kcal)	Fruit/veg (40 kcal)	Protein foods (140 kcal)	Fats (50 kcal)	Dairy foods (90 kcal)	Extras (kcal/day)
1200	5	5	2	1	3	0
1300	5	5	2	2	3	50
1400	5	5	2	2	3	150
1500	6	6	2	2	3	130
1600	6	6	2	3	3	180
1700	7	7	2	3	3	160
1800	8	7	2	3	3	180
1900	8	8	2	3	3	240
2000	8	8	3	3	3	200
2100	9	8	3	3	3	220
2200	9	9	3	3	3	280
2300	9	9	3	3	4	290
2400	10	9	3	4	4	260
2500	10	10	3	4	4	320
2600	11	10	3	4	4	340
2700	12	11	3	4	4	320
2800	13	11	3	4	4	340
2900	14	12	3	4	4	320
3000	15	12	3	4	4	340

Adapted and reproduced with kind permission from NDR-UK Ref: 9262 www.ndr-uk.org

guide to food servings. A comprehensive food portion picture guide is available from nutrition and diet resources (www.ndr-uk.org). Using a behavioural approach, a practitioner can work with individuals to develop individualized meal plans and strategies to monitor and change long-term eating habits.

14.6.1 Recognising the difference between predicted and actual weight loss

According to the calculations above, a 600 kcal deficit diet should result in weekly 0.5 kg weight loss leading to 6-month losses of 10–12 kg. However in reality the observed weight loss is well below predicted values, with individuals typically losing less than half their predicted weight [25]. It has been well documented that conventional dietary treatments including the 600 kcal deficit diet are associated with modest, albeit clinically important, weight loss. Studies consistently show weight losses over a 12-month treatment programme are rarely beyond 5–10 kg [26,27], with lowest weights observed between 26–52 weeks [28,29] often followed by partial or complete weight regain.

The reasons for such a discrepancy between predicted and actual weight losses are important, should be considered in the ongoing adjustment of dietary plans, and highlight the complexity of factors that influence weight change. It is important to recognize the physiological mechanisms linked with energy restriction, with compensatory energy conservation negatively affecting weight loss outcomes. Such mechanisms include a decline in resting energy expenditure mainly due to loss of metabolically active tissue [30], a fall in the energy cost of activity as the size of the body decreases [31] and an increase in appetite. Although a 600 kcal deficit may produce ongoing weight loss for a number of weeks, in time a new energy balance equilibrium will be reached, as energy expenditure falls in response to dieting and may require energy prescriptions to be recalculated and adjusted to account for this decline [32]. Likewise if there is poor weight loss in response to an advised energy prescription it may be helpful to increase the magnitude of the advised energy deficit given the known inaccuracies in energy requirement predictions for some individuals.

14.6.2 Evidence from use of defined energy diets in practice

In a systematic review of obesity treatments in adults, with at least 12 months follow-up, 600 kcal deficit diets were associated with a weight loss of 5.31 kg after one year with improvements in risk factors and weight loss continuing for three years [26]. These findings are markedly different from those observed in anti-obesity drug trials where the 600 kcal deficit diet forms part of the placebo treatment but is not the primary intervention. Higher dropout rates and poorer weight loss outcomes in these placebo groups may reflect differences in the type of participant recruited to such studies with greater numbers of severe and complex individuals suggesting differences in responsiveness to this intervention [33,34].

Limited evidence is available on the comparative effectiveness of defined versus fixed energy diets although there may be some effect on adherence. In a hospital dietetic clinic greater weight losses were found in the tailored energy prescription group compared to those advised on a 1200 kcal diet [2], however this study was limited by its non randomized design and short treatment duration. Fewer programme drop outs and better adherence have been observed in a workplace randomized controlled trial comparing a fixed 1500 kcal diet with tailored energy prescriptions, although no significant difference in weight loss between the groups was observed [35].

14.7   Conclusion

Defined energy prescriptions provide a useful starting point for discussion on portion control and may help patients visualize the extent of dietary change required. They will not suit everyone but may be particularly helpful in those who have tried *ad libitum* dietary approaches with limited success and who need additional guidance on portion size and quantities of food to choose from different food groups. More research is needed to understand the relative effectiveness of defined energy prescriptions versus other dietary treatments and to improve understanding of who does best with this dietary treatment.

References

1. Livingstone MB, Prentice AM, Strain JJ, Coward WA, Black AE, Barker ME, *et al.* Accuracy of weighed dietary records in studies of diet and health. *BMJ* 1990; 300(6726): 708–12.
2. Frost G, Masters K, King C, Kelly M, Hasan U, Heavens P, *et al.* A new method of energy prescription to improve weight loss. *Journal of Human Nutrition and Dietetics* 2007; 20(3): 152–6.
3. Rosado E, Kaippert V, Santiago de Brito R (2013) Energy expenditure measured by indirect calorimetry in obesity. In: A Elkordy (editor) *Applications of Calorimetry, Isothermal Titration Calorimetry and Microcalorimetry.* www.intechopen.com/books/applications-of-calorimetry-in-a-wide-context-differential-scanning-calorimetry-isothermal-titration-calorimetry-and-microcalorimetry/energy-expenditure-measured-by-indirect-calorimetry-in-obesity
4. Ravussin E, Bogardus C. A brief overview of human energy metabolism and its relationship to essential obesity. *American Journal of Clinical Nutrition* 1992; 55(1 Suppl): S242–5.
5. Judges D, Knight A, Graham E, Goff LM. Estimating energy requirements in hospitalised underweight and obese patients requiring nutritional support: a survey of dietetic practice in the United Kingdom. *European Journal of Clinical Nutrition* 2012; 66(3): 394–8.
6. Kross EK, Sena M, Schmidt K, Stapleton RD. A comparison of predictive equations of energy expenditure and measured energy expenditure in critically ill patients. *Journal of Critical Care* 2012; 27(3): 321, e5–12.
7. Foster GD, Wadden TA, Swain RM, Anderson DA, Vogt RA. Changes in resting energy expenditure after weight loss in obese African American and white women. *American Journal of Clinical Nutrition* 1999; 69(1): 13–17.
8. Forman JN, Miller WC, Szymanski LM, Fernhall B. Differences in resting metabolic rates of inactive obese African-American and Caucasian women. *International Journal of Obesity and Related Metabolic Disorders* 1998; 22(3): 215–21.
9. Frankenfield DC, Rowe WA, Smith JS, Cooney RN. Validation of several established equations for resting metabolic rate in obese and nonobese people. *Journal of the American Dietetic Association* 2003; 103(9): 1152–9.
10. Weg M, Watson J, Kleges R, Clemens L, Slawson D, McClanahan B. Development and cross validation of a prediction equation for estimating resting energy expenditure in healthy African-American and European-American women. *European Journal of Clinical Nutrition* 2004; 58: 474–80.
11. Mifflin MD, St Jeor ST, Hill LA, Scott BJ, Daugherty SA, Koh YO. A new predictive equation for resting energy expenditure in healthy individuals. *American Journal of Clinical Nutrition* 1990; 51(2): 241–7.
12. Academy of Nutrition and Dietetics. *Nutrition Care Manual.* www.nutritioncaremanual.org 2011
13. Frankenfield D, Roth-Yousey L, Compher C. Comparison of predictive equations for resting metabolic rate in healthy nonobese and obese adults: a systematic review. *Journal of the American Dietetic Association* 2005; 105(5): 775–89.

14. Weijs PJ. Validity of predictive equations for resting energy expenditure in US and Dutch overweight and obese class I and II adults aged 18–65 y. *American Journal of Clinical Nutrition* 2008; 88(4): 959–70.
15. Weijs PJ, Vansant GA. Validity of predictive equations for resting energy expenditure in Belgian normal weight to morbid obese women. *Clinical Nutrition* 2010; 29(3): 347–51.
16. Wareham NJ, Rennie KL. The assessment of physical activity in individuals and populations: why try to be more precise about how physical activity is assessed? *International Journal of Obesity and Related Metabolic Disorders* 1998; 22 (Suppl 2):S30–8.
17. Westerterp KR. Alterations in energy balance with exercise. *American Journal of Clinical Nutrition* 1998; 68(4): S970–4.
18. Haggarty P, Valencia M, McNeill G, Gonzales N, Moya S. Energy expenditure during heavy work and its interaction with body weight. *British Journal of Nutrition* 1997; 77: 359–73.
19. Vaz M, Karaolis N, Draper A, Shetty P. A compilation of energy costs of physical activities. *Public Health Nutrition* 2005; 8(7A): 1153–83.
20. Schutz Y. Role of substrate utilization and thermogenesis on body-weight control with particular reference to alcohol. *Proceedings of the Nutrition Society* 2000; 59(4): 511–17.
21. Scientific Advisory Committee on Nutrition. *Dietary Reference Values for Energy*. London: TSO, 2011.
22. Subar AF, Kipnis V, Troiano RP, Midthune D, Schoeller DA, Bingham S, *et al.* Using intake biomarkers to evaluate the extent of dietary misreporting in a large sample of adults: the OPEN study. *American Journal of Epidemiology* 2003; 158(1): 1–13.
23. Tooze JA, Schoeller DA, Subar AF, Kipnis V, Schatzkin A, Troiano RP. Total daily energy expenditure among middle-aged men and women: the OPEN Study. *American Journal of Clinical Nutrition* 2007; 86(2): 382–7.
24. Institute of Medicine. *Dietary Reference Intakes for Energy, Carbohydrate, Fibre, Fat, Fatty Acids, Cholesterol, Protein and Amino Acids*. Washington DC: National Academy Press, 2005.
25. Heymsfield SB, Harp JB, Reitman ML, Beetsch JW, Schoeller DA, Erondu N, *et al.* Why do obese patients not lose more weight when treated with low-calorie diets? A mechanistic perspective. *American Journal of Clinical Nutrition* 2007; 85(2): 346–54.
26. Avenell A, Broom J, Brown T. Systematic review of the long term effects and economic consequences of treatments for obesity and implications for health improvement. *Health Technology Assessment* 2004; 8: 1–182.
27. Stunkard A, Mc L-HM. The results of treatment for obesity: a review of the literature and report of a series. *AMA Archives of Internal Medicine* 1959; 103(1): 79–85.
28. Heshka S, Anderson JW, Atkinson RL, Greenway FL, Hill JO, Phinney SD, *et al.* Weight loss with self-help compared with a structured commercial program: a randomized trial. *JAMA* 2003; 289(14): 1792–8.
29. Torgerson JS, Hauptman J, Boldrin MN, Sjostrom L. XENical in the prevention of diabetes in obese subjects (XENDOS) study: a randomized study of orlistat as an adjunct to lifestyle changes for the prevention of type 2 diabetes in obese patients. *Diabetes Care* 2004; 27(1): 155–61.
30. Gallagher D, Belmonte D, Deurenberg P, Wang Z, Krasnow N, Pi-Sunyer FX, *et al.* Organ-tissue mass measurement allows modeling of REE and metabolically active tissue mass. *American Journal of Physiology* 1998; 275(2 Pt 1): E249–58.
31. Levine JA. Non-exercise activity thermogenesis (NEAT). *Nutrition Reviews* 2004; 62 (7 Pt 2): S82–97.

32. Kozusko F. The effects of body composition on setpoint based weight loss. *Math Comput Model* 2002; 35: 973–82.
33. Brown TJ, Avenell A. Adherence to dietary advice in weight-reduction drug trials. *Lancet* 2005; 366(9500): 1847–8.
34. Esposito K, Giugliano D. Effect of Rimonabant on weight reduction and cardiovascular risk. *Lancet* 2005; 366(9483): 367–8; author reply 9–70.
35. Leslie WS, Lean ME, Baillie HM, Hankey CR. Weight management: a comparison of existing dietary approaches in a work-site setting. *International Journal of Obesity and Related Metabolic Disorders* 2002; 26(11): 1469–75.
36. Pietrobelli A, Allison DB, Heshka S, Heo M, Wang ZM, Bertkau A, *et al.* Sexual dimorphism in the energy content of weight change. *IJO* 2002; 26(10): 1339–48.

Meal replacements for the treatment of obesity

P. Clifton
University of South Australia, Adelaide, SA, Australia

15.1   Introduction

A meal replacement is defined as a commercially available, over the counter product (either liquid, powder or snack bar), fortified with minerals and vitamins designed to replace one or two meals per day with at least one meal consumed as normal food, for example meat and vegetables and consumed as part of an energy restricted diet (4200–6600 kJ).

Very low calorie diets (VLCD) or very low energy diets (VLED) are defined as total diet replacements with less than 800 kcal and more than 400 to 450 kcal/d (about 3400–4000 kJ). Diets consisting of between 800 and 1200 kcal/d are classified as low calorie diets or low energy diets (LCD or LED). A variant of the LED is to use 3 meal replacements/day plus 2 snacks as well as 5 serves of fruit and vegetables with no 'normal meals'. For total replacement of normal nutrition one needs to ensure the products contain all the vitamins, minerals and protein required each day. In most countries these are tightly regulated.

VLCDs have been widely used since the 1970s, usually under medical supervision in the USA, but a much more common approach now is the use of partial meal replacement which has been promoted by widespread direct to consumer marketing. This chapter will examine the evidence for the use of VLCDs versus LCDs or partial meal replacement for long-term weight loss with or without intensive follow up, their role in people with Type 2 diabetes and metabolic syndrome and whether the composition and timing of the meal replacement matters.

15.2   Very low calorie diet (VLCD) versus partial meal replacement or controlled diet

The National Institutes of Health National Task Force on the Prevention and Treatment of Obesity in 1991 [1] concluded that VLCD long term was no better than any other form of weight loss method despite initial weight losses of 20 kg over 12–16 weeks but Wim Saris in 2001 [2] wrote after a review of 9 randomised trials: 'There is evidence that a greater initial weight loss using VLCDs with an active

Managing and Preventing Obesity. http://dx.doi.org/10.1533/9781782420996.4.223

follow-up weight-maintenance program, including behavior therapy, nutritional education and exercise, improves weight maintenance' but he found no difference in weight loss between diets containing 400 and 800 kcal. However Tsai and Wadden in 2006 [3] examined trials that compared VLCDs and LCDs and found VLCDs induced greater initial weight loss (16% versus 9.75% of initial weight) but long-term results (>1 year after maximum weight loss) were not statistically different (6.3% vs 5.2%).

In the STOP Regain trial, 186 volunteers who had achieved at least a 10% weight loss over the last 2 years were enrolled in an 18 month trial of face to face, internet or newsletter support. The approaches used were very low calorie diet (VLCD; n=24), commercial program (n=95), or self-guided approach (n=67). At baseline, individuals who had used a VLCD had achieved a weight loss of 24% of their maximum weight within the past 2 years compared to 17% achieved by those who had used the other approaches (P < 0.001). However, individuals who had used a VLCD regained significantly more weight than the other two groups and by 6 months there were no significant differences in overall percent weight loss. In contrast, individuals who had used a self-guided approach maintained their weight losses from baseline through 18 months [4].

In a primary care trial in Sweden 20 men and 57 women completed a VLCD with weight loss of 20 kg and 15.7 kg respectively. At 1 year weight loss was 10.5 kg and after 2 years 5.2 kg with 22 dropouts in total [5]. Vogels and colleagues [6] followed 103 subjects for 2 years after VLCD. Weight loss was relatively small with the VLCD at 7 kg and at 2 years weight loss was only 2 kg but the study had no contrasting control group. Weight regain occurred mostly in those with lower initial fat mass.

In conclusion there has been no recent data to overturn the 1991 NIH conclusion that the cost and inconvenience of VLCD outweigh the long-term benefit in most people and that similar results at 2 years can be achieved with less restrictive methods. In the USA VLCD is usually closely medically supervised whereas in Europe and Australia this does not need to occur and thus VLCD is less costly than in the USA.

15.3   Meal replacement as part of a low calorie diet (LCD) versus conventional diet

We reviewed this area in 2005 [7]. Heysmfield and colleagues [8] pooled 6 studies that compared partial meal replacement with a conventional reduced calorie diet of the same energy level. Body weight reduction was 7–8% in the meal replacement group at 1 year and this was 2.5 kg greater than the recommended diet.

In a general practice setting Wadden and co-workers [9] compared usual care (4 visits/year to discuss weight management) with lifestyle coaching which added monthly counselling to usual care and enhanced lifestyle counselling which added meal replacements or sibutramine or orlistat to the lifestyle coaching. Those using meal replacements with no exposure to sibutramine (n=67) had a weight loss of 4.4 kg at 2 years which was not statistically different from the lifestyle coaching group which had a weight loss of 2.9 kg (n=131). The meal replacements were substituted for 2 meals and one snack for 4 months and then one meal and one snack thereafter.

A variant of the LED is to use 3 meal replacements/day plus 2 snacks as well as 5 serves of fruit and vegetables. With this regime, along with behavioural therapy and exercise a weight loss of 13.7 kg can be achieved at 24 weeks (n=18) compared with 0.7 kg in the control group (n=13) [10]. Long-term data is required for this approach in adults.

In adolescents, use of a regime that incorporates 3 shakes/day plus 1 prepackaged meal and 5 serves of fruit and vegetables/day led to a weight loss of 6.3% compared to 3.8% for a control diet for 4 months, but continued use for the next 8 months did not maintain this difference and at 12 months weight loss was only 3.4% in both [11].

15.4   Type 2 diabetes

There are few studies of meal replacement LCD or VLCD available in this group with or without comparator control groups with follow up for 2 years or more. Both Wing and colleagues [12] and Henry and Gumbiner [13] noted that despite weight regain long-term glucose benefits were seen in people with diabetes using VLCD while Wing and co-workers did not feel the benefit of intermittent VLCD over one year in diabetes justified the cost [14]. People with diabetes however may lose less fat with VLCD than non diabetic subjects even though the same weight loss over 6 months (8.5–9.4 kg) has been achieved [15].

15.4.1 VLCD

Snel and colleagues [16] conducted a 16 week VLCD and VLCD plus exercise study in 27 obese (BMI 37) insulin treated people with type 2 diabetes and followed them up for 18 months. Short-term weight loss was 23–27 kg with more fat mass lost in the exercise group. Insulin-stimulated glucose disposal was more than doubled in both groups and HbA1c fell by 1.3%. Quality of life improved in both groups and in the exercise group at 18 months was no different from lean or obese controls but in the VLCD only group most of the scales were inferior to the controls [17]. At 18 months there was a 12 and 14 kg weight regain with no difference between groups, although IL10 and IL8 remained lower than baseline levels as did pericardial fat volumes [18,19]. In a 5 year study Paisey [20] compared a conventional diet to VLCD and found a weight loss of 8.9 k in the conventional diet group versus 4.8 kg in the VLCD group but the numbers were small (15 in each group commenced–number at 5 years not stated).

15.4.2 LCD

Foster and co-workers [21] compared the effect of a portion controlled diet with 9 sessions of diabetes self management advice to the advice alone and found individuals on the portion controlled diet lost 7.3 kg and their Hba1c was lowered by 0.7% compared with 2.2 kg and 0.4% respectively over a 6 month period. Cheskins and colleagues [22] tested 199 participants with Type 2 diabetes with meal replacements or controlled diet (both with frequent educational sessions) at 75% of estimated energy requirements for 34 weeks with 1 year follow up thereafter. At 34 weeks about 40% achieved >5% weight loss on the meal replacement diet and 12% on the controlled diet (weight loss of 7.3 kg vs 4.7 kg with only 40% still in the study) with better retention and ease of use with the meal replacements. Weight loss at 86 weeks was 5.6 and 4.7 kg but only 20% of participants remained in the study. We performed a 6 month study [23] and found a disappointing result with meal replacements without professional assistance. Consumption of 2 meal replacements for 3 months and 1 meal replacement for the subsequent 3 months led to weight loss of 5.5 kg (5%) and a 0.26% decrease in HbA1c while a diet book group had a weight loss of 3 kg (3%) (p=0.027 for difference between groups) and a decrease in HbA1c of 0.15% (between group ns) in those who completed the 6-month study. There was a high dropout rate in both groups (30%). In a 12-month study [24], in 104 subjects weight loss was 4.6% with meal replacements and 2.3% in the individual diet plan (p < 0.05). HbA1c was 0.5% lower in the meal replacement group (p < 0.05) and a greater number of subjects in this group reduced their medication. Using one meal replacement plus monthly lifestyle advice for 12-months was relatively ineffective with a 1.6 kg weight loss versus 0.6 kg weight loss in the control group in 84 Chinese subjects with abnormal glucose tolerance, although normal glucose tolerance was achieved more often in the meal replacement group [25]. Dichsuneit [26] reported on his group's experience in patients with Type 2 diabetes. After 6 and 12 months, patients in the meal replacement group achieved on average a weight loss of 5.24 and 4.35% of their initial body weight, respectively. In contrast, after 6 and 12 months, patients on the individualised diet plan achieved on average a weight loss of 2.85 and 2.36% of their initial body weight, respectively.

Meal replacements were used in the LOOK Ahead study, (5145 participants with Type 2 diabetes) along with exercise and behavioural modification. Intensive lifestyle participants lost 8.6% of initial weight, compared to 0.7% for standard treatment (p < 0.001). For the year, intensive lifestyle participants attended an average of 35.4 treatment sessions and reported exercising a mean of 136.6 min/week and consuming a total of 361 meal replacement products. Greater self-reported physical activity was the strongest correlate of weight loss, followed by treatment attendance and consumption of meal replacements. After 9.6 years weight loss was 6% compared with 3.5% [27]. Overall there was no difference in cardiac endpoints in the two groups [28].

Meal replacements seem to be useful over 6 months in Type 2 diabetes but apart from the LOOK Ahead study there is little long term data. LOOK Ahead required intensive intervention and would not be replicated in usual care.

VLCD may have persistent effects on glucose metabolism at 2 years despite weight regain.

15.5   Composition of meal replacements

15.5.1 High protein vs normal protein

Meal replacements that deliver 2.2 kg of protein/kg of lean body mass per day were no different in effectiveness compared with isocaloric replacements delivering 1.1 g/kg with a weight loss of 4.3 vs 4.7 kg at 12 months with 1 meal replacement and 1 snack for 3 months followed by 1 meal replacement for 9 months [29]. A similar result was found by Flechtner-Mors and colleagues [30] who delivered 1.34 g/kg/d over 12 months in protein-enriched meal replacements and bars which produced a weight loss of 11.8 kg (n = 31). The control group (n = 43) used conventional diet for 3 months and 1 standard meal replacement for 9 months with a protein intake of 0.8 g/kg/d with a difference in protein intake of about 30 g/d. The weight loss over 12 months was 6.9 kg. The weight change from 3 to 12 months when both groups were using 1 meal replacement was 3 kg in the protein-enriched arm and 2.7 kg in the normal protein arm. Soenen and co-workers [31] also demonstrated similar results over 6 months.

15.5.2 Protein type

In short term studies the protein composition of the meal replacement, i.e. whether soy versus casein, did not matter over 16 weeks [32]. Subjects were instructed to consume 3 shakes, 1 prepackaged entrée, and 5 servings of fruits or vegetables daily to achieve an energy intake of 4.5 to 5.0 MJ/d. Weight loss was 12.8% vs 14%. No difference was seen between milk-based and soy-based meal replacements [33].

15.5.3 Frequency

Williams and colleagues [34] compared a complicated regime of 1 day of VLCD every week for 15 weeks versus 5 days of VLCD every 5 weeks with a 1500–1800 kcal diet at other times versus 1500–1800 kcal continuously in people with Type 2 DM. Greater weight loss occurred in the VLCD groups and better glucose control was obtained in the 5-day VLCD group. There was no long term follow-up after the 20 weeks to see if the advantages persisted.

15.6   Summary

Although the short-term effects of VLCD are excellent with weight losses of 23–27 kg even in people with Type 2 diabetes with sustained reductions in blood glucose, in the latter group long-term results are no different from less intensive regimes of partial meal replacement. However the LOOK Ahead study would suggest that the use of meal replacements leads to better long-term weight loss, especially when combined with exercise, compared with standard dietary advice so meal replacements could be used liberally to aid compliance to a reduced energy diet.

References

1. [No authors listed] Very low-calorie diets. National Task Force on the Prevention and Treatment of Obesity, National Institutes of Health. *JAMA* 1993; 270(8): 967–74.
2. Saris WH. Very-low-calorie diets and sustained weight loss. *Obes Res.* 2001; 9 (Suppl 4): S295–301. Review.
3. Tsai AG, Wadden TA. The evolution of very-low-calorie diets: an update and meta-analysis. *Obesity (Silver Spring)* 2006; 14(8): 1283–93.
4. Marinilli Pinto A, Gorin AA, Raynor HA, Tate DF, Fava JL, Wing RR. Successful weight-loss maintenance in relation to method of weight loss. *Obesity (Silver Spring)* 2008 16(11): 2456–61. doi: 10.1038/oby.2008.364. Epub 14 Aug 2008.
5. Wikstrand I, Torgerson J, Boström KB. Very low calorie diet (VLCD) followed by a randomized trial of corset treatment for obesity in primary care. *Scand J Prim Health Care* 2010; 28(2): 89–94. doi: 10.3109/02813431003778540.
6. Vogels N, Westerterp-Plantenga MS. Successful long-term weight maintenance: a 2-year follow-up. *Obesity (Silver Spring)* 2007; 15(5): 1258–66.
7. Keogh JB, Clifton PM. The role of meal replacements in obesity treatment. *Obes Rev* 2005; 6(3): 229–34. Review.
8. Heymsfield SB, van Mierlo CA, van der Knaap HC, Heo M, Frier HI. Weight management using a meal replacement strategy: meta and pooling analysis from six studies. *Int J Obes Relat Metab Disord* 2003; 5: 537–49.
9. Wadden TA, Volger S, Sarwer DB, Vetter ML, Tsai AG, Berkowitz RI, Kumanyika S, Schmitz KH, Diewald LK, Barg R, Chittams J, Moore RH. A two-year randomized trial of obesity treatment in primary care practice. *N Engl J Med* 2011; 365(21): 1969–79. doi: 10.1056/NEJMoa1109220. Epub 14 Nov 2011.
10. Anderson JW, Reynolds LR, Bush HM, Rinsky JL, Washnock C. Effect of a behavioral/nutritional intervention program on weight loss in obese adults: a randomized controlled trial. *Postgrad Med* 2011 123(5): 205–13. doi: 10.3810/pgm.2011.09.2476.
11. Berkowitz RI, Wadden TA, Gehrman CA, Bishop-Gilyard CT, Moore RH, Womble LG, Cronquist JL, Trumpikas NL, Levitt Katz LE, Xanthopoulos MS. Meal replacements in the treatment of adolescent obesity: a randomized controlled trial. *Obesity (Silver Spring)* 2011; 19(6): 1193–9. doi: 10.1038/oby.2010.288. Epub 9 Dec 2010.
12. Wing RR, Marcus MD, Salata R, Epstein LH, Miaskiewicz S, Blair EH. Effects of a very-low-calorie diet on long-term glycemic control in obese type 2 diabetic subjects. *Arch Intern Med* 1991; 151(7): 1334–40
13. Henry RR, Gumbiner B. Benefits and limitations of very-low-calorie diet therapy in obese NIDDM. *Diabetes Care* 1991; 14(9): 802–23. Review.
14. Wing RR, Blair E, Marcus M, Epstein LH, Harvey J. Year-long weight loss treatment for obese patients with type II diabetes: does including an intermittent very-low-calorie diet improve outcome? *Am J Med* 1994; 97(4): 354–62.
15. Baker ST, Jerums G, Prendergast LA, Panagiotopoulos S, Strauss BJ, Proietto J. Less fat reduction per unit weight loss in type 2 diabetic compared with nondiabetic obese

individuals completing a very-low-calorie diet program. *Metabolism* 2012; 61(6): 873–82. doi: 10.1016/j.metabol.2011.10.017. Epub 5 Dec 2011.

16. Snel M, Gastaldelli A, Ouwens DM, Hesselink MK, Schaart G, *et al.* Effects of adding exercise to a 16-week very low-calorie diet in obese, insulin-dependent type 2 diabetes mellitus patients. *J Clin Endocrinol Metab* 2012; 97(7): 2512–20. doi: 10.1210/jc.2011-3178. Epub 8 May 2012.

17. Snel M, Sleddering MA, Vd Peijl ID, Romijn JA, Pijl H, *et al.* Quality of life in type 2 diabetes mellitus after a very low calorie diet and exercise. *Eur J Intern Med* 2012, 23(2): 143–9. doi: 10.1016/j.ejim.2011.07.004. Epub 17 Aug 2011.

18. Snel M, van Diepen JA, Stijnen T, Pijl H, Romijn JA, *et al.* Immediate and long-term effects of addition of exercise to a 16-week very low calorie diet on low-grade inflammation in obese, insulin-dependent type 2 diabetic patients. *Food Chem Toxicol* 2011; 49(12): 3104–11. doi: 10.1016/j.fct.2011.09.032. Epub 5 Oct 2011.

19. Snel M, Jonker JT, Hammer S, Kerpershoek G, Lamb HJ, *et al.* Long-term beneficial effect of a 16-week very low calorie diet on pericardial fat in obese type 2 diabetes mellitus patients. *Obesity (Silver Spring).* 2012; 20(8): 1572–6. doi: 10.1038/oby.2011.390. Epub 26 Jan 2012 .

20. Paisey RB, Frost J, Harvey P, Paisey A, Bower L, *et al.* Five year results of a prospective very low calorie diet or conventional weight loss programme in type 2 diabetes. *J Hum Nutr Diet* 2002; 15(2): 121–7.

21. Foster GD, Wadden TA, Lagrotte CA, Vander Veur SS, Hesson LA, *et al.* A randomized comparison of a commercially available portion-controlled weight-loss intervention with a diabetes self-management education program. *Nutr Diabetes* 2013; 3: e63. doi: 10.1038/nutd.2013.3

22. .Cheskin LJ, Mitchell AM, Jhaveri AD, Mitola AH, Davis LM, *et al.* Efficacy of meal replacements versus a standard food-based diet for weight loss in type 2 diabetes: a controlled clinical trial. *Diabetes Educ* 2008; 34(1): 118–27. doi: 10.1177/0145721707312463.

23. Keogh JB, Clifton PM Meal replacements for weight loss in type 2 diabetes in a community setting. *J Nutr Metab* 2012; 2012: 918571. doi: 10.1155/2012/918571. Epub 2 Oct 2012.

24. Li Z, Hong K, Saltsman P, DeShields S, Bellman M, *et al.* Long-term efficacy of soy-based meal replacements vs an individualized diet plan in obese type II DM patients: relative effects on weight loss, metabolic parameters, and C-reactive protein. *Eur J Clin Nutr* 2005; 59(3): 411–8.

25. Xu DF, Sun JQ, Chen M, Chen YQ, Xie H, *et al.* Effects of lifestyle intervention and meal replacement on glycaemic and body-weight control in Chinese subjects with impaired glucose regulation: a 1-year randomised controlled trial. *Br J Nutr* 2012; 5: 1–6 (Epub ahead of print).

26. Ditschuneit HH Do meal replacement drinks have a role in diabetes management? *Nestle Nutr Workshop Ser Clin Perform Programme* 2006; 11: 171–9; discussion 179–81.

27. Wadden TA, West DS, Neiberg RH, Wing RR, Ryan DH, *et al.*, for the Look AHEAD Research Group. One-year weight losses in the Look AHEAD study: factors associated with success. *Obesity (Silver Spring)* 2009; 17(4): 713–22. doi: 10.1038/oby.2008.637. Epub 29 Jan 2009.

28. The Look AHEAD Research Group: Wing RR, Bolin P, Brancati FL, Bray GA, Clark JM, Coday M *et al.* Cardiovascular effects of intensive lifestyle intervention in Type 2 diabetes. *N Engl J Med* 2013; 369(2): 145–54. doi: 10.1056/NEJMoa1212914. Epub 24 Jun 2013.

29. Li Z, Treyzon L, Chen S, Yan E, Thames G, Carpenter CL. Protein-enriched meal replacements do not adversely affect liver, kidney or bone density: an outpatient randomized controlled trial. *Nutr J.* 2010; 9: 72. doi: 10.1186/1475-2891-9-72

30. Flechtner-Mors M, Boehm BO, Wittmann R, Thoma U, Ditschuneit HH. Enhanced weight loss with protein-enriched meal replacements in subjects with the metabolic syndrome. *Diabetes Metab Res Rev* 2010; 26(5): 393–405. doi: 10.1002/dmrr.1097.

31. Soenen S, Hochstenbach-Waelen A, Westerterp-Plantenga MS. Efficacy of α-lactalbumin and milk protein on weight loss and body composition during energy restriction. *Obesity (Silver Spring)* 2011; 19(2): 370–9. doi: 10.1038/oby.2010.146. Epub 24 Jun 2010.

32. Anderson JW, Fuller J, Patterson K, Blair R, Tabor A. Soy compared to casein meal replacement shakes with energy-restricted diets for obese women: randomized controlled trial. *Metabolism* 2007; 56(2): 280–8.

33. Anderson JW, Hoie LH. Weight loss and lipid changes with low-energy diets: comparator study of milk-based versus soy-based liquid meal replacement interventions. *J Am Coll Nutr* 2005; 24(3): 210–6.

34. Williams KV, Mullen ML, Kelley DE, Wing RR. The effect of short periods of caloric restriction on weight loss and glycemic control in type 2 diabetes. *Diabetes Care* 1998; 21(1): 2–8.

Very-low-calorie diets (VLCDs) for the treatment of obesity

P. Sumithran, J. Proietto
University of Melbourne, Melbourne, VIC, Australia

16.1   Introduction

Very-low-calorie diets (VLCDs) are diets containing 3350 kilojoules (800 kilo-calories) or less per day (National Task Force on the Prevention and Treatment of Obesity, 1993). They generally take the form of meal replacement formulations, which may be used as the sole source of nutrition during a weight loss programme, and provide between 1700–3350 kilojoules (450–800 kilocalories) per day. The purpose of VLCDs is to enable rapid, substantial weight loss while maintaining an adequate intake of required nutrients. As such, they should contain at least 0.8–1.0 gram per kilogram of ideal body weight per day of high-quality protein, as well as the recommended daily allowances of essential vitamins, minerals, electro-lytes and fatty acids. A daily minimum of 50 g protein and 55 g carbohydrate has been suggested to minimise loss of lean mass during weight loss (SCOOP-VLCD Task 7.3, 2002).

16.2   Indications and contraindications for the use of very-low-calorie diets (VLCDs)

16.2.1   Indications

VLCDs may be used for the treatment of obesity (body mass index [BMI] $\geq$30 kg/ m^2) in adults, when less restrictive dietary approaches have not been successful. They may also be considered in people with BMI > 27 kg/m^2 who have medical conditions likely to improve with weight loss, such as Type 2 diabetes or obstruct-ive sleep apnoea. Although in many countries the products are widely available in pharmacies without prescription, expert panels and clinical practice guidelines recommend that VLCDs only be used under medical supervision, as part of an obesity treatment programme, which includes nutritional education and modification of lifestyle and behaviour (NH&MRC 2003, SCOOP-VLCD Task 7.3, 2002, National Task Force on the Prevention and Treatment of Obesity, 1993; Tsigos *et al.*, 2008).

Managing and Preventing Obesity. http://dx.doi.org/10.1533/9781782420996.4.231

16.2.2 Contraindications

VLCDs are contraindicated in people with increased nutritional requirements, including pregnant or lactating women, or those with a significant illness, such as systemic infection, active malignancy or severe renal or hepatic impairment. They should not be used within 3 months of major cardiovascular events, or in people with malignant arrhythmias, cerebrovascular disease, electrolyte disorders, porphyria or hereditary metabolic diseases, unstable psychiatric disorders, alcohol or drug dependence, or a history of anorexia nervosa (Mustajoki and Pekkarinen, 2001, National Task Force on the Prevention and Treatment of Obesity, 1993). VLCDs should not be used by normal weight people, as excessive lean body mass may be lost.

Relative contraindications to VLCDs include use in people with Type 1 diabetes, cholelithiasis, renal stones or gout. They are also not recommended for persons under 18 years, as children and adolescents have increased nutritional requirements. There is little information about the safety of VLCDs in people aged over 65 years, who may be at risk of losing excessive lean body mass. Furthermore, the relative increase in health risks associated with excess weight declines with age (Stevens *et al.*, 1998; Diehr *et al.*, 1998; Dey *et al.*, 2001), and it is uncertain whether weight loss is beneficial in older adults, particularly those without severe obesity (Wannamethee *et al.*, 2005). The position statement of the American Society of Nutrition and NAASO recommends against the use of VLCDs in persons ≥65 years (Villareal *et al.*, 2005). However, if the benefits of rapid weight loss are thought to outweigh the potential risks for people in the above-mentioned situations, VLCDs may be used with caution, under the supervision of a medical practitioner experienced in their use (National Task Force on the Prevention and Treatment of Obesity, 1993; Pi-Sunyer, 1992).

16.3   How to use VLCDs

VLCD products are commonly formulated as a powder to be mixed with water to make a 'milkshake', but various other presentations, including bars, soups and desserts are available. A full VLCD programme usually consists of 3 sequential phases:

1. During the *intensive* phase, the formulation is taken in place of breakfast, lunch and dinner, with an additional 2 cups per day of low-starch vegetables, to provide fibre and help satisfy the social aspect of eating. The addition of 7–10 grams of fat per day is recommended, to stimulate gallbladder contraction and reduce the risk of gallstone formation (Saris, 2001; SCOOP-VLCD TASK 7.3, 2002), and at least 2 litres of water (or calorie-free fluids) daily is advised.
2. The intensive phase is followed by a *transition*, in which regular foods are gradually reintroduced, ideally under the supervision of a dietician. Initially, 1 meal is reintroduced and 2 VLCD products continued, followed by 2 meals and one VLCD product per day.
3. The VLCD treatment is completed by reintroducing a third daily meal (*maintenance* phase).

The duration of VLCD treatment is variable, but typically ranges from 8–16 weeks for the intensive phase, and 3–8 weeks for the transition (Mustajoki and Pekkarinen, 2001; Tsai and Wadden, 2005).

In our clinical experience, patients rarely adhere to a prolonged VLCD regimen which replaces all 3 meals, and our usual practice is to use VLCD products to replace 2 meals, with a third daily meal consisting of lean protein and 2 cups of low-starch vegetables.

16.3.1 Concomitant medications

In people with Type 2 diabetes, careful self-monitoring of blood glucose is recommended, and for those treated with sulfonylureas or insulin, we usually advise a dose reduction of 50% upon commencement of the VLCD, to reduce the risk of hypoglycaemia. To minimise the risk of hypotension and electrolyte disturbances, it is recommended that diuretics are discontinued for the duration of the VLCD (Mustajoki and Pekkarinen, 2001; National Task Force on the Prevention and Treatment of Obesity, 1993).

16.4 Efficacy of VLCDs

16.4.1 Short term

Several literature reviews and meta-analyses have shown that compared with low-calorie diets (LCDs, usually containing 3350–5000 kJ (800–1200 kcal/d)), VLCDs are associated with greater initial weight loss, in the order of 1.5–2.5 kg per week (compared to 0.4–0.5 kg per week with LCDs), equating to around 12–35 kg during an 8–16 week treatment period (Mustajoki and Pekkarinen, 2001; National Task Force on the Prevention and Treatment of Obesity, 1993; NH&MRC, 2003; Tsai and Wadden 2006; Anderson et al., 1992). Since VLCDs provide a fixed energy content, there is significant inter-individual variation in the amount of weight lost, as differences in energy requirements, gender, body mass and composition are not taken into account. The majority ($\geq$75%) of weight lost using either VLCDs or LCDs is fat mass (Barrows and Snook, 1987; Burgess, 1991; Rossner and Flaten, 1997; SCOOP-VLCD TASK 7.3, 2002). There appears to be no clinical advantage in reducing the daily energy content of a VLCD below 3350 kJ (800 kcal) (Foster et al. 1992; Lin et al., 2009).

16.4.2 Long term

In the long-term, diet-induced weight loss is poorly maintained. There are conflicting reports regarding the relative success of VLCDs compared with other dietary approaches. In its 1998 report (NHLBI, 1998) (currently being updated), the National Heart Lung and Blood Institute expert panel recommended the use of LCDs for the treatment of obesity, based on data from 4 randomised controlled trials which showed no difference between VLCDs and LCDs in weight loss beyond 1 year, despite greater initial weight loss on VLCDs. This is supported by the conclusion of a more recent meta-analysis of 6 randomised controlled trials, some of which were included in the NHLBI expert panel report, comparing VLCDs and LCDs with at least 1 year follow-up after maximum weight loss (Tsai and Wadden, 2006). Studies were conducted in the US (4) and Scandinavia (2), and published between 1989 and 1997. Participants used VLCDs for 8–24 weeks followed by LCDs, or LCDs alone (containing 4200–7500 kJ (1000–1800 kcal)/d), and all programmes included behaviour therapy, with or without exercise, for 6 to 26 months. Attrition was not different between the VLCD and LCD groups. Participants lost significantly more weight using VLCDs (mean difference 6.4 kg over 12.7 weeks), but after an average of 1.9 years follow-up, weight loss was not significantly different between groups (mean 6.3 ± 3.2 vs. $5.0 \pm 4.0\%$ for VLCDs and LCDs respectively).

In contrast, a number of reviews of the published data have concluded that greater initial weight loss, including that induced by VLCDs, is associated with better maintenance of weight loss (Anderson et al., 2001; Astrup and Rossner, 2000), provided that there is a subsequent programme of behavioural modification and supportive follow-up (Ayyad and Andersen, 2000). In a meta-analysis examining 29 predominantly non-randomised studies of structured weight loss programme involving a VLCD (13 studies), low-calorie diet (14 studies) or both (2 studies), with follow-up of at least 2 years, participants maintained greater weight loss after a VLCD compared with a LCD (16.1 vs. 7.2% weight loss at 1 year, and 6.2 vs. 2% at 5 years for VLCDs and LCDs respectively) (Anderson et al., 2001).

16.4.3 Benefits of VLCDs

VLCD-induced weight loss has beneficial effects on several obesity-related conditions, including dyslipidaemia (reduction in total cholesterol, low-density lipoprotein and triglycerides), hypertension, insulin resistance, Type 2 diabetes, hepatic steatosis and obstructive sleep apnoea (Anderson et al., 1992; Lewis et al., 2006; Suratt et al., 1987). Although these benefits are common to most methods of weight reduction, there may be certain advantages in using a VLCD. In one study (Wing et al., 1991), obese participants with Type 2 diabetes underwent a 20-week programme of behaviour modification and a hypocaloric diet 4200–6300 kJ (1000–1500 kcal)/d, and were randomly assigned to include a VLCD or not from weeks 5–12. They were instructed to continue the hypocaloric diet for a further 52 weeks, unless goal weight was reached prior. The VLCD group lost significantly more weight during the first 20 weeks (18.6 ± 9.5 vs. 10.1 ± 4.3 kg). At one year, although there was no significant difference in weight loss between groups (8.6 ± 9.2 vs. 6.8 ± 6.9 kg), the VLCD group had significantly greater improvements in fasting glucose and HbA1c (Wing et al., 1991). Other advantages of VLCDs include the motivating effect of rapid weight loss, the convenience of meal replacement formulations, which may improve dietary adherence compared with a conventional diet (Noakes et al., 2004), and a mild ketosis due to the relatively low carbohydrate intake, which may reduce appetite (Sumithran et al., 2013). In one study, participants reported less hunger, despite a significantly lower energy intake, on a VLCD compared with a balanced LCD (Wadden et al., 1985).

16.5   Safety of VLCDs

Minor adverse effects commonly experienced while using VLCDs are generally self-limiting and transient, and include cold intolerance, dry skin, hair loss, constipation, dizziness, headaches, and fatigue (National Task Force on the Prevention and Treatment of Obesity, 1993).

More serious adverse effects are less common, and can include gallstones, hyperuricemia, and reduction in bone mineral density. Obesity itself is a risk factor for cholelithiasis and gout. The risk of cholelithiasis is further increased by rapid weight loss, whether induced by VLCDs or other means, such as bariatric surgery (Everhart, 1993), and may be mitigated by slowing the rate of weight loss to <1.5 kg/wk (Weinsier *et al.*, 1995), administration of ursodeoxycholic acid (Shiffman *et al.*, 1995), or increasing the fat content of the diet (Festi *et al.*, 1998).

Weight loss is generally accompanied by a reduction in serum uric acid (Zhu *et al.*, 2010), but levels may increase during VLCD treatment, and rarely, gout may be precipitated, usually in persons previously affected. Liberalisation of carbohydrate intake or treatment with allopurinol has been suggested for patients with marked hyperuricemia (>590 pmol/L) or symptomatic gout (National Task Force on the Prevention and Treatment of Obesity, 1993).

Weight loss of 5% or more is associated with a reduction in bone mineral density and increased fracture risk (Langlois *et al.*, 2001; Meyer *et al.*, 1995). The reduction in BMD is proportional to the amount of weight loss (Schwartz *et al.*, 2012; Villalon *et al.*, 2011), and has been demonstrated following mild to moderate dietary restriction (3800 to 6700 kJ/d), VLCDs, and bariatric surgery (Andersen *et al.*, 1997; Schwartz *et al.*, 2012; Hinton *et al.*, 2012; Fleischer *et al.*, 2008) in middle-aged and older men and women (Ensrud *et al.*, 2005; Langlois *et al.*, 2001; Salamone *et al.*, 1999), but has not been consistently found in younger people (Redman *et al.*, 2008; Hamilton *et al.*, 2013; Shapses *et al.*, 2001; Hinton *et al.*, 2012; Fogelholm *et al.*, 2001). Exercise may help ameliorate bone loss in the elderly during dietary weight loss (Shah *et al.*, 2011), but seems not to affect changes in BMD and bone turnover markers during diet-induced weight loss in younger people (Hamilton *et al.*, 2013; Hinton *et al.*, 2012; Fogelholm *et al.*, 2001). Increasing dietary intake of calcium, vitamin D and protein have been reported to attenuate changes in bone density or turnover markers during weight reduction in some (Thorpe *et al.*, 2008; Sukumar *et al.*, 2011; Josse *et al.*, 2012) but not all (Hinton *et al.*, 2010) studies.

Rarely, electrolyte disturbances (particularly in people taking diuretics), a transient increase in liver function tests, or mild hepatic portal inflammation and fibrosis may occur during VLCD use (Andersen *et al.*, 1991).

Concern about the cardiovascular safety of VLCDs arose after the occurrence of more than 60 sudden deaths in the 1970s among users of a liquid protein diet composed of collagen or gelatine hydrolysates (Wadden *et al.*, 1983). Many of the deaths occurred in people with pre-existing medical conditions (Wadden *et al.*, 1983), however, 17 people who died (16 of whom were women), were relatively young (median age 35 years) and healthy apart from their severe obesity (mean BMI 40.6 kg/m^2). They had lost a mean of 35% initial weight over an average of 5 (range

2–8) months on diets containing 1250–1700 kJ (300–400 kcal/d) (Sours *et al.*, 1981), and post-mortem findings were consistent with the cardiac effects of protein-calorie malnutrition, which include myocardial atrophy, QT prolongation and ventricular arrhythmias (Isner *et al.*, 1979). Of note, 4 of the 17 deceased had supplemented or replaced the liquid protein diet with a dairy- or egg-based protein source, therefore although the precise mechanism of death is not certain, it cannot be attributed solely to the use of low-quality protein products (Sours *et al.*, 1981). In 1984, the FDA concluded that the level of energy restriction was likely to be of greater importance than the protein quality, and established label warning requirements alerting consumers of potential hazards of using protein-based VLCDs containing 1700 kJ (400 kcal) or less per day (FDA, 1984).

Newer VLCDs are required to provide at least 1880 kJ (450 kcal) per day (SCOOP-VLCD TASK 7.3, 2002) and include high-quality protein (generally dairy-, soy- or egg-based), and appear to be safe (Mustajoki and Pekkarinen, 2001; Moyer *et al.*, 1989). A review of the scientific literature as well as reports in the public domain regarding nutritionally complete VLCDs found no fatalities which could be attributed to the VLCD (SCOOP-VLCD TASK 7.3, 2002), although there is a paucity of data regarding the safety of prolonged (>16 weeks) exclusive use of a VLCD. We have reported the case of a severely obese man (BMI 47 kg/m2) who replaced all 3 daily meals with a VLCD for 5 months under medical supervision, and continued on a modified VLCD for 12 months with no apparent adverse effects (Sumithran and Proietto, 2008), and Rossner reported a patient who consumed only a VLCD preparation for 46 weeks without medical supervision, in whom no adverse events occurred other than cholelithiasis and one episode of palpitations with no documented ECG abnormality (Rossner, 1998). Greenway and colleagues reported no changes in QT interval in obese men and women who undertook VLCDs containing 1700–2500 kJ (400–600 kcal)/d for up to 20 weeks (Greenway *et al.*, 1994), and others have reported no significant abnormalities during cardiac monitoring in patients on VLCDs containing 2700–3350 kJ (660–800 kcal)/d for 6 to 12 weeks (Moyer *et al.*, 1989; Seim *et al.*, 1995). However, a recent case report described the occurrence of recurrent episodes of torsades de pointes in an obese, otherwise well woman under 40 years of age, who had lost 57 kg over the preceding 6 months using a nutritionally complete VLCD, providing 2210 kJ (530 kcal)/day, including 50 g each of carbohydrate and high-quality protein, under medical supervision (Crawford and Cochran, 2009).

16.6   Monitoring required during the diet

Everyone who undertakes a VLCD should have an initial evaluation by a medical practitioner familiar with its use, including a medical history, physical examination, and assessment of weight-related health risks. Thereafter, review should occur at least fortnightly during the VLCD and re-feeding for assessment of weight, pulse and blood pressure, along with glycaemic control in people with diabetes (National Task Force on the Prevention and Treatment of Obesity, 1993). We and others advocate baseline testing of full blood count, electrolytes, renal and liver function, fasting glucose and lipids, iron studies and uric acid (National Task Force on the Prevention and Treatment of Obesity, 1993). We suggest repeating electrolyte and creatinine levels after 6 weeks on the VLCD, or earlier in people who require more careful monitoring (such as those with renal impairment or who are taking diuretics). In people who continue the VLCD for more than 12 weeks, we advise repeating the baseline tests at least every 2 months. There is minimal information on which to base recommendations for biochemical monitoring before and during VLCD treatment, and some physicians suggest that blood tests are only necessary if indicated by clinical evaluation, or in the presence of a specific condition which requires monitoring (Mustajoki and Pekkarinen, 2001). Increased frequency of monitoring of blood levels/parameters is required in people taking medications whose metabolism may be affected by VLCD treatment, such as lithium or warfarin. (Mustajoki and Pekkarinen, 2001, National Task Force on the Prevention and Treatment of Obesity, 1993). The National Task Force on the Prevention and Treatment of Obesity recommends performing an ECG at baseline, considering cardiology consultation for patients with QTc > 0.44 msec prior to starting a VLCD, regular monitoring of ECG and electrolytes during the VLCD and re-feeding periods, and that medications which lengthen QT intervals (such as phenothiazines and tricyclic antidepressants) be used with extreme caution in patients on VLCDs (National Task Force on the Prevention and Treatment of Obesity, 1993).

16.7 Future trends

The majority of obese people who lose weight by dietary restriction regain weight over the long-term. Diet-induced weight loss is accompanied by numerous physiological changes which encourage weight regain, including alterations in energy expenditure, substrate metabolism, and hormone pathways involved in appetite regulation, many of which are persistent well beyond the initial weight loss period (Sumithran et al., 2011; Sumithran and Proietto, 2013). It has been shown that over 6 months, people using a VLCD can achieve equivalent weight loss to those undergoing laparoscopic adjustable gastric banding (O'Brien et al., 2006). However, there are currently no non-surgical treatments available which counteract these physiological changes, and at present, bariatric surgery is the most effective long-term treatment option for people with moderate to severe obesity (Sjostrom et al., 2004; O'Brien et al., 2006). Studies involving sibutramine and rimonabant (which are no longer on the market) indicate that pharmacotherapy may be at least partially effective in facilitating maintenance of diet-induced weight loss (Apfelbaum et al., 1999; Mathus-Vliegen 2005; Pi-Sunyer et al., 2006). Two appetite suppressants were approved by the U.S. Food and Drug Administration in 2012 for the treatment of obesity: lorcaserin (a serotonin 2C receptor agonist) and the combination of phentermine and topiramate. Other pharmacological agents currently undergoing clinical trials for the treatment of obesity include the GLP-1 analogue liraglutide and the combination of naltrexone and bupropion (Astrup et al., 2009; Greenway et al., 2009). Studies examining whether these medications can improve maintenance of VLCD-induced weight loss safely and effectively over the long-term will be of interest.

References

Andersen T, Gluud C, Franzmann MB and Christoffersen P (1991). Hepatic effects of dietary weight loss in morbidly obese subjects. *Journal of Hepatology*, 12: 224–229.

Andersen RE, Wadden TA and Herzog RJ (1997). Changes in bone mineral content in obese dieting women. *Metabolism: Clinical and Experimental*, 46: 857–861.

Anderson JW, Hamilton CC and Brinkman-Kaplan V (1992). Benefits and risks of an intensive very-low-calorie diet program for severe obesity. *Am J Gastroenterol*, 87: 6–15.

Anderson JW, Konz EC, Frederich RC and Wood CL (2001). Long-term weight-loss maintenance: a meta-analysis of US studies. *Am J Clin Nutr*, 74: 579–584.

Apfelbaum M, Vague P, Ziegler O, Hanotin C, Thomas F and Leutenegger E (1999). Long-term maintenance of weight loss after a very-low-calorie diet: a randomized blinded trial of the efficacy and tolerability of sibutramine. *American Journal of Medicine*, 106: 179–184.

Astrup A and Rossner S (2000). Lessons from obesity management programmes: greater initial weight loss improves long-term maintenance. *Obesity Reviews*, 1: 17–19.

Astrup A, Rossner S, Van Gaal L, Rissanen A, Niskanen L, Al Hakim M, *et al.* (2009). Effects of liraglutide in the treatment of obesity: a randomised, double-blind, placebo-controlled study. *Lancet*, 374: 1606–1616.

Ayyad C and Andersen T (2000). Long-term efficacy of dietary treatment of obesity: a systematic review of studies published between 1931 and 1999. *Obesity Reviews*, 1: 113–119.

Barrows K and Snook JT (1987). Effect of a high-protein, very-low-calorie diet on body composition and anthropometric parameters of obese middle-aged women. *Am J Clin Nutr*, 45: 381–390.

Burgess NS (1991). Effect of a very-low-calorie diet on body composition and resting metabolic rate in obese men and women. *Journal of the American Dietetic Association*, 91: 430–434.

Crawford EJT and Cochran D (2009). Recurrent torsades de pointes in association with a very low calorie diet. *Anaesthesia*, 64: 903–907.

Dey DK, Rothenberg E, Sundh V, Bosaeus I and Steen B (2001). Body mass index, weight change and mortality in the elderly. A 15y longitudinal population study of 70y olds. *Eur J Clin Nutr*, 55: 482–492.

Diehr P, Bild DE, Harris TB, Duxbury A, Siscovick D and Rossi M (1998). Body mass index and mortality in nonsmoking older adults: the Cardiovascular Health Study. *American Journal of Public Health*, 88: 623–629.

Ensrud KE, Fullman RL, Barrett-Connor E, Cauley JA, Stefanick ML, *et al.* (2005). Voluntary weight reduction in oldermen increases hip bone loss: the Osteoporotic Fractures in Men study. *J Clin Endocrinol Metab*, 90: 1998–2004.

Everhart JE (1993). Contributions of obesity and weight loss to gallstone disease. *Annals of Internal Medicine*, 119: 1029–1035.

Festi D, Colecchia A, Orsini M, Sangermano A, Sottili S, Simoni P, *et al.* (1998). Gallbladder motility and gallstone formation in obese patients following very low calorie diets. Use it (fat) to lose it (well). *Int J Obes*, 22: 592–600.

Fleischer J, Stein EM, Bessler M, Della Badia M, Restuccia N, Olivero-Rivera L, *et al.* (2008). The decline in hip bone density after gastric bypass surgery is associated with extent of weight loss. *J Clin Endocrinol Metab*, 93: 3735–3740.

FDA (Food and Drug Administration) (1984). Food Labeling; Protein Products; Warning Labeling. Final rule. Federal Register, 21 CFR Part 101, Vol. 49, no 68.

Fogelholm GM, Sievanen HT, Kukkonen-Harjula TK and Pasanen ME (2001). Bone mineral density during reduction, maintenance and regain of body weight in premenopausal, obese women. *Osteoporos Int*, 12: 199–206.

Foster GD, Wadden TA, Peterson FJ, Letizia KA, Bartlett SJ and Conill AM (1992). A controlled comparison of three very-low-calorie diets: effects on weight, body composition, and symptoms. *Am J Clin Nutr*, 55: 811–817.

Greenway FL, Raum WJ and Atkinson RL (1994). Higher calorie content preserves myocardial electrical activity during very-low-calorie dieting. *Obesity Research*, 2: 95–99.

Greenway FL, Dunayevich E, Tollefson G, Erickson J, Guttadauria M, Fujioka K, *et al.* (2009). Comparison of combined bupropion and naltrexone therapy for obesity with monotherapy and placebo. *J Clin Endocrinol Metab*, 94: 4898–4906.

Hamilton KC, Fisher G, Roy JL, Gower BA and Hunter GR (2013). The effects of weight loss on relative bone mineral density in premenopausal women. *Obesity (Silver Spring)*, 21: 441–448.

Hinton PS, Rector RS, Donnelly JE, Smith BK and Bailey B (2010). Total body bone mineral content and density during weight loss and maintenance on a low- or recommended-dairy weight-maintenance diet in obese men and women. *Eur J Clin Nutr*, 64: 392–399.

Hinton PS, Rector RS, Linden MA, Warner SO, Dellsperger KC, Chockalingam A, *et al.* (2012). Weight-loss-associated changes in bone mineral density and bone turnover after partial weight regain with or without aerobic exercise in obese women. *Eur J Clin Nutr*, 66: 606–612.

Isner JM, Sours HE, Paris AL, Ferrans VJ and Roberts WC (1979). Sudden, unexpected death in avid dieters using the liquid-protein-modified-fast diet. Observations in 17 patients and the role of the prolonged QT interval. *Circulation*, 60: 1401–1412.

Josse AR, Atkinson SA, Tarnopolsky MA and Phillips SM (2012). Diets higher in dairy foods and dietary protein support bone health during diet- and exercise-induced weight loss in overweight and obese premenopausal women. *J Clin Endocrinol Metab*, 97: 251–260.

Langlois JA, Mussolino ME, Visser M, Looker AC, Harris T and Madans J (2001). Weight loss from maximum body weight among middle-aged and older white women and the risk of hip fracture: the NHANES I Epidemiologic Follow-Up Study. *Osteoporos Int*, 12: 763–768.

Lewis M, Phillips M, *et al.* (2006). Change in liver size and fat content after treatment with Optifast very low calorie diet. *Obes Surg*, 16: 697–701.

Lin W-Y, Wu C-H, Chu N-F and Chang C-J (2009). Efficacy and safety of very-low-calorie diet in Taiwanese: a multicenter randomized, controlled trial. *Nutrition*, 25: 1129–1136.

Mathus-Vliegen EMH (2005). Long-term maintenance of weight loss with sibutramine in a GP setting following a specialist guided very-low-calorie diet: a double-blind, placebo-controlled, parallel group study. *Eur J Clin Nutr*, 59 (Suppl 1): S31–38.

Meyer HE, Tverdal A and Falch JA (1995). Changes in body weight and incidence of hip fracture among middle-aged Norwegians. *BMJ*, 311: 91–92.

Moyer CL, Holly RG, Amsterdam EA and Atkinson RL (1989). Effects of cardiac stress during a very-low-calorie diet and exercise program in obese women. *Am J Clin Nutr*, 50: 1324–1327.

Mustajoki P and Pekkarinen T (2001). Very low energy diets in the treatment of obesity. *Obes Rev*, 2: 61–72

NH and MRC (National Health and Medical Research Council) (2003). *Clinical Practice Guidelines for the Management of Overweight and Obesity in Adults*. Canberra.

NHLBI (National Heart Lung and Blood Institute) (1998). 'Clinical Guidelines on the Identification, Evaluation, and Treatment of Overweight and Obesity in Adults–The Evidence Report.' *Obesity Research*, 6 (Suppl 2): S51–209.

National Institutes of Health. Obesity research, 6 (Suppl 2):51S–209S.

National Task Force on the Prevention and Treatment of Obesity (1993). Very low-calorie diets. *JAMA*, 270: 967–974.

Noakes M, Foster PR, Keogh JB and Clifton PM (2004). Meal replacements are as effective as structured weight-loss diets for treating obesity in adults with features of metabolic syndrome. *J Nutr*, 134: 1894–1899.

O'Brien PE, Dixon JB, Laurie C, Skinner S, Proietto J, McNeil J, *et al* (2006). Treatment of mild to moderate obesity with laparoscopic adjustable gastric banding or an intensive medical program: a randomized trial. *Ann Intern Med*, 144: 625–633.

Pi-Sunyer F (1992). The role of very-low-calorie diets in obesity. *Am J Clin Nutr*, 56: S240–243.

Pi-Sunyer FX, Aronne LJ, Heshmati HM, Devin J and Rosenstock J (2006). Effect of rimonabant, a cannabinoid-1 receptor blocker, on weight and cardiometabolic risk factors in overweight or obese patients: RIO-North America: a randomized controlled trial. *JAMA*, 295: 761–775.

Redman LM, Rood J, Anton SD, Champagne C, Smith SR and Ravussin E. (2008). Calorie restriction and bone health in young, overweight individuals. *Arch Intern Med*, 168: 1859–1866.

Rossner S and Flaten H (1997). VLCD versus LCD in long-term treatment of obesity. *Int J Obes*, 21: 22–26.

Rossner S (1998). Effects of 46 weeks of very-low-calorie-diet treatment on weight loss and cardiac function–a case report. *Obes Res*, 6: 462–463.

Salamone LM, Cauley JA, Black DM, Simkin-Silverman L, Lang W, *et al.* (1999). Effect of a lifestyle intervention on bone mineral density in premenopausal women: a randomized trial. *Am J Clin Nutr*, 70: 97–103.

Saris WH (2001). Very-low-calorie diets and sustained weight loss. *Obes Res*, 9 (Suppl 4): S295–301.

Schwartz AV, Johnson KC, Kahn SE, Shepherd JA, Nevitt MC, Peters AL, *et al.* (2012). Effect of 1 year of an intentional weight loss intervention on bone mineral density in type 2 diabetes: results from the Look AHEAD randomized trial. *J Bone Miner Res*, 27: 619–627.

SCOOP-VLCD Task 7.3 (2002). Collection of data on products intended for use in very-low-calorie-diets. Reports on tasks for scientific cooperation. http://ec.europa.eu/food/fs/scoop/7.3_en.pdf

Seim HC, Mitchell JE, Pomeroy C and de Zwaan M (1995). Electrocardiographic findings associated with very low calorie dieting. *Int J Obes*, 19: 817–819.

Shah K, Armamento-Villareal R, Parimi N, Chode S, Sinacore DR, Hilton TN, *et al.* (2011). Exercise training in obese older adults prevents increase in bone turnover and attenuates decrease in hip bone mineral density induced by weight loss despite decline in bone-active hormones. *J Bone Miner Res*, 26: 2851–2859.

Shapses SA, Von Thun NL, Heymsfield SB, Ricci TA, Ospina M, *et al.* (2001). Bone turnover and density in obese premenopausal women during moderate weight loss and calcium supplementation. *J Bone Miner Res*, 16: 1329–1336.

Shiffman ML, Kaplan GD, Brinkman-Kaplan V and Vickers FF (1995). Prophylaxis against gallstone formation with ursodeoxycholic acid in patients participating in a very-low-calorie diet program. *Annals of Internal Medicine*, 122: 899–905.

Sjostrom L, Lindroos A-K, Peltonen M, Torgerson J, Bouchard C, Carlsson B, *et al.* (2004). Lifestyle, diabetes, and cardiovascular risk factors 10 years after bariatric surgery. *N Engl J Med*, 351: 2683–2693.

Sours HE, Frattali VP, Brand CD, Feldman RA, Forbes AL, Swanson RC, *et al.* (1981). Sudden death associated with very low calorie weight reduction regimens. *Am J Clin Nutr*, 34: 453–461.

Stevens J, Cai J, Pamuk ER, Williamson DF, Thun MJ and Wood JL (1998). The effect of age on the association between body-mass index and mortality. *N Engl J Med*, 338: 1–7.

Sukumar D, Ambia-Sobhan H, Zurfluh R, Schlussel Y, Stahl TJ, *et al.* (2011). Areal and volumetric bone mineral density and geometry at two levels of protein intake during caloric restriction: a randomized, controlled trial. *J Bone Miner Res*, 26: 1339–1348.

Sumithran P and Proietto J (2008). Safe year-long use of a very-low-calorie diet for the treatment of severe obesity. *Med J Aust*, 188: 366–368.

Sumithran P, Prendergast LA, Delbridge E, Purcell K, Shulkes A, Kriketos A and Proietto J. (2011). Long-term persistence of hormonal adaptations to weight loss. *N Engl J Med*, 365: 1597–1604.

Sumithran P, Prendergast LA, Delbridge E, Purcell K, Shulkes A, Kriketos *et al.* (2013). Ketosis and appetite-mediating nutrients and hormones after weight loss. *Eur J Clin Nutr*, 67: 759–764.

Sumithran P and Proietto J (2013). The defence of body weight: a physiological basis for weight regain after weight loss. *Clinical Science*, 124: 231–241.

Suratt PM, McTier RF, Findley LJ, Pohl SL and Wilhoit SC (1987). Changes in breathing and the pharynx after weight loss in obstructive sleep apnea. *Chest*, 92: 631–637.

Thorpe MP, Jacobson EH, Layman DK, He X, Kris-Etherton PM and Evans EM (2008). A diet high in protein, dairy, and calcium attenuates bone loss over twelve months of weight loss and maintenance relative to a conventional high-carbohydrate diet in adults. *J Nutr*, 138: 1096–1100.

Tsai AG and Wadden TA (2005). Systematic review: an evaluation of major commercial weight loss programs in the United States. *Ann Intern Med*, 142: 56–66.

Tsai AG and Wadden TA (2006). The evolution of very-low-calorie diets: an update and meta-analysis. *Obesity (Silver Spring)*, 14: 1283–1293.

Tsigos C, Hainer V, Basdevant A, Finer N, Fried M, Mathus-Vliegen E, *et al.* (2008) Management of obesity in adults: European clinical practice guidelines. *Obesity Facts*, 1: 106–116.

Villalon KL, Gozansky WS, Van Pelt RE, Wolfe P, Jankowski CM, *et al.* (2011). A losing battle: weight regain does not restore weight loss-induced bone loss in postmenopausal women. *Obesity (Silver Spring)*, 19: 2345–2350.

Villareal DT, Apovian CM, Kushner RF and Klein S (2005). Obesity in older adults: technical review and position statement of the American Society for Nutrition and NAASO, The Obesity Society. *Obesity Research*, 13: 1849–1863.

Wadden TA, Stunkard AJ and Brownell KD (1983). Very low calorie diets: their efficacy, safety, and future. *Ann Intern Med*, 99: 675–684.

Wadden TA, Stunkard AJ, Brownell KD and Day SC (1985). A comparison of two very-low-calorie diets: protein-sparing-modified fast versus protein-formula-liquid diet. *Am J Clin Nutr*, 41: 533–539.

Wannamethee SG, Shaper AG and Lennon L (2005). Reasons for intentional weight loss, unintentional weight loss, and mortality in older men. *Archives of Internal Medicine*, 165: 1035–1040.

Weinsier RL, Wilson LJ and Lee J (1995). Medically safe rate of weight loss for the treatment of obesity: a guideline based on risk of gallstone formation. *American Journal of Medicine*, 98: 115–117.

Wing RR, Marcus MD, Salata R, Epstein LH, Miaskiewicz S and Blair EH (1991). Effects of a very-low-calorie diet on long-term glycemic control in obese type 2 diabetic subjects. *Arch Intern Med*, 151: 1334–1340.

Zhu Y, Zhang Y and Choi HK (2010). The serum urate-lowering impact of weight loss among men with a high cardiovascular risk profile: the Multiple Risk Factor Intervention Trial. *Rheumatology*, 49: 2391–2399.

Commercial weight loss programs and their effectiveness in managing obesity

N. R. Fuller, M. Fong, N. S. Lau
University of Sydney, Sydney, NSW, Australia

17.1 Introduction

Excess weight and obesity is a global epidemic and is a major public health issue in many countries, accounting for 44% of the global burden of diabetes, 23% of ischemic heart disease and 7–41% of certain cancers (WHO, 2009). A modest weight loss of 5–10% (commonly achieved by behavioural modification programs incorporating diet and exercise) is associated with clinically significant health benefits including a reduction in risk factors for diabetes and cardiovascular disease (Knowler *et al.*, 2002, Caterson *et al.*, 2011), with more improvement in these risk factors found with greater degree of sustained weight loss (Goldstein, 1992).

The unfortunate truth is that no single approach will bring down overweight and obesity rates on its own. Of particular impact in clinical weight loss management are the role of commercial weight loss programs. The cost of these programs is not insubstantial, with the annual amount spent in Australia on commercial weight loss products and programs $AUD 644 million (IBISWorld, Aug 2013). Commercial weight loss programs have, and always will exist, so it is important to determine not only which ones are efficacious, but also cost-effective, particularly as these programs can carry associated costs such as program-related food products and endorsements.

Traditionally commercial weight loss programs aim to educate and motivate participants to lose weight by promoting a hypocaloric diet, balanced eating, increased physical activity, and group support. They often include frequent weekly meetings that focus on intensive behavioural therapy and cognitive restructuring through means of goal setting, problem solving, stimulus control, and relapse prevention. Such programs can produce clinically significant weight loss which may reduce the risk of chronic diseases such as Type 2 diabetes and cardiovascular disease.

While there are an abundance of commercial weight loss programs available exclusively online, this chapter will focus on the still popular and traditional 'face to face' programs, with or without an online component.

Managing and Preventing Obesity. http://dx.doi.org/10.1533/9781782420996.4.243

17.2 Commonly available commercial weight loss programs

There are multitudes of commercial weight loss programs available worldwide. Each differs in their program support, staff qualifications, diet prescription, exercise instruction, behaviour modification, and country availability. Several of these programs are also available online and therefore potentially available to countries even where the program has no physical presence. The international increase in overweight and obesity, coupled with the lack of a strict regulatory regimen to oversee commercial weight loss programs has led to the rapid increase in the size of the industry. However the focus of this chapter is on the largest and most widely available programs, which are listed in Table 17.1.

While not listed in this table, specific mention is warranted for Overeaters Anonymous (OA). OA is among the most widely internationally available programs, is aimed at people with disordered food intake and utilises a 12-step, spiritually orientated approach. However as OA is a not-for-profit organisation and is not obesity focused, it was not included in this review.

17.3 Efficacy of commercial weight loss programs: a summary of available evidence

As demonstrated in Table 17.2, there is both a general paucity of clinical data supporting the efficacy of commercial weight loss programs and even less available from high quality randomised controlled trials (RCTs). Of clinical importance, this lack of evidence contributes to the difficulties faced by health care professionals and individuals in deciding on an appropriate and effective commercial weight loss program.

To date, the majority of research within the commercial program sector has been conducted with Weight Watchers, followed by Slimming World and Rosemary Conley respectively. The results from these studies are discussed below.

Four large quality RCTs have been conducted internationally with the Weight Watchers program to examine its clinical efficacy against active comparator weight loss programs (Table 17.2). The most recent multisite RCT involved 772 overweight and obese adults and was conducted across three countries (Australia, the United Kingdom and Germany). This RCT demonstrated that compared to participants who received standard care (primary care physician led lifestyle management), those randomised to the Weight Watchers program achieved significantly greater weight loss over 12 months (5.1 vs. 2.3 kg) (Jebb et al., 2011). The results proved robust regardless of the method of dealing with drop-out participants and the weight loss achieved in all three countries was comparable. Between the four published RCTs for Weight Watchers, the weight loss results at 12 months for their program are similar (Table 17.2). As Weight Watchers is a widely available commercial weight loss program offered in 20 countries, it stands to reason that the results from these studies may broadly be generalised to other countries where the program is offered.

Table 17.1 Structure and content of commonly available commercial weight loss programs

Program	Program support	Staff qualifications	Diet prescription	Exercise instruction	Behaviour modification	Country availability
Weight Watchers	Weekly group meetings, online support, mobile support, optional one-on-one consultations via phone or face to face contact	Successful program completer selected through interview process	ProPoints® plan, member prepares own meals, option to purchase Weight Watchers supermarket products	Recommendations provided by company trained counsellors, members encouraged to wear ProPoints® pedometer	Behavioural weight control methods	Australia, UK, US, Bahamas, Belgium, Brazil, Canada, China, Denmark, Germany, Spain, France, Hong Kong, Ireland, Netherlands, NZ, Austria, Switzerland, South Africa, Sweden Online membership available in all countries
Jenny Craig	Weekly individual session with counsellor, home delivery of pre-prepared Jenny Craig meals, online support	Company trained counsellor	Low calorie diet of pre-packaged Jenny Craig meals	Recommendations provided by company trained counsellors	Manual on weight loss strategies provided	Australia, NZ, US, Canada, France, UK, Puerto Rico Online membership available in all countries
Take off Pounds Sensibly	Weekly group meetings, online support	Group leader elected by local chapter	Food Exchange System and MyPlate model, member prepares own meals	Members make plan with their health care provider	Included in curriculum	Canada, US
Lite & Easy	Home delivery of pre-prepared Lite & Easy meals supplemented with member's own food	Meals designed by qualified dietitian	Members select Lite & Easy meals to be delivered as part of a calorie controlled diet plan	Recommendations from dietitian available online	None	Australia

(Continued overleaf)

Table 17.1 Continued

Program	Program support	Staff qualifications	Diet prescription	Exercise instruction	Behaviour modification	Country availability
Slimming World	Weekly meetings, online support	Successful program completer selected through interview process	Low calorie diet and recipes, member prepares own meals, focus on 'Food Optimising' where energy dense foods are replaced with low kilojoule options	'Body Magic' exercise program	Weekly IMAGE (Individual Motivation And Group Experience) meetings, provision of motivational tool kit from consultant, motivating articles available online	UK, US Online membership available in all countries
Rosemary Conley	Weekly group classes, optional home delivery of pre-packaged 'Solo Slim' foods, optional weekly group exercise sessions, online support	Varied, may be successful slimmers, exercise classes conducted by qualified instructors	'Fat Attack Booster Diet', weight loss recipes available online, member prepares own meals with option of having pre-packaged 'Solo Slim' products home delivered	Optional weekly group exercise sessions	Provided by company trained counsellor	UK Online membership available in all countries
LA Weight Loss	Weekly individual sessions, optional home delivery of LA Weight Loss food products	Company trained counsellor	Low calorie diet, member prepares own meals	Optional walking videotape	Included in counselling sessions, provision of food diary and support materials	US Online membership available in all countries

US – United States; UK – United Kingdom; NZ – New Zealand
Adapted from Tsai and Wadden (2005) as published in *Annals of Internal Medicine*

Table 17.2 Efficacy of commercial weight loss programs

Commercial weight loss program	Evidence supporting efficacy	Type of evidence	Weight loss outcomes at 12 months (unless otherwise specified)			Weight loss outcomes at 24 months	
			kg	%	cm	kg	%
Weight Watchers	Yes	RCT (Jebb et al., 2011; Holzapfel et al., 2013)	−5.1 LOCF −4.1 BOCF −6.7 completers	−5.8 LOCF −4.7 BOCF −7.7 completers	−5.6 LOCF −4.1 BOCF −6.9 completers	−4.1 LOCF −1.3 BOCF −4.8 completers	−4.8 LOCF −1.5 BOCF −5.5 completers
		RCT (Jolly et al., 2010)	−4.4 LOCF −3.5 BOCF −4.4 completers	−4.7 LOCF −3.7 BOCF −4.7 completers	N/A	N/A	N/A
		RCT (Truby et al., 2006)	−6.6 BOCF at 6 months −9.1 at 12 months completers	−7.3 BOCF At 6 months −10.3 at 12 months completers	−8.3 BOCF at 6 months	N/A	N/A
		RCT (Heshka et al., 2003)	−4.3 LOCF −5.0 completers	−4.6 LOCF −5.3 completers	−4.1 LOCF −4.9 completers	−2.9 LOCF −3.0 completers	−3.1 LOCF −3.2 completers
Jenny Craig	Yes	RCT (Rock et al., 2007)	−6.6 BOCF −7.3 completers	−7.1 BOCF −7.8 completers	−8.2 BOCF −9.0 completers	N/A	N/A

(Continued overleaf)

Table 17.2 Continued

Commercial weight loss program	Evidence supporting efficacy	Type of evidence	Weight loss outcomes at 12 months (unless otherwise specified)			Weight loss outcomes at 24 months	
			kg	%	cm	kg	%
Take off Pounds Sensibly	Yes	Retrospective cohort analysis (Mitchell et al., 2011)	−6.7 completers	−6.1 completers	N/A	−7.6 completers (−7.3 at 36 months for completers)	−6.9 completers (−6.7 at 36 months for completers)
Lite & Easy	No	N/A	N/A	N/A	N/A	N/A	N/A
Slimming World	Yes	Retrospective cohort analysis (Stubbs et al., 2012)	−8.9 LOCF at 24 weeks −6.3 LOCF non completers only at 24 weeks −9.6 completers at 24 weeks	−8.6 LOCF at 24 weeks −6.2 LOCF non completers only at 24 weeks −9.3 completers at 24 weeks	N/A	N/A	N/A
		RCT (Jolly et al., 2010)	−3.3 LOCF −1.9 BOCF −3.1 completers	−3.5 LOCF −2.0 BOCF −3.3 completers	N/A	N/A	N/A
		Simple intervention (Lavin et al., 2006)	−5.4 completers at 12 weeks −11.1 completers at 24 weeks	−6.4 completers at 12 weeks −11.3 completers at 24 weeks	N/A	N/A	N/A

Rosemary Conley	Yes	RCT (Jolly et al., 2010)	−3.2 LOCF −2.1 BOCF −3.3 completers −6.3 BOCF at 6 months −10.9 completers at 12 months	−3.4 LOCF −2.3 BOCF −3.5 completers −7.0 BOCF at 6 months −13.1 completers at 12 months	N/A	N/A	N/A
		RCT (Truby et al., 2006)	N/A	N/A	N/A	N/A	N/A
LA Weight Loss	No	N/A	N/A	N/A	N/A	N/A	N/A

RCT – Randomised controlled trial; LOCF – last observation carried forward; BOCF – baseline observation carried forward; N/A – no data available

Weight Watchers is one of the few commercial programs to have published any longer-term follow-up data. Participants followed up one year after a 12 month intervention (i.e. to two years) were shown to still weigh 3 to 4 kg less than their baseline weight, depending on the statistical method adopted to deal with drop-out participants (Holzapfel *et al.*, 2013). These 24-month results were also similar to that reported by Heshka and colleagues where a 2.9 kg weight loss was reported after two years of Weight Watchers intervention (Heshka *et al.*, 2003).

Interestingly, the international RCT of the Weight Watchers program (Jebb *et al.*, 2011) utilised a shared care approach, whereby participants were initially recruited into the study by their primary care physicians before being randomised into the Weight Watchers or standard care groups. These results suggest that referral by primary health-care physicians to commercial weight loss programs can be a clinically effective and realistic intervention for weight management in overweight and obese people and can be delivered at scale.

A large amount of research surrounding the efficacy of the Slimming World program has also been published. However, the majority of these studies were descriptive retrospective cohort analyses of the Slimming World program, utilising routine data collected within the program's referral pathways. A single prospective study was identified, which investigated the feasibility of building commercial weight management referral into primary care. This showed that participants who completed 12 and 24 weeks of the Slimming World program lost significant amounts of weight (5.4 kg and 11.1 kg at 12 and 24 weeks, respectively) (Lavin *et al.*, 2006). Only one single RCT that used this program was identified and this is discussed below. There is a lack of long-term follow-up of the Slimming World programs' efficacy, so it remains unclear how much weight loss is achieved or maintained in these participants beyond one year.

Although efficacious, the aforementioned weight loss programs rely on their clients having a certain level of cooking literacy and sufficient time to prepare meals. To overcome issues of poor cooking literacy and time constraints, there are a number of programs that offer home delivery of calorie controlled meals. These programs have been shown to produce greater weight loss than standard care, as seen in a small RCT (n = 70) conducted by Rock *et al.* (2007). Participants allocated to the commercial program were provided with pre-prepared Jenny Craig meals as part of a reduced calorie diet and also encouraged to increase their physical activity. At 12 months, those in the Jenny Craig group lost 6.6 kg, or 7.1% of their starting body weight, which is greater than that reported for all the other commercial programs. The larger weight loss with the Jenny Craig program may be attributed to the prescriptive nature of meal delivery weight loss programs. Reducing food choice and controlling meal portions may help to create the energy deficit required for weight loss.

There is data from RCTs that have compared commercial weight loss programs to standard treatments. The BBC 'diet trials' study randomised overweight and obese participants to the Weight Watchers or Rosemary Conley's commercial programs, to the Akins diet, to a commercial low calorie meal replacement program, or to a clinician-run lifestyle orientated weight loss program (Truby *et al.*, 2006). While all treatment groups lost weight, for the primary outcome, weight loss at six months program's end, there were no differences between groups. Twelve-month data was limited by drop out but participants from all programs maintained clinically significant weight loss.

The Lighten Up study is the second RCT that compared the efficacy of multiple commercial weight loss programs with other weight loss strategies (Jolly *et al.*, 2010). In contrast to Truby and colleagues, this RCT involved more programs and had a greater number of overweight and obese participants. Participants were recruited through their primary care physicians and randomised to one of eight groups: one of three commercial weight loss programs (Weight Watchers, Slimming World or Rosemary Conley), a community run weight loss group (Size Down) that was based on a national program, two primary care programs (general practise or community pharmacy), a 'self select' group where participants chose their treatments, or a minimal intervention 'exercise only' comparator group. All programs achieved weight loss at 12 weeks but only participants in the Weight Watchers and Rosemary Conley programs achieved statistically greater weight loss than the comparator program. By 12 months, all programs except the two primary care programs had maintained weight loss. There were no differences in weight loss between those randomly allocated to a weight loss program or those who had a choice. However, only participants from the Weight Watchers group still had significantly greater weight loss than the comparator group. Furthermore, the primary care based programs were the most costly to run (Jolly *et al.*, 2010).

It has been noted that attendance rate is higher in commercial weight loss groups compared to those receiving standard care (Jolly *et al.*, 2010), and therefore the efficacy of a commercial program may lie simply in the ongoing and regular support that is offered (Truby *et al.*, 2006). With respect to weight loss maintenance, future studies should compare commercial programs with other methods of weight loss such as the work done by Pinto and colleagues, who assessed the effects of the methods of weight loss (very low calorie diet, commercial programs and self-directed lifestyle modification) on long term weight loss and maintenance (Pinto *et al.*, 2008).

17.4 Internet-based weight loss programs

With the expansion of the global online community, many are turning to the anonymity of the internet for weight management treatment. Commercial internet-based weight loss programs have developed to offer round the clock services such as online forums and bulletin boards, which participants use to cultivate social support. Web-based programs also mitigate travel and time demands that may contribute to the attrition rates of traditional 'face to face' programs. For these reasons, one could assume that a commercial internet weight loss program may be efficacious in terms of weight loss when compared to a traditional 'face to face' program.

However, a recent meta-analysis of web-based weight loss and maintenance programs found few studies suitable for analysis, which were of such significant heterogeneity that no conclusions regarding weight loss efficacy could be drawn (Neve *et al.*, 2010). Furthermore, an RCT conducted by Womble *et al.*, (2004) found that the participants in a web-based weight loss group lost significantly less weight than those in a self-help comparator group at weeks 16 and 52. The investigators reported that although online resources were constantly available, participants made minimal use of these resources and on average only logged into the online program approximately once per week (Womble *et al.*, 2004). The reduced weight loss was also attributed to the structure of the online program. Unlike traditional programs that follow a logical progression and provide 'face to face' support, web–based programs allow participants to move back and forth between modules. This may reduce the time spent on individual lifestyle components. Additionally, as there is no direct contact between web-based group leaders and participants, rapport is harder to establish and individuals using such programs may feel less accountable. Although exclusively online commercial weight loss programs may not be effective, what is less clear is the value of on-line support supplementing established commercial weight loss providers and whether this has any effect on weight loss and maintenance. Finally, the continued and rapid evolution of information technologies has resulted in the development of even more novel approaches for weight loss, such as using social media to deliver weight loss programs and a multitude of smart phone applications. The clinical efficacy of these newer approaches is an open question.

17.5   The cost-effectiveness of commercial weight loss programs

To alleviate the burden on health care resources it is imperative that weight loss strategies are cost-effective. It is important for governments to know whether it is more cost-effective to fund and develop novel programs, to support those already in place or subsidise others including extant commercial programs. However the evidence examining the cost-effectiveness of commercial weight loss programs is sparse. Weight Watchers is currently the only commercial program with evidence of its cost-effectiveness. From a within-trial cost-effectiveness analysis, the cost per kilogram of weight loss for Weight Watchers was shown to be lower than standard care in Australia and the United Kingdom, although this was not reported for Germany (Fuller *et al.*, 2013). Despite its efficacy possibly being attributed to the more frequent meetings, Weight Watchers was still cost-effective even after the extra participant travel costs were included in the analyses. The incremental cost-effectiveness ratios reported (expressed as the cost per quality adjusted life year – QALY) were below the commonly accepted threshold for cost-effectiveness of £20,000 in the UK, and US $50,000 in Australia and Germany (Fuller *et al.*, 2013). In contrast, another cost-effectiveness analysis of the Weight Watchers program reported a much higher cost per QALY figure, more than double the $50,000 threshold. However this analysis was smaller in scale and based on a limited data set that did not include complete measures of physical activity or food intake. The authors readily acknowledged that these factors may have contributed to the decreased cost-effectiveness (Cobiac *et al.*, 2010).

Other commercial providers that require the purchase of pre-prepared meals, such as Jenny Craig, are even less unlikely to be cost-effective as food products significantly increase program costs. Despite this assumption, there is no data surrounding the cost-effectiveness of any of the other commercial weight loss programs.

17.6   Applications in the treatment of overweight and obesity

Primary health-care professionals often do not have the time, training or resources to effectively deal with weight management in the primary care setting and therefore it is often neglected. It is highly likely that many of their patients have used commercial weight loss programs. However, health professionals should inform themselves about the efficacy and cost-effectiveness of these programs, to enable them to have evidence-based discussions and recommendations with their patients. It is also important for patients to know about the effectiveness of the larger commercial programs and to know what is expected from each provider in terms of regularity of visits as well as food products and supplemental material that may make up the total cost of any program.

17.7   Conclusions

In summary, while the overall quality of studies into commercial weight loss programs is variable, several of the largest providers have been the subject of higher quality research. From the current available RCTs, the results suggest that the Weight Watchers, Slimming World, Rosemary Conley and Jenny Craig programs produce clinically significant weight loss results over a one-year period. However, no follow-up data exists for any program except for Weight Watchers. The greater availability and evidence base to support the Weight Watchers program suggests that it is effective and may be deliverable on a large scale through primary health-care referrals. Research into their cost-effectiveness is even scanter than their efficacy with only Weight Watchers having been studied. However more large-scale quality RCTs reporting on efficacy and cost-effectiveness need to be conducted with all commercial programs (perhaps apart from Weight Watchers) before clinicians will feel confident in referring their patients to these programs.

Disclosures: Nicholas R Fuller and Namson S Lau were contributing authors on several of the referenced articles that relate to the Weight Watchers program. Weight Watchers International provided funding for the investigator-initiated clinical trial through a grant to the UK Medical Research Council. However neither author received direct or indirect payments from Weight Watchers International. The authors report no other conflicts of interest.

References

Caterson, I. D., Finer, N., Coutinho, W., Van Gaal, L. F., Maggioni, A. P., *et al.* (2011). Maintained intentional weight loss reduces cardiovascular outcomes: results from the Sibutramine Cardiovascular OUTcomes (SCOUT) trial. *Diabetes, Obesity and Metabolism*, 14, 523–553.

Cobiac, L., VOS, T. and Veerman, L. (2010). Cost-effectiveness of Weight Watchers and the Lighten Up to a Healthy Lifestyle program. *Australian and New Zealand Journal of Public Health*, 34, 240–247.

Fuller, N. R., Colagiuri, S., Schofield, D., Olson, A. D., Shrestha, R., *et al.* (2013). A within-trial cost-effectiveness analysis of primary care referral to a commercial provider for weight loss treatment, relative to standard care – an international randomised controlled trial. *International Journal of Obesity*, 37, 828–834.

Goldstein, D. J. (1992). Beneficial health-effects of modest weight-loss. *International Journal of Obesity*, 16, 397–415.

Heshka, S., Anderson, J. W., Atkinson, R. L. *et al.* (2003). Weight loss with self-help compared with a structured commercial program: a randomized trial. *JAMA*, 289, 1792–1798.

Holzapfel, C., Cresswell, L., Ahern, A. L., Fuller, N. R., Eberhard, M. I., *et al.* (2013). The challenge of two year follow-up after intervention for weight loss in primary care. *International Journal of Obesity*, published online 13 Sep: doi:10.1038/ijo.2013.180.

IBISWorld. (Aug 2013). *Weight Loss Services in Australia: Market Research Report. ANZSIC S9512* [Online]. Available: http://www.ibisworld.com.au/industry/default. aspx?indid=1704 [accessed 16 September 2013].

Jebb, S. A., Ahern, A. L., Olson, A. D., Aston, L. M., Holzapfel, C., *et al.* (2011). Primary care referral to a commercial provider for weight loss treatment versus standard care: a randomised controlled trial. *The Lancet*, 378, 1485–1492.

Jolly, K., Daley, A., Adab, P., Lewis, A., Denley, J., *et al.* (2010). A randomised controlled trial to compare a range of commercial or primary care led weight reduction programs with a minimal intervention control for weight loss in obesity: the Lighten Up trial. *BMC Public Health*, 10, 439.

Knowler, W. C., Barrett-Connor, E., Fowler, S. E., Hamman, R. F., Lachin, J. M., *et al.* and Diabetes Prevention Program Res, G. (2002). Reduction in the incidence of type 2 diabetes with lifestyle intervention or metformin. *New England Journal of Medicine*, 346, 393–403.

Lavin, J. H., Avery, A., Whitehead, S. M., Rees, E., Parsons, J., *et al.* (2006). Feasibility and benefits of implementing a Slimming on Referral service in primary care using a commercial weight management partner. *Public Health*, 120, 872–881.

Mitchell, N. S., Dickinson, L. M., Kempe, A. and Tsai, A. G. (2011). Determining the effectiveness of Take Off Pounds Sensibly (TOPS), a nationally available nonprofit weight loss program. *Obesity*, 19, 568–573.

Neve, M., Morgan, P. J., Jones, P. R. and Collins, C. E. (2010). Effectiveness of web-based interventions in achieving weight loss and weight loss maintenance in overweight and obese adults: a systematic review with meta-analysis. *Obesity Reviews*, 11, 306–321.

Pinto, A. M., Gorin, A. A., Raynor, H. A., Tate, D. F., Fava, J. L. and Wing, R. R. (2008). Successful weight-loss maintenance in relation to method of weight loss. *Obesity*, 16, 2456–2461.

Rock, C. L., Pakiz, B., Flatt, S. W. and Quintana, E. L. (2007). Randomized trial of a multi-faceted commercial weight loss program. *Obesity*, 15, 939–949.

Stubbs, R. J., Brogelli, D. J., Pallister, C. J., Whybrow, S., Avery, A. J. and Lavin, J. H. (2012). Attendance and weight outcomes in 4754 adults referred over 6 months to a primary care/commercial weight management partnership scheme. *Clinical Obesity*, 2, 6–14.

Truby, H., Baic, S., Delooy, A., Fox, K. R., Livingstone, M. B. E., *et al.* (2006). Randomised controlled trial of four commercial weight loss programmes in the UK: initial findings from the BBC 'diet trials'. *BMJ*, 332, 1309–1314.

Tsai, A. G. and Wadden, T. A. (2005). Systematic review: an evaluation of major commercial weight loss programs in the United States. *ACC Current Journal Review*, 14, 15.

WHO (World Health Organization) (2009). Global health risks: mortality and burden of disease attributable to selected major risks. *In:* Press, W. (ed.), *World Health Organization.*

Womble, L. G., Wadden, T. A., Mcguckin, B. G., Sargent, S. L., Rothman, R. A. and Krauthamer-Ewing, E. S. (2004). A randomized controlled trial of a commercial internet weight loss program. *Obesity Research*, 12, 1011–1018.

Popular diets and over-the-counter dietary aids and their effectiveness in managing obesity

18

R. Stanton
University of New South Wales, NSW, Australia

18.1 Introduction: why diets are best sellers

In the days when few people were obese, weight loss and dieting were not issues that received attention. Popular diet books were more likely to promote specific 'health' food diets with claims they would improve looks and energy levels. Gayelord Hauser, a self-styled American nutritionist who sold many diet books in the 1930s, 1940s and 1950s, for example, touted the value of five 'wonder' foods – yoghurt, skim milk powder, wheatgerm, brewer's yeast and blackstrap molasses. Like others, he paid little attention to body fat levels. Books promoting 'super' foods are still popular, but to make the best seller lists, popular diet books now make weight loss their major focus.

Health authorities emphasise the health risks of excess body fat and while most popular diets also mention health benefits from weight loss, they place even greater emphasis on appearance. Fashion fervently favours slenderness for women and low body fat levels with high levels of musculature for men, so this is what many diets promote. Before and after photos of successful dieters are particularly popular in diets published in magazine and newspapers and on Internet sites. Products sold over the counter or online and diets and products sold by gyms, fitness centres and personal trainers also push the body beautiful image more than the avoidance or correction of health problems associated with obesity.

Celebrities are 'gold' to promoters of popular diets and over-the-counter weight loss aids. Personal experience of having lost weight with a particular diet may be a motivator for some film stars or sportspeople to write a diet book; many others endorse particular diets. Such backing can increase sales throughout the world. The Dukan Diet, written by a French doctor some years previously, soared in popularity when it was reputedly followed by the Duchess of Cambridge's mother before the royal wedding to Prince William. Whether the rumours were correct or not, the story was picked up eagerly by the popular press and millions of copies of the diet sold. Psychologists note that many people follow plans endorsed by singers, actors or other celebrities because they want to identify with, or look like the star involved.

Managing and Preventing Obesity. http://dx.doi.org/10.1533/9781782420996.4.257

18.2   Claims that 'the science is wrong'

Many diets achieve notoriety by claiming a breakthrough in medical science, often insisting that past scientists and current guidelines have 'got it wrong'. This trend gained great prominence in the early 1970s when Dr Robert Atkins first published his popular diet, claiming that fats of all kinds were not the cause of obesity, but the major problem was carbohydrate. The initial stages of his original diet prohibited fruit and even some vegetables, as well as forbidding grains, legumes, milk and yoghurt. Because they had virtually no carbohydrate, cream and butter were permitted in unlimited quantities. More recent versions of the Atkins Diet continue to exclude foods containing carbohydrates, but now claim their diet has only one third of the fat as saturated fat and that this results in an increase only in larger and less atherogenic LDL particles.[1] The references cited for this claim[2] have been challenged by others.[3, 4] Although the company that distributed his branded food products filed for bankruptcy in 2005,[5] the company bearing his name continues with its high protein/high fat/low carbohydrate diet. Among the many products they sell is a new range of low carbohydrate foods that include shakes, drinks and confectionery bars.

A number of studies have compared weight loss on an Atkins Diet with a more typical low fat diet (1200–1800 Cal/day, with 25–30% of energy from fat). Short-term (3–6 months), the low carbohydrate diets may produce a slightly greater weight loss, explainable by a greater deficit in energy, but by 12 months, there is no difference in loss.[6] With a larger group and adding a behaviour intervention program to an Atkins Diet or a low fat diet produced no differences in weight loss or body composition at 1 and 2 years or at earlier time points. During the first 6 months, the low fat group had greater decreases in LDL cholesterol while the low carbohydrate group had greater decreases in triglyceride levels. None of these differences were apparent at 12 or 24 months.[7]

While much of the fame for high protein/low carbohydrate diets may be due to the publicity afforded Dr Atkins over the last 40 years, his diet has spawned many other similar diets and they continue to be popular, in spite of high drop-out rates.

The Dukan Diet has been one of the most popular of the high protein, low carbohydrate diets, but unlike the Atkins Diet, it is also low in fat. Designed by Frenchman Dr Pierre Dukan the diet begins with a highly restricted 'attack phase' of only lean low fat meat, chicken and fish, selected non-fat dairy products and 1.5 tablespoons of oat bran. In phase two, the 'cruise phase', you add non-starchy vegetables every second day until you reach your goal weight. This may last for months. In the 'consolidation phase', fruit, cheese, starchy foods and occasional treats are reintroduced. The final phase, 'stabilisation', allows you to return to eating what you like, as long as you have one day every week where you eat only protein. The diet has been criticised by dieticians as unbalanced because it lacks sufficient dietary fibre and several nutrients.[8]

A major advocate of the 'science is wrong' approach has been journalist Gary Taubes who writes that scientists have misled us by blaming the increasing problems of obesity and Type 2 diabetes on overeating and sedentary behaviour. Taubes writes persuasively and backs the theory espoused by Dr Atkins and at least eight other authors of best-selling popular diets that a low fat, high carbohydrate diet is responsible for obesity, heart disease and other chronic diseases. Like Dr Atkins and the diet authors of similar books, Taubes thinks we have been wrong to give advice against saturated fat when we should have been concentrating on the uniquely fattening properties of carbohydrates, specifically sugar, flour, white rice and maybe beer.

Taubes and other critics of dietary guidelines ignore the fact that few people actually follow dietary guidelines. One study in Australia found that out of 10,561 middle-aged women, only two followed all the dietary guidelines.[9] Claiming that the proportion of energy from fat has decreased in the United States ignores the fact that the National Health and Nutrition Examination Survey (NHANES) data showed that the number of grams of fat consumed did not change between 1971 and 2000, but overall energy intake rose – by 22% in women and 7% in men.[10] The increase in calories was mainly due to an increase in carbohydrate consumption. Protein consumption for both men and women did not change over this period. The Global Burden of Diseases Nutrition and Chronic Diseases Expert Group (NutriCoDE) also notes that saturated fat intake in many countries, including 'Australasia', barely changed between 1990 and 2010.[11]

Rather than dismissing the science, it would help if diet book authors gave more thought to the way science is interpreted, or misinterpreted. Dietary guidelines called for a reduction in fat, especially saturated fat with suggestions to trim meat and avoid fatty meats as well as using fat-reduced dairy products. They also recommended more foods naturally low in fat such as fruits, vegetables, legumes and grains (preferably wholegrains). The processed food industry, however, saw a marketing opportunity and produced a wide range of energy-dense, nutrient-poor, low-fat processed foods. Some of the fat was removed from many foods, but replaced with sugars and refined starches. A large range of fat-reduced, highly processed food products have been marketed, especially in the United States. Australian research found that a high intake of foods labelled as fat-reduced could lead to a relatively energy-dense diet and thus promote weight gain.[12] Dietary studies in Australia have also found that energy-dense, nutrient-poor 'extra' foods now contribute 41% of children's and 35% of adults' energy intake.[13] Similar levels are found in children in the United States.[14] In social situations where marketing urges us to consume so many of these foods, in direct contravention of dietary guidelines, it is not surprising that obesity flourishes.

18.3   All or nothing approaches

The low carbohydrate diets continue to be popular, with some specifically concentrating on fructose or sucrose as the prime cause of obesity. Dietary guidelines in many countries, including Australia, have always included advice about refined sugar consumption, with the most recent guidelines released in 2013 specifically recommending limiting sugar-sweetened beverages as well as confectionary, biscuits and cakes (also sources of saturated fat). No dietary guidelines have recommended avoiding all sugar, presumably because there is a lack of evidence to support such a ban and it would be impractical. The approach of 'limiting' the quantity consumed does not suit some diet authors who prefer an all or nothing approach. Some authors do not support any restrictions on saturated fat, but ask for a total ban on sugar.

There are also claims that sugars pose dangers to health that justify controlling them like alcohol.[15] Dr Robert Lustig argues that fructose exerts toxic effects on the liver similar to those of alcohol. To help reduce excessive sugar consumption, Lustig suggests extra taxes on sugar-sweetened foods and drinks as well as controls over licensing requirements for vending machines and snack bars in schools and workplaces – approaches that are supported by those working in public health. However, while Lustig's published papers take a line that fits with the limits suggested by dietary guidelines, the take-up by media and other diet book authors extrapolates this approach to recommending absolutely no sugar. Some object even to the sugars present naturally in fruit and some vegetables, while others permit a small intake of fruit, but no fruit juice or any processed food containing any added sugar. In their push against fructose, some diet book authors recommend using powdered or liquid glucose in place of sucrose in baking and put no restrictions on food sources of fat or protein. Since much of our sugar intake comes from processed foods, and few people do much home baking, promoting the use of glucose may present few problems in practice. However, it is not valid to argue that the energy content of glucose – and that provided by fats – is unimportant.

Two popular examples of this approach include I Quit Sugar, by Australian journalist, television host and health coach Sarah Wilson, who lost 12 kg on her diet, and Sweet Poison, by Australian, ex-lawyer David Gillespie, who lost 40 kg when he gave up sugar. In her books and blogs, Sarah Wilson claims that sugar causes 'leaky gut' and thus triggers autoimmune disorders, prevents white blood cells destroying toxins (which she claims starts 30 minutes after consumption), causes insulin surges that can destroy the thyroid gland and increases production of cortisol which then suppresses the action of the pituitary gland. She also states that her diet will result in a loss of 'bulk' especially around the face and abdomen which she claims is where the liver holds the weight gained from excess sugar consumption. Wilson's blog attracts many comments from her fans and she has also written several popular recipe books which include sweet treats using 'safe' sweeteners such as rice malt syrup instead of sugar. Her book of chocolate recipes features fructose-free cakes, fudges, truffles and brownies, smoothies, cheesecakes and desserts. Many of the recipes are high in saturated fat which arises from ingredients such as coconut butter, coconut oil and coconut cream as well as chocolate.

David Gillespie has also added to his original book with *Sweet Poison Quit Plan* and a *Quit Plan Cookbook* as well as *Big Fat Lies: How the diet industry is making you sick, fat and poor* and *Toxic oil: Why Vegetable Oil Will Kill You & How to Save Yourself.* These and various guides to the sugar content in different categories of branded foods are available from his websites, along with recipe books and the opportunity to ask questions and discuss a range of diet-related issues. Powdered glucose is recommended as a substitute for sucrose and since Mr Gillespie believes saturated fat is harmless, he recommends no restriction on foods such as bacon, butter and fatty meats. His main target is fructose, which he claims causes hormonal dysfunction that leads to excess weight. Mr Gillespie also maintains that fructose causes 'a massive decrease in nitric oxide production', contributing to erectile dysfunction. His reference for this comes from a study of rats given a diet with 65% fructose in which the resulting insulin resistance was found to impair the nitric oxide vasodilation in strips taken from their aortas.[16] Gillespie also claims that bodies such as the World Health Organisation and various cancer authorities give 'useless prevention advice'. On his website, he claims that 'vegetable oil makes you exceedingly vulnerable to cancer' and that 'every extra mouthful of vegetable oil you consume takes you one step closer to a deadly (and irreversible) outcome'.

These authors quote limited evidence in support of their various claims and are critical of the nutrition advice provided by reputable national and international bodies. The weight of opinion amongst researchers in the field continues to be critical of targeting any one food or ingredient as the primary cause of what is a complex problem and supportive of a balanced dietary approach to weight management combined with exercise.[17–19]

18.4   Claims to more moderate diets

Some 'no sugar' diets offer a little more balance by permitting a wider range of foods and noting adverse effects of saturated fats. The latest version of the popular Sugar Busters! (whose authors include three physicians) continues to ban all kinds of sugar and foods containing it, and also forbids white flour, white rice, potatoes, parsnips, sweet corn, beetroot, watermelon, ripe bananas and pineapple. However, it does recommend low-fat dairy products and lean meats and permits nuts, olive and canola oils, brown rice, oatmeal and wholegrain wheat flour.

Dr Gott's No Flour, No Sugar Diet, authored by American family medical doctor Peter Gott MD and Robin Donovan advises followers to stop eating sugar and flour (which means no bread, pizza, pasta, cakes, confectionary and biscuits), but does not limit grains such as oats, barley and rice or starchy vegetables such as sweet corn and potatoes. It also promotes fruit, lean meats, low-fat dairy products and recommends increasing exercise. Dr Gott supports slow steady weight loss, backs choices from the food groups and his recipe book helps readers understand healthier carbohydrate choices.

SOS (Stop Only Sugar) Diet: You Won't Even Know You're on a Diet, by digestive health expert Dr James Surrell, is a relatively simple approach designed for slow and sustainable weight loss of 2–3kg/month. Although it claims to have no rules apart from low sugar and high fibre, it does not permit foods such as bananas, grapes, carrots, beetroot and potatoes even though they contain dietary fibre along with some natural sugars. Milk, white flour and white rice are also out, although wholegrains are heartily recommended. Dr Surrell notes that excess sugar pushes the pancreas to release insulin which causes sugar to be stored as fat and the liver to manufacture cholesterol which will increase the risk of heart disease. This may be correct, but

Dr Surrell does not clearly define 'excess' sugar and does not emphasise the need for physical activity which could prevent storage of sugar as fat. He is in favour of artificial sweeteners and fibre supplements.

The South Beach Diet, designed by cardiologist Dr Arthur Agatston and dietitian Marie Almon some years ago, remains popular. It emphases no sugar and a higher protein intake, but recommends 'good carbs' such as low glycaemic index whole-grains and legumes and 'good fats' such as olive oil, avocado and nuts – in moderate quantities. Accepting the heart health risks posed by saturated fats, the South Beach Diet advises only lean meats, skinless poultry and no bacon, butter, cheese and cream. However, as in the Atkins Diet, the South Beach Diet starts with two extremely strict weeks which eliminate all sugar and foods containing carbohydrates, including fruit and some vegetables. This produces a rapid initial weight loss which is unlikely to be sustained.

The Zone Diet, originally written in 1995 by biochemist Dr Barry Sears, recommends three carefully-timed meals and two snacks a day, each designed to provide 40% of energy from carbohydrates, 30% from protein and 30% from fats. Keeping to this 40:30:30 ratio of macronutrients is more protein and less carbohydrate than most people would normally consume, and applying these ratios to each meal and snack increases the difficulty. Dr Sears' rationale is that a ratio of 30:40 between protein and carbohydrates will stimulate an ideal production of the hormones insulin and glucagon and lead to an anti-inflammatory response and increased oxidation of fats. Sears believes that excess cellular inflammation is the basic cause of weight gain as well as being responsible for chronic disease, ageing and poor physical, emotional, and mental health. Sears has published a description of his theory, but there is little evidence the diet is effective for any reason other than its overall restriction of energy intake.[20] To assist the anti-inflammatory response, Sears also recommends his own brand of patented fish oil supplements, and his online 'shop' offers a selection of meal replacements, snack foods, polyphenol supplements and various 'zone' books. Residents of the US and Canada can also buy a finger prick test and send it for analysis which is supposed to assist with appropriate dietary changes. The Zone diet has more carbohydrate than the Atkins style diets, but prefers these to come from colourful fruits and vegetables. The list of 'unfavourable' foods includes potatoes, bananas, raisins, corn and carrots. Fatty meats and egg yolks are also out of favour, with fats restricted to 'good' ones such as olive oil, nuts and avocado. Moderate exercise is also recommended. Unless the meal replacement products are purchased, the Zone Diet is not easy to follow. It deserves some credit for promoting healthy sources of fat, for recommending some carbohydrate as essential and promoting daily consumption of 1200 to 1600 Calories (5000 to 6700 kJ). Dr Sears and colleagues have also published results of a small study comparing a very low carbohydrate (ketogenic) diet with one that is less restricted, reporting equal loss of body weight but several adverse effects from the diet with minimal carbohydrate.[21]

The CSIRO Total Wellbeing Diet by Dr Peter Clifton and Dr Manny Noakes was released in Australia in 2005, later followed by a second version and a recipe book. The diet was based on studies by CSIRO scientists comparing low fat diets that differed in their content of protein and carbohydrate. Neither diet was extreme. In each study, no significant differences occurred in weight loss. Over the long-term, it was also noted that the group on a lower protein intake increased their intake of protein while those who started on a higher intake decreased their intake. By 68 weeks, there was no significant difference between the diets for the two groups.[22] The CSIRO Total Wellbeing Diet deserves praise for recommending plenty of vegetables, fruit, low fat dairy products, lean meats and wholegrain products in preference to more refined grains. The accompanying recipe book also promoted home cooking instead of fast foods and ready-to-eat meals. The major criticisms concern recommendations for a higher intake of protein from red and processed meats, even though their trials reported no difference in weight loss with the high meat diet. In both diets, weight loss was due entirely to loss of body fat and both significantly increased HDL cholesterol and decreased fasting insulin and insulin resistance. The high content of red meat and processed meats (the latter were reduced but not eliminated in the second version) also raised concern in view of the World Cancer Research Fund stating that evidence was convincing that consumption of red meat and processed meat (such as contained in this diet) are causes of colorectal cancer.[23] The fact that Meat and Livestock Australia (MLA) provided financial support for the CSIRO's high protein diet studies and MLA promoted the diet also provoked criticism of the Total Wellbeing Diet.[24,25]

18.5   Unconventional diets

18.5.1   Palaeolithic diets

Palaeolithic diets have a large following, come in various forms and are often promoted on websites run by fitness coaches and body builders. The first of the popular Palaeolithic diets (dubbed the Stone-Age or Caveman Diet) was published in 1975 by Dr Walter Voegtlin, a gastroenterologist. Dr Voegtlin believed that humans had teeth more like a dog than a sheep and should therefore follow a largely carnivorous diet. He recommended more meat, including its fat, but no dairy products or salt and also advised minimising any plant foods, especially grains and sugar.

In the late 1980s, Dr Boyd Eaton published a version of the paleo diet, based largely on the diet of our East African ancestors. This paleo diet was low in saturated fat in keeping with the lean flesh of wild animals, with a 1:1 ratio of energy from plant and animal foods. Fruits, roots and shoots supplied moderate amounts of carbohydrate.[26] Dr Eaton has since worked closely with Dr Loren Cordain, an exercise physiologist whose website claims he is the founder of the Paleo Diet Movement. Cordain's version of the paleo diet is based on grass-fed meat, poultry, eggs, seafood, fruits and non-starchy vegetables. Fats are not restricted, but grains, legumes, potatoes, dairy products and sugar are all off the table, resulting in a diet that is high in protein and low in carbohydrate. Cordain claims our ancestors were not only lean but also had no cardiovascular disease, Type 2 diabetes, cancer, autoimmune diseases, osteoporosis, acne, myopia, varicose veins, gastric reflux or gout. He and others attribute this to their lack of grains, legumes, dairy products and potatoes.

Palaeolithic diets can be commended for their criticism of the processed foods rich in sugar, saturated fats and salt that dominate the modern Western diet. However, these diets ignore the benefits of plant based foods such as wholegrains and legumes, and push a pattern far removed from that of our ancestors. Even when domesticated animals are grass-fed, their flesh is unlike that of wild animals. Free range poultry do not rely on foraging for food, but are fed grains – unlike wild birds. Wild-caught fish are an option, but world stocks are limited and many are in crisis. Modern fruits and vegetables are also unlike those consumed in palaeolithic times.

Some paleo enthusiasts' websites cite several relatively recent studies to justify their recommendations, but all are short-term trials involving only small numbers of subjects. They do not constitute adequate proof of benefit or balance.

Anthropological experts also dispute the claims of the paleo diets. In her book *Paleofantasy*, evolutionary biologist Professor Marlene Zuk debunks many myths, well summarised in a recent review.[27] Anthropologist Dr Christina Warinner from the University of Oklahoma and the Molecular Research Group at the Centre for Evolutionary Medicine at the University of Zurich, notes that most versions of the paleo diet are closer to an early 20th century affluent farmer's diet than that of our Palaeolithic ancestors.[28] Another highly respected anthropologist, Katherine Milton, also notes that much of what has been ascribed to hunter gatherer populations is inaccurate and does not reflect the different dietary patterns among groups living in different parts of the world.[29]

18.5.2   Blood type diets

The Eat Right for Your Type Diet, authored by naturopath Peter D'Adamo, claims that the body interacts adversely with lectins in foods according to the consumer's blood type, leading to weight gain and other health problems. D'Adamo theorises that eating foods matching one's blood type will enable weight loss and greater energy. Those with blood group Type O have the original blood type of hunters and gatherers and should follow a low carbohydrate diet with plenty of red meat, seafood, liver, spinach and broccoli. Grains, dairy products, legumes and coffee are banned, as are cauliflower, beans and cucumber. Those with blood group Type A have supposedly adapted to agriculture and are prescribed a vegetarian diet that can include oatmeal and other grains (except wheat), legumes (except kidney or Lima beans), nuts, seeds and coffee. Dairy products, meat, oranges, bananas, tomatoes, potatoes, cabbage, capsicum and eggplant are off the table. D'Adamo claims blood group Type B represents an adaptation to pastoral life and can enjoy an omnivorous diet that includes dairy products, meat (but not chicken or pork), eggs and legumes, but excludes avocado, tomato, corn, legumes, peanuts, sesame and wheat. The small number of people with blood group Type AB can enjoy a more balanced diet with dairy products, fish, eggs, tofu, most grains, lamb, rabbit and turkey (but not chicken or beef) and most fruits and vegetables, with the exception of oranges, bananas, avocado, corn and capsicum. Like many diet promoters, D'Adamo has created an entire brand around his specialty diet, offering more than 20 books, plus protein powders, multivitamins, skin products, food bars and shakes, blood typing kits, videos and software.

No studies (or rationale) support his proposed link between weight, blood groups and reaction to lectins. Experts have also pointed out the error in his claim that blood Type O is the original blood group.[30] One study that suggested potential benefits from adherence to the vegetarian diet recommended for Type A and the diet recommended for Type AB found the benefits were independent of blood group.[31]

All followers of the blood type diets are also asked to avoid sugar and highly processed foods and all except the four percent of the population with Type AB must avoid wheat. In practice, all four versions of the diet restrict so many foods that energy intake will inevitably fall.

18.5.3   The Fast Diet (commonly dubbed the 5:2 diet)

Developed by Dr Michael Mosely, a medical doctor and British television journalist, this diet swept the world in 2013. The 'fast' in the title does not refer to the rate of weight loss but to the diet's regimen of 'normal' eating for five days a week with two days devoted to a semi-fast. There are no restrictions for the five 'normal' days of the week. On each of the two 'fast' days, men can consume 600 Cals (2500 kJ) and women 500 Cals (2100 kJ) – both values representing about a quarter of normal energy needs. Mosely's co-author, Mimi Spencer, has written a companion book of calorie-counted recipes that may be used throughout the week. Both authors lost 10 kg on the program. Dr Mosely has also written Fast Exercise, in which 'fast' does refer to time, with claims people can get fitter, stronger and better toned in just a few minutes of ultra-short bursts of high intensity exercise each day.

The 5:2 plan does not promote any special mix of macronutrients and does not dispute that 'calories count'. No food need be banned but Dr Mosely clearly states that success depends on not over-eating on the 'normal' days. On the 'fast' days, the diet book gives suggestions for appropriate meals with their calorie content as well as a calorie count per 100 g (or 100 mL) for over 500 foods. These lists could play a useful educational role, although in countries where kilojoules are the official unit of energy, translating the values may reduce the educational value.

The obvious questions concern whether people can stick to such an eating plan long-term and whether they will eat more the evening before a 'fast' day. A small study has shown that fat oxidation may increase with intermittent fasting. However, hunger on the fasting days suggested that subjects were unlikely to continue with such a pattern for an extended period and the authors suggested that a small meal on fasting day (as recommended by Mosely) may make this type of dietary restriction more acceptable.[32]

Several small, short-term studies provide some evidence that intermittent fasting may be as effective as daily caloric restriction[33,34] as has one somewhat larger, longer trial (107 obese women over a 6-month period).[35] However, further studies are needed, as one group reported the benefits may only occur with a low intake of dietary fat[36] and a rodent study found that intermittent fasting induced obesity and diabetes and worsened spontaneous atherosclerosis in mice with genetic hypercholesterolaemia.[37]

Without long term studies, it is not possible to rate this dietary pattern. Those motivated to follow it could discover they can accommodate occasional feelings of hunger without harm and this could be of value in reducing snacking. Lessons about energy values of different foods would also be useful and followers would discover that large servings of vegetables come at a small energy cost. Greater use of vegetables could also improve the overall nutritional value of the total diet. Those who use their 'normal' days to eat more will soon find the diet does not work and will abandon it.

18.5.4   Further unusual diets

Over the years, we have seen many diets come and go: the Drinking Man's Diet, the Grapefruit Diet, the Israeli Army Diet (no connection with the Israeli Army), the Mayo Clinic Diet (disowned by the Mayo Clinic), food-combining diets, detox diets, the HCG Diet, the Cabbage Soup Diet, the Hollywood Diet, the Lemon Diet, the Flat Belly Diet, the Lunch Box Diet, the Cookie Diet, the Watermelon Diet, Fit for Life and the Drunkorexia Diet are some examples. The ultimate example of a foolish fad diet – the Breatharian Diet – in which you are supposed to live on air and sunlight alone fortunately does not attract too many followers.

These diets, like many of the diets already discussed, and those that occur in magazines and weekend newspaper supplements, promise rapid weight loss. They fail, however, to disclose that much of the loss will be water, glycogen from muscle stores and lean tissue and that fat cannot be lost fast. Fortunately, most of these extremely restrictive diets are so boring or unpleasant they are short-lived. At least this means their inevitable nutritional inadequacies do not have time to incur serious harm.

18.6   Evaluation of promised time-scales

Among all popular diets, the most consistent feature is the promised speed of weight loss – usually at least 1 kg/week and often up to 4 kg/week. A continued loss of even 1 kg a week is beyond weight loss shown in any long-term studies. Even those promoting the Atkins Diet only report losses of less than 1 kg/month over a 12-month period,[38] with almost half that regained over the following 12 months. The initial rapid loss usually reflects a low level of carbohydrate which results in rapidly depleted stores of muscle glycogen and associated water, together responsible for about 2 kg.[39] High protein diets also claim to induce greater loss of body fat with preservation of lean body tissue, although several studies show this not to be the case.[40,41] Only small short term studies have supported the theory.[42]

Support for high protein diets for weight loss has been the subject of a number of papers. Short term studies show a greater initial weight loss with low carbohydrate/ high protein diets, but long term studies reveal no difference in weight loss due to changes in macronutrient intake.[43–45] A recent meta-analysis of long-term randomised control trials, reported that such diets have neither specific beneficial nor detrimental effects on outcome markers of obesity, cardiovascular disease or glycaemic control.[46] Others disagree – at least in mice[47,48] and in results of cohort studies. Two cohort studies from the United States have reported that a low carbo-hydrate diet, high in animal protein was associated with higher all-cause mortality in both men and women, but not if the protein was mainly from plant sources.[49] A large Swedish cohort study reported that low carbohydrate-high protein diets, used on a regular basis and without consideration of the nature of carbohydrates or the source of proteins, are associated with increased risk of cardiovascular disease[50] while a review of cohort studies concluded that low carbohydrate diets were associated with a significantly higher risk of all-cause mortality, but not with increased risk of cardiovascular mortality or incidence.[51] There is also concern over colonic health with a study showing that a low carbohydrate diet (which also means a low intake of dietary fibre) significantly decreased faecal cancer-protective metabolites and increased concentrations of hazardous metabolites.[52] For weight maintenance, more conventional energy-restricted diets may have an edge with evidence from a random-ised controlled trial showing that while those following a low carbohydrate diet/high protein diet maintained most of their initial weight loss, those on a conventional diet continue to lose weight over the long-term.[53]

18.7 Evaluation of claims to simplicity

Theories espoused in popular diets change from time to time, but some themes recur over the years. The idea that you can eat as much as you like – but only of selected foods – crops up often. Reading the fine print reveals the flaws in 'eat more, lose weight' claims. For example, diets may claim they allow unlimited quantities of fatty foods such as butter or cream but then forbid the bread, pasta, potatoes, biscuits, cakes and desserts that would normally be vehicles for the fats. One diet claimed followers could eat as much pasta as they desired, but the details revealed that nothing could accompany the pasta, which had to be consumed on its own. In prac-tice, whenever the range of foods is strictly limited, overall kilojoule intake is almost certain to fall.

Popular diets usually emphasise the simplicity of their solution to obesity. If these fast, easy diets were successful, we might expect a lessening of the incidence and extent of obesity, or at least a lower number of new diets. No such luck!

In contrast to the popular diet promoters, researchers and clinicians understand that complex factors are involved in weight gain and also in successful long-term reduc-tions in body fat.[54] Individual differences are important, relating to family history and dynamics, genetic factors and social and cultural contexts. Weight loss recommenda-tions need a multi-faceted approach that includes appropriate dietary strategies, skills and educational materials as well as back-up counselling and support to assist with long-term maintenance of appropriate and health-promoting changes in eating and exercise habits. Those marketing various popular diets and over-the-counter weight loss products, on the other hand, offer a one-size-fits-all solution that ignores the complexities.

18.8 Over-the-counter weight loss aids

Pharmacies, health food stores, supermarkets and internet sites sell many products that claim to induce rapid weight loss. As well as meal replacements and associated food products, they include herbal supplements which may 'work' by inducing increased laxation or diuresis. Marketers emphasise rapid results, with items such as 7-day weight loss pills or 5-day programs that are supposed to 'detoxify' the body, 'ignite metabolism', 'remove stubborn belly fat' or 'strip away' or even 'melt' unwanted fat. Most also claim they will suppress appetite.

The ingredients credited with these 'slimming' abilities may include caffeine, chromium picolinate, green tea extract, phaseolus vulgaris (a bean extract), chitosan (derived from the shells of crustaceans), glycine max (from soy bean leaves), garcinia cambogia (a small, pumpkin-shaped fruit containing hydroxycitric acid), Irvingia gabonensis (African mango seeds), usnic acid (isolated from types of lichen), guggul tree extracts (from the sap of a small flowering tree grown in north India), glucomannan (usually extracted from the root of the konjac plant), conjugated linoleic acid (a component of dairy fats), senna leaf (from a flowering leguminous plant), Arctostaphylos (sometimes called bearberry), buchu leaf (a herbal plant), olive leaf and various other herbs. Some warn the products will increase bowel movements and increase urine output – both seen as ways to 'flush away waste and toxins'. Such effects should be expected from known laxatives in senna, or the diuretic properties of plant compounds such as Arctostaphylos, uva ursi and buchu leaf.

Some of the ingredients in these so-called weight loss aids have been subjected to research, usually showing no real benefits and sometimes with indications of potential harm. Studies have all been short-term and usually involve small numbers of subjects.[55] In some studies quoted as reporting benefits, no records are kept of dietary intake or exercise levels, making any claimed results useless. Other studies are published in unusual journals or in those journals where the author pays for publication.

Before recommending any supplements, considerations of efficacy and safety are paramount. Websites and pamphlets may make claims that are not backed by good research studies or they may refer to studies in reputable journals that have involved only animals or may simply be laboratory findings that the claimed ingredient is present in the supplement. A lack of benefit for weight loss has been found with many ingredients in supplements, including Garcinia cambogia,[56,57] chromium picolinate,[58] phaseolus vulgaris,[59] Irvingia gabonensis,[60] chromium,[61] glucomannan,[62] green tea[63] and conjugated linoleic acid.[64] Safety aspects for any of these compounds require special attention, as some cause severe toxicity reactions.[65–68]

Many products sold by mail order may escape official scrutiny. However, pharmacies, health food stores and supermarkets also sell supplements carrying weight loss claims with no evidence of efficacy. Unfortunately, many of these products and their claims are only investigated if an individual or consumer group makes a specific complaint. Health authorities need to give more publicity to the fact that no product will 'blast fat' and, although ubiquitous, the process of 'detoxing' has no basis for health or weight loss.

18.9 Discussion

Over the last 40 or 50 years, millions of books and magazines have promoted different diets and diet products that claim to be able to reverse obesity. More recently, almost every popular diet book or weight loss product has also spawned websites (the plural is intentional here) with glowing testimonials, 'before and after' photographs as well as a 'shop' from which you make online purchases of associated products. These range from books to meal replacements and exotic juices, snack bars, shakes, soups and supplements as well as recipes, detox products, blood test kits and exercise programs. Many sites also include a forum for customers to discuss their hopes, aspirations and progress. Celebrities feature on some sites and draw in customers. Overall, online opportunities have boosted the potential for diets and products promising weight loss to become more widely known and make money for their promoters.

Apart from the inevitable testimonials from satisfied users identified only by their first name or initials, there is little proof that any of these popular diets and products can solve the world's obesity crisis. Virtually none of the popular diets can back its claims with evidence of long-term success. If any diet or product *could* provide a single universal solution for obesity, we might have expected to see a decrease in the incidence of excess body fat. Instead, obesity continues to increase and has now spread to populations where it was previously uncommon.

In spite of those who maintain that science has 'got it wrong', no one has yet disproved the laws of thermodynamics,[69] although some have tried.[70] Those who claim their diet confers metabolic advantages due to a low content of carbohydrate or a high content of protein lack proof. Reviews of the literature show little or no effect, or small differences detectable only under the precision of metabolic ward conditions for short periods of time. None are relevant to free-living people consuming a varied diet over time. Obesity remains an imbalance between energy intake and output with weight loss requiring energy output to be greater than energy input. The important addendum, however, is to note that many complex factors govern energy intake and output. Research continues to look at the multiple genes involved, prenatal and early childhood environment, psychosocial factors, and the increasing influence of our 'obesogenic' environment.[71]

Long-term studies of successful weight loss interventions are rare. The National Weight Control Registry in the United States notes that only 20% of those who intentionally lose at least 10% of their weight maintain the loss for at least a year.[72] This may be sufficient to correct metabolic abnormalities associated with obesity[73] but in a climate where many have been led to expect instant success, it is not a message that is likely to outdo sales of popular diets.

For those who grow despondent looking at the low levels of success, it is worth checking the habits of over 10,000 members listed in the National Weight Control Registry who lost an average of 33 kg and maintained their losses for more than 5 years. Almost all modified their food intake, eating a low kilojoule, low fat diet, consuming breakfast regularly, maintaining a consistent eating pattern across weekdays and weekends, monitoring their weight and increasing their physical activity to at least an hour a day. Many report that weight loss maintenance has become easier over time, with those who have successfully maintained their loss for 2 to 5 years increasing their chance of longer-term success.[74]

Perhaps the best we can do is to issue a guide to those who are looking for a popular diet. Signs that a diet should be rejected:

1. Anything that promises weight loss will be rapid or easy.
2. Any product/diet that relies on testimonials rather than research published in a reputable journal.
3. Any diet that claims to be new or revolutionary.
4. Any diet that cuts out one or more entire food groups.
5. Any diet that claims you can eat unlimited quantities of any food (except vegetables).
6. Any diet that claims calories (or kilojoules) do not count.
7. Any program that claims exercise is unnecessary.
8. Anything that claims you can eat whatever you like as long as you use a particular pill, injection or supplement.
9. Any diet that claims superiority even if scientists have rejected its claims.
10. Any diet or supplement that sounds too good to be true.

18.10   Sourcing unbiased information

The best sources of unbiased information are available from reputable scientific research organisations. In Australia, the National Health and Medical Research Council produces *Dietary Guidelines*[75] and clinical practice guidelines for the management of obesity in adults, adolescents and children in Australia.[76] In general, Departments of Health, recognised medical groups and organisations such as the World Obesity Federation (previously the International Association for the Study of Obesity), offer reliable advice.

References

1. http://www.atkins.com/Science/Articles—Library/Fats/Atkins-Position-on-Saturated-Fat-.aspx, accessed February 2014.
2. Dreon DM, Fernstrom HA, Williams PT, Krauss RM. A very low-fat diet is not associated with improved lipoprotein profiles in men with a predominance of large, low-density lipoproteins. *Am J Clin Nutr* 1999; 69(3): 411–18.
3. Kenney JJ, Barnard RJ, Inkeles S. Very low fat diets do not necessarily promote small dense LDL particles. *Am J Clin Nutr* 1999; 70(3): 423–4.
4. Grant WB. Low-fat, high-sugar diet and lipoprotein profiles. *Am J Clin Nutr* 1999; 70(6): 1111–1112.
5. Webb, M. *The Washington Post*, 2 August 2005, available at http://www.washingtonpost.com/wp-dyn/content/article/2005/08/02/AR2005080200276.html. Accessed February 2014.
6. Foster GD, Wyatt HR, Hill JO, McGuckin BG, Brill, C, *et al.* A randomized trial of a low-carbohydrate diet for obesity. *N Engl J Med* 2003; 348: 2082–90. doi: 10.1056/NEJMoa022207.

7. Foster GD, Wyatt HR, Hill JO, Makris AP, Rosenbaum DL, *et al.* Weight and metabolic outcomes after 2 years on a low-carbohydrate versus low-fat diet: a randomized trial. *Ann Intern Med* 2010; 153(3): 147–57. doi: 10.7326/0003-4819-153-3-201008030-00005.

8. (British Dietetic Association News Nov 2013, available at https://web.archive.org/web/20140209081959/http://bda.uk.com/news/131125BadDiets.html, accessed May 26 2014).

9. Ball K, Mishra GD, Thane CW, Hodge A. How well do Australian women comply with dietary guidelines? *Public Health Nutr* 2004: 7(3): 443–452.

10. *Trends in Intake of Energy and Macronutrients, United States, 1971–2000*, available at http://www.cdc.gov/nchs/index.htm accessed February 2014. CDC. Trends in intake of energy and macronutrients—United States, 1971–2000. *MMWR* 53: 80–2. 2004.

11. Micha R, *et al.* Global, regional and national consumption levels of dietary fats and oils in 1990 and 2010: a systematic analysis including 266 country-specific nutrition surveys. *BMJ* 2014; 348: g2272.

12. La Fontaine HA, Crowe TC, Swinburn BA, Gibbons CJ. Two important exceptions to the relationship between energy density and fat content: foods with reduced-fat claims and high-fat vegetable-based dishes. *Public Health Nutr* 2004; 7(4): 563–8.

13. Rangan AM *et al.* Consumption of 'extra' foods by Australian children: types, quantities and contribution to energy and nutrient intakes. *Eur J Clin Nutr* 2008; 62(3): 356–64.

14. Poti JM, Slining MM, Popkin BM. Where are kids getting their empty calories? Stores, schools, and fast-food restaurants each played an important role in empty calorie intake among US children during 2009–2010. *J Acad Nutr Diet* 2013. pii: S2212-2672(13)01336-1. doi: 10.1016/j.jand.2013.08.012.

15. Lustig RH, Schmidt LA, Brindis CD. Public health: the toxic truth about sugar. *Nature* 2012; 482(7383): 27–9. doi: 10.1038/482027a.

16. Shinozaki K, Kashiwagi A, Nishio Y, Okamura T, Yoshida Y, Masada M, Toda N, Kikkawa R. Abnormal biopterin metabolism is a major cause of impaired endothelium-dependent relaxation through nitric oxide/O2-imbalance in insulin-resistant rat aorta. *Diabetes* 1999; 48(12): 2437–45. doi: 10.2337/diabetes.48.12.2437.

17. Bleich S, Cutler D, Murray C, Adams A. Why is the developed world obese? *Annu Rev Public Health*, 2008; 29: 273–95. doi: 10.1146/annurev.publhealth.29.020907.090954.

18. Hall KD, Sacks G, Chandramohan D, Chow CC, Wang YC, Gortmaker SL, Swinburn BA. Quantification of the effect of energy imbalance on body weight. *Lancet*, 2011; 378(9793): 826–37. doi: 10.1016/S0140-6736(11)60812-X.

19. Swinburn BA, Sacks G, Lo SK, Westerterp KR, Rush EC, Rosenbaum M, Luke A, Schoeller DA, DeLany JP, Butte NF, Ravussin E. Estimating the changes in energy flux that characterize the rise in obesity prevalence. *Am J Clin Nutr* 2009; 89(6): 1723–1728. doi: 10.3945/ajcn.2008.27061.

20. Sears B, Ricordi C. Role of fatty acids and polyphenols in inflammatory gene transcription and their impact on obesity, metabolic syndrome and diabetes. *Eur Rev Med Pharmacol Sci* 2012; 16(9): 1137–54.

21. Johnston CS, Tjonn SL, Swan PD, White A, Hutchins H, Sears B, Ketogenic low-carbohydrate diets have no metabolic advantage over nonketogenic low-carbohydrate diets. *Am J Clin Nutr* 2006; 83(5): 1055–61.

22. Brinkworth GD1, Noakes M, Keogh JB, Luscombe ND, Wittert GA, Clifton PM. Long-term effects of a high-protein, low-carbohydrate diet on weight control and cardiovascular risk markers in obese hyperinsulinemic subjects. *Int J Obes Relat Metab Disord* 2004; 28(5): 661–70.

23. http://www.wcrf.org/cancer_research/cup/key_findings/colorectal_cancer.php, accessed February 2014

24. Stanton R, Crowe T. Risks of a high-protein diet outweigh the benefits. *Nature* 2006; 440(7086): 868.

25. Stanton R, Scrinis G. Total Wellbeing or too much meat? *Australasian Science* 72: 37–8.

26. Eaton SB.Humans, lipids and evolution. *Lipids* 1992; 27(10): 814–20.

27. Jabr F. How to really eat like a hunter-gatherer: why the paleo diet is half-baked. *Scientific American*, June 3, 2013, available at http://www.scientificamerican.com/article.cfm?id=why-paleo-diet-half-baked-how-hunter-gatherer-really-eat, accessed February 2014.

28. http://tedxtalks.ted.com/video/Debunking-the-Paleo-Diet-Christ, accessed February 2014.

29. Milton K, Hunter-gatherer diets – a different perspective. *Am J Clin Nutr* 2000; 71(3): 665–7.

30. Saitou N, Yamamoto Y. Evolution of primate ABO blood group genes and their homologous genes. *Mol Biol Evol* 1997; 14(4): 399–411.

31. Wang J, García-Bailo, Nielsen DE, El-Sohemy. ABO genotype, 'blood-type' diet and cardiometabolic risk factors. *PLoS One* 2014; 9(1): e84749. doi:10.1371/journal.pone.0084749.

32. Heilbronn LK, Smith SR, Martin CK, Anton SD, Ravussin E. Alternate-Day fasting in non-obese subjects: effects on body weight, body composition and energy metabolism. *Am J Clin Nutr* 2005; 81(1): 69–73.

33. Varady KA. Intermittent versus daily calorie restriction: which diet regimen is more effective for weight loss. *Obes Rev* 2011; 12(7): e593–601. doi: 10.1111/j.1467–789X.2011.00873.x

34. Varady KA, Bhutani S, Klempel MC, Kroeger CM, Trepanowski JF, *et al.* Alternate day fasting for weight loss in normal weight and overweight subjects: a randomized controlled trial. *Nutr J* 2013; 12(1): 146. doi: 10.1186/1475-2891–12–146.

35. Harvie MN, Pegington M, Mattson MP, Frystyk J, Dillon B, *et al.* The effects of intermittent or continuous energy restriction on weight loss and metabolic disease risk markers: a randomized trial in young overweight women. *Int J Obes (Lond)* 2011; 35(5): 714–27. doi:10.1038/ijo.2010.171.

36. Klempel MC, Kroeger CM, Norkeviciute E, Goslawski M, Phillips SA, Varady KA. Benefit of a low-fat over high-fat diet on vascular health during alternate day fasting. *Nutr Diabetes* 2013; 3:e71. doi: 10.1038/nutd.2013.14.

37. Dorighello GG, Rovani JC, Luhman CJF, Paim BA, Raposo HF, Vercesi AE, Oliveira HCF. Food restriction by intermittent fasting induces diabetes and obesity and aggravates spontaneous atherosclerosis development in hypercholesterolaemic mice. *British Journal of Nutrition*, available on CJO2013. doi:10.1017/S0007114513003383.

38. Foster GD, Wyatt HR, Hill JO, Makris AP, Rosenbaum DL, *et al.* Weight and metabolic outcomes after 2 years on a low-carbohydrate versus low-fat diet: a randomized trial. *Ann Intern Med* 2010; 153(3): 147–57. doi: 10.7326/0003–4819–153–3–201008030–00005.

39. Kreitzman SN, Coxon AY, Szaz KF. Glycogen storage: illusions of easy weight loss, excessive weight regain, and distortions in estimates of body composition. *Am J Clin Nutr* 1992; 56: 292S–3S.

40. Skov AR, Toubro S, Ronn B, Holm L, Astrup A. Randomized trial on protein vs carbohydrate in ad libitum fat reduced diet for the treatment of obesity. *Int J Obes Relat Metab Disord* 1999; 23: 528–36.

41. Brehm BJ, Seeley RJ, Daniels SR, D'Alessio DA. A randomized trial comparing a very low carbohydrate diet and a calorie-restricted low fat diet on body weight and cardiovascular risk factors in healthy women. *J Clin Endocrinol Metab* 2003; 88: 1617–23.

42. Layman DK, Boileau RA, Erickson DJ, *et al.* A reduced ratio of dietary carbohydrate to protein improves body composition and blood lipid profiles during weight loss in adult women. *J Nutr* 2003; 133: 411–17.

43. Fogelholm M, Anderssen S Gunnarsdottir I, Lahti-Koski M. Dietary macronutrients and food consumption as determinants of long-term weight change in adult populations: a systematic literature review. *Food Nutr Res* 2012; 56. doi:10.3402/fnr.v56i0.19103.

44. Sacks FM, Bray GA, Carey VJ, Smith SR, Ryan DH, *et al.* Comparison of weight-loss diets with different compositions of fat, protein, and carbohydrates. *N Engl J Med* 2009; 360: 859–73. doi: 10.1056/NEJMoa0804748.

45. de Souza RJ, Bray GA, Carey VJ, Hall KD, LeBoff MS, *et al.* Effects of 4 weight-loss diets differing in fat, protein, and carbohydrate on fat mass, lean mass, visceral adipose tissue, and hepatic fat: results from the POUNDS LOST trial. *Am J Clin Nutr* 2012; 95(3): 614–25. doi: 10.3945/ajcn.111.026328.

46. Schwingshackl L, Hoffmann G. Long-term effects of low-fat diets either low or high in protein on cardiovascular and metabolic risk factors: a systematic review and meta-analysis. *Nutr J* 2013; 12: 48. doi: 10.1186/1475-2891-12-48.

47. Foo SY, Heller ER, Wykrzykowska J, Sullivan CJ, Manning-Tobin JJ, *et al.* Vascular effects of a low-carbohydrate high-protein diet. *Proc Natl Acad Sci USA* 2009; 106(36): 15418–23. doi: 10.1073/pnas.0907995106

48. Kostogrys RB, Franczyk-Żarów M, Maślak E, Gajda M, Mateuszuk L, Jackson CL, Chłopicki S. Low carbohydrate, high protein diet promotes atherosclerosis in apolipoprotein E/low-density lipoprotein receptor double knockout mice (apoE/LDLR(-/-)). *Atherosclerosis* 2012; 223(2): 327–31. doi: 10.1016/j.atherosclerosis.2012.05.024

49. Fung TT, van Dam RM, Hankinson SE, Stampfer M, Willett WC, Hu FB. Low-carbohydrate diets and all-cause and cause-specific mortality: two cohort studies. *Ann Intern Med* 2010; 153: 289–98. doi:10.1059/0003–4819–153–5–201009070–00003.

50. Lagiou P, Sandin S, Lof M, Trichopoulos D, Adami HO, Weiderpass E. Low carbohydrate-high protein diet and incidence of cardiovascular diseases in Swedish women: prospective cohort study. *BMJ* 2012; 344: e4026. doi: 10.1136/bmj.e4026.

51. Noto H, Goto A, Tsujimoto T, Noda M. Low-carbohydrate diets and all-cause mortality: a systematic review and meta-analysis of observational studies. *PLoS One* 2013; 8(1): e55030. doi: 10.1371/journal.pone.0055030

52. Russell WR, Gratz SW, Duncan SH, Holtrop G, Ince J, *et al.* High-protein, reduced-carbohydrate weight-loss diets promote metabolite profiles likely to be detrimental to colonic health. *Am J Clin Nutr* 2011; 93(5): 1062–72. doi: 10.3945/ajcn.110.002188.

53. Stern L, Iqbal N, Seshadri, Chicano KL, Daily DA *et al.* The effects of low-carbohydrate versus conventional weight loss diets in severely obese adults: one-year follow-up of a randomized trial. *Ann Intern Med* 2004; 140(10): 778–785. doi:10.7326/0003–4819–140–10–200405180–00007.

54. Jebb SA, Kopelman PG, Butland B. Foresight tackling obesities: future choices project. *Obesity Reviews* 8: Issue Supplement s1, vi–ix, March 2007. doi:10.1111/j.1467–789X.2007.00344.x

55. Egras AM, Hamilton WR, Lenz TL, Monaghan MS. An evidence-based review of fat modifying supplemental weight loss products. *J Obes* 2011; 2011: 297315. doi: 10.1155/2011/297315.

56. Ji-Eun Kim, Seon-Min Jeon, Ki Hun Park, Woo Song Lee, Tae-Sook Jeong, *et al.* Does *Glycine max* leaves or *Garcinia Cambogia* promote weight-loss or lower plasma cholesterol in overweight individuals? a randomized control trial. *Nutr J* 2011; 10: 94. doi:10.1186/1475-2891-10-94.

57. Onakpoya I, Hung SK, Perry R, Wider B, Ernst E. The use of *Garcinia cambogia* (hydroxycitric acid) as a weight loss supplement: a systematic review and meta-analysis of randomised clinical trials. *J Obes* 2011; 2011: 509038. doi: 10.1155/2011/509038

58. Tian H, Guo X, Wang X, He Z, Sun R, Ge S, Zhang Z. Chromium picolinate supplementation for overweight or obese adults. *Cochrane Database Syst Rev* 2013; 11: CD010063. doi: 10.1002/14651858.CD010063.pub2.

59. Onakpoya I, Aldaas S, Terry R, Ernst E. The efficicy of phaseolus vulgaris as a weight loss supplement: a systematic review and meta analysis of randomised clinical trials. *Br J Nutr* 2011; 106(2): 196–202.

60. Onakpoya I, Davies L, Posadzki P, Ernst E. The efficacy of Irvingia gabonensis supplementation in the management of overweight and obesity: a systematic review of randomised controlled trials. *Diet Suppl* 2013; 10(1): 29–38. doi: 10.3109/19390211.2012.760508.

61. Onakpoya I, Posadzki P, Ernst E. Chromium supplementation in overweight and obesity: a systematic review and meta-analysis of randomised clinical trials. *Obes Rev* 2013; 14(6): 496–507. doi: 10.1111/obr.1202.

62. Onakpoya I, Posadzki P, Ernst E. The efficacy of glucomannan supplementation in overweight and obesity: a systematic review and meta-analysis of randomised clinical trials. *J Am Coll Nutr* 2014; 33(1): 70–8. doi: 10.1080/07315724.2014.870013.

63. Jurgens TM, Whelan AM, Killian L, Doucette S, Kirk S, Foy E. Green tea for weight loss and weight maintenance in overweight or obese adults. *Cochrane Database Syst Rev* 2012; 12: CD008650. doi: 10.1002/14651858.CD008650.pub2.

64. Onakpoya I, Posadzki PP, Watson LK, Davies LA, Ernst E. The efficacy of long-term conjugated linoleic acid supplementation on body composition in overweight and obese individuals: a systematic review and meta-analysis of randomised clinical trials. *Eur J Nutr* 2012; 51(2): 127–34. doi: 10.1007/s00394–011–0253–9.

65. Yellapu RK, Mittal V, Grewal P, Fiel MI, Schiano T. Acute liver failure caused by 'fat burners' and dietary supplements. A case report and literature review. *Can J Gastroenterol* 2011; 25(3): 157–60.

66. Dietz BM, Bolton JL. Biological reactive intermediates formed from botanical dietary supplements. *Chem Biol Interact* 2011; 192(0): 72–80. doi: 10.1016/j.cbi.2010.10.007.

67. Pawar RS, Tamta H, Ma J, Krynitsky AJ, Grundel E, Wamer WG, Rader JI. Updates on chemical and biological research on botanical ingredients in dietary supplements. *Anal Bioanal Chem* 2013; 405(13): 4373–84. doi: 10.1007/s00216–012–6691–2.

68. Bunchorntavakul C, Reddy KR. Review article: herbal and dietary supplements hepatotoxicity. *Aliment Pharmacol Ther* 2013; 37(1): 3–17. doi: 10.1111/apt.12109.

69. Buchholz AC, Schoeller DA. Is a calorie a calorie?1'2'3'4. *Am J Clin Nutr* 2004; 79 (5): 899S–906S.

70. Manninen AH. Is a calorie really a calorie? Metabolic advantages of low-carbohydrate diets. *J Int Soc Sports Nutr* 2004; 1(2): 21–26.

71. Swinburn BA, Sacks G, Hall KD, McPherson K, Finegood DT, Moodie ML, Gortmaker SL. The global obesity pandemic: shaped by global drivers and local environments. *Lancet* 2011; 377: 804–14.

72. Wing RR, Phelan S. long term weight maintenance. *Am J Clin Nutr* 2005; 82(1): 222S–225S.

73. Korczak D, Kister C. Overweight and obesity: The efficacy of diets for weight maintenance after weight loss. *GMS Health Technol Assess* 2013; 9: Doc06. doi: 10.3205/hta000112.

74. http://www.nwcr.ws/Research/published%20research.htm, accessed Feburary 2014.

75. www.eatforhealth.gov.au, accessed February 2104.

76. http://www.nhmrc.gov.au/_files_nhmrc/publications/attachments/n57_obesity_guidelines_130531.pdf, accessed February 2014.

Part Five

Government and industry interventions in the prevention of obesity

Regulatory strategies for preventing obesity and improving public health

C. A. Roberto[1], J. Soo[1], L. Pomeranz[2]
[1]Harvard School of Public Health, Boston, MA, USA; [2]Temple University, Philadelphia, PA, USA

19.1 Introduction

For the past thirty years, the prevalence of obesity has been rising in the United States and across the globe (Center for Disease Control; World Health Organization). Attempts at reducing obesity have historically focused on treatment, despite relatively little progress in developing safe and affordable weight loss programs or medications that produce sustained weight loss (Dansinger *et al.*, 2007; Christensen *et al.*, 2007; Curioni and Lourenco, 2005; Glazer 2001; Heshka *et al.*, 2003; Surapaneni *et al.*, 2011; Tsai and Wadden, 2005). Although an individual's weight is in part influenced by genetics, the rapid rise in obesity over the last thirty years cannot be explained by genetic changes at the population level. Instead, the more likely drivers of worldwide obesity have been global changes in food and physical activity environments (Finucane *et al.*, 2011). Nutrient poor, energy-dense foods are highly palatable, widely available, inexpensive, served in large portions, inadequately labeled, and heavily marketed, all of which promote overconsumption. Environmental changes have also encouraged more sedentary behaviors in occupational, recreational, transportation and household settings (Sallis *et al.*, 2006). In addition, cultural, social, and economic factors contribute to obesity (Christakis and Fowler, 2007; McCabe *et al.*, 2011). Despite educational efforts and the strong desire of many individuals to weigh less, obesity remains a major public health problem, suggesting a need for policy interventions that will address environmental drivers of the problem. In this chapter, we discuss five policy strategies for improving diet: (1) restriction of food marketing to children, (2) altering school food environments, (3) food taxes; (4) nutrition labeling, and (5) placing limits on restaurant portion sizes.

19.2 Restricting child-targeted food marketing

The food industry spends billions of dollars each year marketing their products to young consumers to increase sales and create lifelong brand loyalty (Harris *et al.*,

2009a). Although television remains the most popular medium for advertising (Federal Trade Commission (US), 2007), other forms of marketing abound including food and beverage product placement in movies, television shows, and video games, food company sponsorships of sporting and entertainment events, and in-store product cross-promotions with other items (Calvert, 2008). In addition, companies market through online advergames, videos, and social marketing (Cheyne *et al.*, 2013, Brady *et al.*, 2010). This ubiquitous marketing is concerning because most of the foods advertised are low in nutrients and high in calories, fat, sugar, and/or sodium (Folta *et al.*, 2006, Powell *et al.*, 2011, Kelly *et al.*, 2008). Further, food marketing has been found to influence children's food preferences, short-term eating behaviors, and purchases (Cairns *et al.*, 2013; Harris *et al.*, 2009a, 2009b; Institute of Medicine, 2006; Roberto *et al.*, 2010a).

In the United States, the First Amendment protects companies' right to advertise. This makes it difficult to restrict food advertising in media and the retail environment even when the goal is to protect children (*Lorillard v. Reilly*, 2001). Although never tested in court, there is a valid argument that marketing directed at young children is deceptive and should be restricted because those under 8 are too young to fully comprehend the nature and purpose of advertising (National Research Council, 2006). This makes children a vulnerable population who cannot differentiate between factual information and advertising intended to persuade them (Harris and Graff, 2012; Pomeranz, 2010). However, the broad reach of most advertising makes it difficult to tailor such a restriction without impinging on protected speech to teens and adults. The one clear exception to this challenge involves advertising directed at children on school grounds. Government may reserve the school space for its educational purpose and restrict advertising on school property by, for example, prohibiting all marketing or prohibiting ads for products not permitted to be sold on school grounds (Pomeranz, 2012).

Policies to limit or regulate food marketing to children have been implemented in other countries, mostly focused on television advertising. Child-directed food advertisements have been banned during children's television programming in Sweden (since 1991), Norway (since 1992), and Quebec, Canada (since 1980). In addition, over 30 countries, including many in Europe, Australia, and the Republic of Korea, have national laws setting specific restrictions on television advertising to children, such as limits on advertising at certain times or on certain programs, or limits on specific marketing techniques such as the use of cartoon characters (Hawkes, 2004).

In 2006, the food industry in the United States launched its own voluntary, self-regulatory program, the Children's Food and Beverage Advertising Initiative (CFBAI), designed to modify the mix of food advertising primarily directed to children to encourage more nutritious dietary choices and healthier lifestyles. The Initiative addresses marketing on traditional media (television, radio, print, and the Internet), along with new and emerging media (mobile technology and video games). Significantly, this does not apply in the retail environment where purchasing decisions are actually made. However, in 2009, Congress directed representatives from four federal agencies to form the Interagency Working Group (2011), and recommended voluntary guidelines for industry self-regulation of food marketing. In April 2011, the Interagency Working Group (IWG) released sound recommendations that took into consideration both positive and negative nutritional attributes of foods. The food industry refused to adopt the government-backed standards, affirming that they would continue to abide by the industry-generated CFBAI, led by the Better Business Bureau (Watson, 2011).

In the absence of a policy to restrict marketing, 18 food companies are members of the voluntary CFBAI. However, the pledges apply only to certain types of marketing. For example they exclude the retail environment, and define 'child-directed' advertising as only including programming where children less than 12 years old comprise at least 35% of the audience (Harris *et al.*, 2013). Further, the nutrition criteria for foods that can be marketed are significantly weaker than the IWG standards (Center for Science in the Public Interest, 2009). Finally, networks that are not members of the CFBAI, like Nickelodeon, do not restrict the placement of unhealthy food advertisements on their children's programming, websites, and mobile apps (Bachman, 2013). Despite the CFBAI efforts, there has also been little observed improvement in the nutritional content of advertised foods and beverages (Center for Science in the Public Interest., 2010). In addition, children continue to see large numbers of unhealthy food and beverage advertisements on programs that are not considered child-specific (Harris *et al.*, 2013).

Many challenges exist in future efforts to regulate food marketing to children. Countries, food companies, and researchers all differ in their definition of a child (Lobstein *et al.*, 2011). Comprehensive bans on advertising are also difficult to enforce especially across borders. Advertisements targeted to children can be difficult to distinguish from those intended for the entire family or for adults. Currently, self-regulatory programs have focused on media or programs which have a certain percentage of children users or viewers; however, many forms of media predominantly used by adults can also be seen by large numbers of children. In addition, although the nutrition criteria developed by the CFBAI are an important step toward consistency as to what products can be advertised, the adherence by individual companies to these guidelines remains to be determined. Finally, newer forms of media entertainment are constantly becoming available, such as media streamed in from other countries via the Internet or satellite television, and policymakers will have to decide which forms of media will need to be regulated, and how to enforce the legislation.

19.3 Improving the school environment

Data from the U.S. indicate that children spend more time in school than in any other place away from home (Story *et al.*, 2009), and consume 35% of their daily calories at school (Gleason and Suitor, 2001). Thus, the school environment represents a promising opportunity for the implementation of a broad range of nutrition and wellness policies. Several countries have taken action to improve school food environments. Schools in France are not permitted to have vending machines that sell food and drink (Mercer, 2005) and the United Kingdom has restricted the sale of certain foods in schools (United Kingdom Department of Education, 2013). In addition, six provinces in Canada have implemented guidelines for school food (Hawkes, 2007).

In the United States, several federal-, state-, and district-level school policies have been passed to address nutrition education and wellness. At the federal level, the U.S. Department of Agriculture (USDA) announced changes to the school meal program, to improve nutrition standards. Such changes include making potable water available and free of charge during meal services, increasing the amount and variety of fruits and vegetables offered, and reducing the amount of fat and saturated fat in meals. However, outside of school meal times, students are presented with numerous other opportunities to purchase foods of poor nutritional quality through vending machines, fundraisers, a la carte items during lunch, and at school stores. Such foods are increasingly prevalent in schools, and often lack nutrients in favor of fat, sugar, and sodium (Gordon and Fox, 2007). The increased availability of these snack foods in schools has been shown to be associated with increased consumption (Neumark-Sztainer et al., 2005), as well as inversely associated with fruit and vegetable intake, and positively associated with fat intake (Kubik et al., 2003).

In June 2013, the USDA announced the 'Smart Snacks in School' standards, setting nutrition criteria for snack foods sold on school campus during the school day. These standards are designed to limit salt, sugar and fat in such foods, and to increase whole grains, low fat dairy, fruits, vegetables and lean protein (Food and Nutrition Service, 2013). The regulations are to take effect in July 2014, and while they will not apply to foods sold during after-school sporting events or other activities, or foods consumed as part of birthday celebrations or fundraisers, they nevertheless represent a critical step toward improving the nutrition profile of many foods eaten on school campuses.

State-level school nutrition policies also provide ample opportunity for improving the food environment, as many often surpass federal policies in their regulatory stringency (Trust for America's Health, 2009, Boehmer et al., 2008). One recent, controversial state policy was the implementation of BMI report cards, which identify children at high risk for obesity, and alert parents to modify the child's eating and activity patterns (Nihiser et al., 2009). About a quarter of U.S. states currently have some sort of BMI screening and surveillance program, beginning with Arkansas in 2003, and the majority of the states notify parents of the results (Vogel, 2011). However, evidence is still inconclusive as to the effectiveness of the report cards. Furthermore, there is concern that the report cards may increase stigma toward overweight children or encourage them to adopt unhealthy eating behaviors (Ikeda et al., 2006), although early research in Arkansas seems to suggest that the possible negative consequences of teasing, use of diet pills, or excessive concerns about weight have not materialized (Thompson and Card-Higginson, 2009).

Finally, district-level regulation can provide additional guidelines tailored to the needs of the specific location and the demographics of its students. Examples of policies that could cultivate healthier school food environments include modifying the scheduling and duration of lunch periods, as research has shown that a later lunch was associated with lower a la carte sales (Probart et al., 2006), implementing zoning laws that would restrict fast-food vendors from operating near schools (Mair et al., 2005), eliminating open-campus policies (Neumark-Sztainer et al., 2005), or prohibiting parents or students from bringing food into cafeterias from local fast-food establishments (Probart *et al.*, 2006). Overall, school policies represent powerful tools with which to tackle and reverse childhood obesity.

19.4   Food and beverage taxes

A policy option receiving increasing attention is taxation of certain foods or beverages. Some countries, particularly in Europe, have legislated taxes on soft drinks or other unhealthy foods, with varying results. In October 2011, Denmark introduced the world's first so-called 'fat tax' on butter, milk, cheese, pizza, meat, oil, and other processed foods containing more than 2.3% saturated fat (BBC, 2011). However, one year later lawmakers repealed the tax, claiming that it failed to change the Danes' eating habits, encouraged cross-border purchases in Sweden and Germany, put Danish jobs at risk, and was extremely difficult to implement and enforce. At the same time, the Danish tax ministry also canceled plans for a proposed sugar tax (BBC, 2012, Strom, 2012).

In 2012, France implemented a tax on sugar-sweetened beverages, amounting to about 9 cents per liter (Harless, 2012) and Hungary implemented taxes targeting energy drinks and packaged foods with certain amounts of salt or sugar to combat obesity, reduce salt consumption, and fund their health care system. (Daley, 2013). Additional countries, including Finland, Britain, Ireland, and Romania, have also implemented some form of food tax, or are discussing doing so. Most recently, in 2013 Mexico successfully passed a tax of 8% on processed foods such as potato chips, and a tax of one peso (about eight U.S. cents) per liter on sugary beverages, a tax of about 10% (Boseley, 2014).

In the United States, the most common proposal has been an excise tax of a penny per ounce for any beverages with added sugar, with revenue allocated to child nutrition or obesity prevention programs. Research has suggested that such a tax would generate $14.9 billion in the first year nationally (Brownell *et al.*, 2009), $79 billion over five years, and reduce sugar-sweetened beverage consumption by 24% (Andreyeva *et al.*, 2011). Other studies have projected similar reductions in caloric intake and weight as a result of a sugar-sweetened beverage tax (Finkelstein *et al.*, 2010), and consumer support for such a tax appears to be increasing (Rivard *et al.*, 2012).

Although this penny-per-ounce tax has been debated in numerous states and cities in the United States, none so far have successfully enacted legislation. Some states have implemented smaller taxes on sugar-sweetened beverages, amounting to about a 5% increase in price, but research suggests the prices must increase 10–20% to meaningfully affect consumption (Andreyeva *et al.*, 2010). Although data suggest tobacco taxes have been effective at reducing consumption (Wisotzky *et al.*, 2004), the effectiveness of taxes on sugar-sweetened beverages has been questioned (Fletcher *et al.*, 2010). It is possible that a tax on sugar-sweetened beverages for example would simply encourage consumers to switch to sweet foods or other unhealthy beverages not included in the tax (Fletcher *et al.*, 2013). In response, more comprehensive taxation schemes have been proposed, including taxes combined with a subsidy for water to encourage healthier behavior, or a tax that taxes all caloric sweeteners at the manufacturer level (Miao *et al.*, 2012). Although the effects of these taxes on consumer behavior and on health outcomes is not well understood yet, taxation represents a compelling policy option for incentivizing behavior change.

19.5   Nutrition labeling

19.5.1   Calorie labelling at restaurants

Menu labeling is a policy introduced in the United States that requires chain restaurants to post calorie information for their menu items so that it is visible at the point of purchase. Several U.S. states and cities have already implemented menu labeling and it will be implemented nationally as part of the Patient Protection and Affordable Care Act (Nutr. Label. Stand. Menu Items Chain Restaur., 2010). Existing research on menu labeling is mixed; some studies find that it has not influenced consumers to purchase fewer calories (Elbel *et al.*, 2009, Finkelstein *et al.*, 2011; Harnack *et al.*, 2008), while other studies have found that it promotes ordering and/or consumption of fewer calories when dining out (Dumanovsky *et al.*, 2011; Bollinger *et al.*, 2011; Roberto *et al.*, 2010b; Krieger *et al.*, 2013)

19.5.2   Front-of-package nutrition labeling

In addition to posting calorie information on restaurant menus, there is growing interest in placing labels on the front of packaged foods to quickly alert consumers to the nutritional quality of food products. There are a variety of existing front-of-package labeling systems. In the United States, the food industry recently introduced Facts Up Front, a label that includes information about calories, saturated fat, sodium and sugars per serving as well as percent daily value. The label also highlights up to two nutrients to encourage (i.e. potassium, fiber, Vitamin A). In the United Kingdom, the Food Standards Agency developed a multiple traffic light system used by some food manufacturers (Food Standards Agency, 2010). This system uses red, yellow, and green traffic lights to indicate high, medium, and low amounts of saturated fat, sodium, and sugar. Ecuador recently announced a mandate for a nutritional label system based on the traffic light system (Gara, 2013). Some countries such as the Netherlands have adopted the 'Choices' (Choices Program, 2010), which is placed on products meeting a scientific standard for healthfulness. Chile also has a new labeling system in effect as of early 2014, requiring food makers to put warning labels on packages if foods are high in sugar, salt, calories or fat (Bodzin, 2014).

Although research suggests that labeling systems like the multiple traffic light and Choices symbol are fairly well understood by consumers (Hawley *et al.*, 2013), more studies are needed examining how front-of-package nutrition labels influence food purchases and/or consumption. Related research on shelf-tag labeling systems in supermarkets has found that these kinds of labeling systems increase the sales of foods promoted by the labels (Sutherland *et al.*, 2010; Levy *et al.*, 1985). In addition to influencing consumer behavior, calorie labels on restaurant menus and front-of-package food labels have the potential to encourage food companies to reformulate products to improve the nutritional composition of foods. Evidence following the implementation of the Choices symbol in the Netherlands suggests reformulation is happening (Vyth *et al.*, 2010) and data following calorie labeling implementation in Seattle also suggests restaurants are responding with some reformulation (Bruemmer *et al.*, 2012).

19.6   Limiting portion sizes of sugar-sweetened beverages

Research has consistently demonstrated that large portion sizes increase short-term energy intake among both adults and children (Fisher and Kral, (2008); Rolls *et al.*, 2002, 2003, 2004a, 2004b, 2007). However, most restaurants serve large portions as a default, despite significant public health concern about obesity (Young and Nestle, 2002). Although some consumers desire smaller portions, people have a tendency to stick with default options presented to them (Samuelson and Zeckhauser, 1988), and so few customers spontaneously ask for smaller portions, regardless of their preference (Schwartz *et al.*, 2012). To address large portion sizes of sugary drinks, the New York City Board of Health adopted a regulation limiting the permissible serving size of sugary beverages available for sale and self-service in the city's food service establishments. The 2012 ordinance established a maximum cup size of sixteen ounces due to the association between excessive consumption of sugary beverages and weight gain, obesity, diabetes and cardiovascular disease (Ebbeling *et al.*, 2006, 2012; Pan *et al.*, 2013). The serving size limit alters the default to a smaller portion, but preserves freedom by enabling consumers to purchase as many drinks as desired and retailers to offer free refills. In New York City, retailers, the beverage industry, and other groups, sued the city to prevent enforcement of the ordinance. Although two lower courts ruled against the city, the state's highest court accepted the city's appeal in October 2013. At the time of this writing the legality of New York City's ordinance was under consideration. However, research into portion limit policies is still necessary to understand how they influence consumer purchase decisions and whether there are unanticipated or unintended consequences, such as consumers purchasing multiple drinks or switching to other beverages (e.g., alcohol) not subject to a restriction. Although the outcome of the lawsuit in New York City applies in New York State only, this innovative policy might be considered in other places in the United States or the world.

19.7   Conclusion

Obesity continues to be a major threat to worldwide public health, but there is reason for hope. In this chapter, we have described a number of promising policies that have been implemented or are being considered across the world with respect to restricting child-targeted food marketing, improving school food environments, implementing food taxes, requiring better disclosure of nutrition information for restaurant and packaged foods, and limiting the portion sizes of sugar-sweetened beverages in restaurants. Such policies have the potential to curb obesity and improve the world' diet.

References

Andreyeva, T., Chaloupka, F. J. and Brownell, K. D. (2011). Estimating the potential of taxes on sugar-sweetened beverages to reduce consumption and generate revenue. *Prev Med*, 52, 413–16.

Andreyeva, T., Long, M. W. and Brownell, K. D. (2010). The impact of food prices on consumption: a systematic review of research on the price elasticity of demand for food. *Am J Public Health*, 100, 216–22.

BBC. (2011). Denmark introduces world's first food fat tax. *BBC News*. Available from: http://www.bbc.com/news/world-europe-15137948. Accessed February 2014.

BBC. (2012). Denmark to abolish tax on high-fat foods. *BBC News*. Available from: http://www.bbc.com/news/world-europe-20280863. Accessed February 2014.

Bodzin, S. (2014). Label it: Chile battles obesity. *The Christian Science Monitor*.

Boehmer, T. K., Luke, D. A., Haire-Joshu, D. L., Bates, H. S. and Brownson, R. C. (2008). Preventing childhood obesity through state policy. Predictors of bill enactment. *Am J Prev Med*, 34, 333–40.

Bollinger, B., Leslie, P. and Sorensen, A. (2011). Calorie posting in chain restaurants. *Am. Econ. J. Econ. Policy*, 3, 91–128.

Boseley, S. (2014). Mexico enacts soda tax in effort to combat world's highest obesity rate. *The Guardian*. Available from: http://www.theguardian.com/world/2014/jan/16/mexico-soda-tax-sugar-obesity-health. Accessed Feb 2014.

Brady, J., Mendelson, R., Farrell, A. and Wong, S. (2010). Online marketing of food and beverages to children: a content analysis. *Can J Diet Pract Res*, 71, 166–71.

Brownell, K. D., Farley, T., Willett, W. C., Popkin, B. M., Chaloupka, F. J., *et al.* (2009). The public health and economic benefits of taxing sugar-sweetened beverages. *N Engl J Med*, 361, 1599–1605.

Bruemmer, B., Krieger, J., Saelens, B.E., and Chan, N. (2012). Energy, saturated fat, and sodium were lower in entrees at chain restaurants at 18 months compared with 6 months following the implementation of mandatory menu labeling in King County, Washington. *J Acad Nutr Diet*, 12, 1169–76.

Cairns, G. Angus, K., Hastings, G. and Caraher, M. (2013). Systematic reviews of the evidence on the nature, extent and effects of food marketing to children. A retrospective summary. *Appetite*, 62, 209–15.

Calvert, S. L. (2008). Children as consumers: advertising and marketing. *Future Child*, 18, 205–34.

Center for Science in the Public Interest (2009). Summary of Polls on Nutrition Labeling in Restaurants. Available from: http:www.cspinet.org/new/pdf/census_menu_board_question.pdf. Accessed February 2014.

Center for Science in the Public Interest (2010). Report Card on Food-Marketing Policies: An Analysis of Food and Entertainment Company Policies Regarding Food and Beverage Marketing to Children. Washington, DC.

Cheyne, A. D., Dorfman, L., Bukofzer, E. and Harris, J. L. (2013). Marketing sugary cereals to children in the digital age: a content analysis of 17 child-targeted websites. *J Health Commun*, 18, 563–82.

Choices Program (2010). Healthy Choices Made Easy. Brussels, Belgium: Choices Int. Found.

Christakis, N.A., and Fowler, J.H. (2007). The spread of obesity in a large social network over 32 years. *N Engl J Med*, 357, 370–9.

Christensen, R., Kristensen, P. K., Bartels, E. M., Bliddal, H. and Astrup, A. (2007). Efficacy and safety of the weight-loss drug rimonabant: a meta-analysis of randomised trials. *Lancet*, 370, 1706–13.

Curioni, C. C. and Lourenco, P. M. (2005). Long-term weight loss after diet and exercise: a systematic review. *Int J Obes (Lond)*, 29, 1168–74.

Daley, S. (2013). Hungary tries a dash of taxes to promote healthier eating habits. *The New York Times*. Available from: http://www.nytimes.com/2013/03/03/world/europe/hungary-experiments-with-flood-tax-to-coax-healthier-habits.html?pagewanted=all&_r=0. Accessed February 2014.

Dansinger, M. L., Tatsioni, A., Wong, J. B., Chung, M. and Balk, E. M. (2007). Meta-analysis: the effect of dietary counseling for weight loss. *Ann Intern Med*, 147, 41–50.

Dumanovsky, T., Huang, C. Y., Nonas, C. A., Matte, T. D., Bassett, M. T. and Silver, L. D. (2011). Changes in energy content of lunchtime purchases from fast food restaurants after introduction of calorie labelling: cross sectional customer surveys. *BMJ*, 343, d4464.

Ebbeling, C. B., Feldman, H. A., Chomitz, V. R., Antonelli, T. A., Gortmaker, S. L., *et al.* (2012). A randomized trial of sugar-sweetened beverages and adolescent body weight. *N Engl J Med*, 367, 1407–16.

Ebbeling, C. B., Feldman, H. A., Osganian, S. K., Chomitz, V. R., Ellenbogen, S. J. and Ludwig, D. S. (2006). Effects of decreasing sugar-sweetened beverage consumption on body weight in adolescents: a randomized, controlled pilot study. *Pediatrics*, 117, 673–80.

Elbel, B., Kersh, R., Brescoll, V. L. and Dixon, L. B. (2009). Calorie labeling and food choices: a first look at the effects on low-income people in New York City.. *Health Aff. (Millwood)*, 28, w1110–21.

Finkelstein, E. A., Strombotne, K. L., Chan, N. L. and Krieger, J. (2011). Mandatory menu labeling in one fast-food chain in King County, Washington. *Am J Prev Med*, 40, 122–7.

Finkelstein, E. A., Zhen, C., Nonnemaker, J. and Todd, J. E. (2010). Impact of targeted beverage taxes on higher- and lower-income households. *Arch Intern Med*, 170, 2028–34.

Finucane, M.M., Stevens, G.A., Cowan, M.J., Danaei, G., Lin, J.K., *et al.* (2011). National, regional, and global trends in body mass index since 1980: Systematic analysis of health examination surveys and epidemiological studies with 960 country-years and 9.1 million participants. *Lancet*, 377, 557–67.

Fisher, J. O. and Kral, T. V. (2008). Portion sizes and obesity: response of fast-food companies. *Physiology and Behavior*, 94, 39–47.

Fletcher, J., Frisvold, D. and Tefft, N. (2013). Substitution patterns can limit the effects of sugar-sweetened beverage taxes on obesity. *Prev Chronic Dis*, 10, E18.

Fletcher, J. M., Frisvold, D. and Tefft, N. (2010). Taxing soft drinks and restricting access to vending machines to curb child obesity. *Health Aff (Millwood)*, 29, 1059–66.

Folta, S. C., Goldberg, J. P., Economos, C., Bell, R. and Meltzer, R. (2006). Food advertising targeted at school-age children: a content analysis. *J Nutr Educ Behav*, 38, 244–8.

Food and Nutrition Service, U. (2013). National School Lunch Program and School Breakfast Program: nutrition standards for all foods sold in school as required by the Healthy, Hunger-Free Kids Act of (2010). Interim final rule. *Fed Regist*, 78, 39067–120.

Food Standards Agency. (2010). *Traffic light labeling* [Online]. Available: http://www.eatwell.gov.uk/foodlabels/trafficlights/.

Gara, T. (2013). After Bloomberg, Latin America Steps Up in War on Junk Food. *The Wall Street Journal*. Available from: http://blogs.wsj.com/corporate-intelligence/2013/12/27/latin-america-steps-up-where-bloomberg-failed/. Accessed January 2014.

Glazer, G. (2001). Long-term pharmacotherapy of obesity 2000: a review of efficacy and safety. *Arch Intern Med*, 161, 1814–24.

Gleason, P. and Suitor, C. (2001). Food for Thought: Children's Diets in the 1990s. Princeton, NJ: Mathematica Policy Res.

Gordon, A. and Fox, M. K. (2007). School Nutrition Dietary Assessment Study-III: Summary of Findings. Alexandria, VA: U.S. Dep. Agric. Food Nutr. Serv.

Grocery Manufact. ASSOC. (2011). Nutrition Keys Front-of-Pack Labeling Initiative. Washington, DC: Grocery Manufact. Assoc.

Harnack, L.J., French, S.A., Oakes, J.M., Story, M.T., Jeffery, R.W., and Rydell, S.A. (2008). Effects of calorie labeling and value size pricing on fast food meal choices: Results from an experimental trial. *Int J Behav Nutr Phys Act*, 5, 63.

Harless, W. (2012). Taxes on unhealthy foods gain traction in Europe. *PBS Newshour*. Available from: http://www.pbs.org/newshour/rundown/while-soda-tax-debate-continues-in-the-us-taxes-on-unhealthy-foods-gain-traction-in-europe/. Accessed January 2014.

Harris, J. L., Pomeranz, J. L., Lobstein, T. and Brownell, K. D. (2009a). A crisis in the market-place: how food marketing contributes to childhood obesity and what can be done. *Annu Rev Public Health*, 30, 211–25.

Harris, J.L., Bargh, J.A., Brownell, K. D. (2009b). Priming effects of television food advert-ising on eating behavior. *Health Psychol*, 28, 404–13.

Harris, J. L. and Graff, S. K. (2012). Protecting young people fron junk food advertising: implications of psychological research for First Amendment law. *Am J Public Health*, 102, 214–22.

Harris, J. L., Sarda, V., Schwartz, M. B. and Brownell, K. D. (2013). Redefining 'child-directed advertising' to reduce unhealthy television food advertising. *Am J Prev Med*, 44, 358–64.

Hawkes, C. (2004). Marketing food to children: the global regulatory environment. Geneva: World Health Organization.

Hawkes, C. (2007). Regulating food marketing to young people worldwide: Trends and policy drivers. *Am J Pub Health*, 97, 1962–1973.

Hawley, K. L., Roberto, C. A., Bragg, M. A., Liu, P. J., Schwartz, M. B. and Brownell, K. D. (2013). The science on front-of-package food labels. *Public Health Nutr*, 16, 430–9.

Heshka, S., Anderson, J. W., Atkinson, R. L., Greenway, F. L., Hill, J. O., Phinney, S. D., Kolotkin, R. L., Miller-Kovach, K. and Pi-Sunyer, F. X. (2003). Weight loss with self-help compared with a structured commercial program: a randomized trial. *JAMA*, 289, 1792–8.

Holt D. J., Ippolito, P. M., Desrochers, D. M., Kelley, C. R. (2007). Children's exposure to TV advertising in 1977 and 2004. Federal Trade Commission (US), Bureau of Economics Staff Report.

Ikeda, J. P., Crewford, P. B. and Woodward-Lopez, G. (2006). BMI screening in schools: helpful or harmful. *Health Educ Res*, 21, 761–9.

Inst. Med. Comm. Food Market. Diets Children Youth. (2006). *Food Marketing to Children and Youth: Threat or Opportunity?* Washington, DC: Natl. Acad. Press. 516 pp.

Kelly, B., Bochynska, K., Kornman, K. and Chapman, K. (2008). Internet food marketing on popular children's websites and food product websites in Australia. *Public Health Nutr*, 11, 1180–7.

Krieger, J.W., Chan, N.L., Saelens, B.E., Ta, M.L., Solet, D., and Fleming, D.W. (2013). Menu labeling regulations and calories purchased at chain restaurants. *Am J Prev Med*, 44, 595–604.

Kubik, M. Y., Lytle, L. A., Hannan, P. J., Perry, C. L. and Story, M. (2003). The association of the school food environment with dietary behaviors of young adolescents. *Am J Public Health*, 93, 1168–73.

Levy, A. S., Mathews, O., Stephenson, M., Tenney, J. E. and Schucker, R. E. (1985). The impact of a nutrition information program on food purchases. *J. Public Policy Mark,* 4 1–13.

Lobstein, T., Parn, T. and Aikenhead, A. (2011). A Junk-Free Childhood: Responsible Standards for Marketing Foods and Beverages to Children. London: Int. Assoc. Study Obes.

Lorillard v. Reilly, 533 U.S. 525 (2001).

Mair, J. S., Pierce, M. W. and Teret, S. P. (2005). The use of zoning to restrict fast food outlets: a potential strategy to combat obesity. *The Center for Law and the Public's Health at Johns Hopkins and Georgetown Universities.*

McCabe, M.P., Mavoa, H., Ricciardelli, L.A., Schultz, J.T., Waqa, G., and Fotu, KF. (2011). Sociocultural agents and their impact on body image and body change strategies among adolescents in Fiji, Tonga, Tongans in New Zealand and Australia. *Obes Rev,* 12 Suppl 2, 61–7.

Mercer, C. (2005). France launches controversial school vending machine ban. NUTRAaingredients.com. Retrieved from: http://www.nutraingredients.com/Regulation/France-launches-controversial-school-vending-machine-ban.

Miao, Z., Beghin, J. C. and Jensen, H. H. (2012). Taxing sweets: sweetener input tax or final consumption tax? *Contemp Econ Policy* 30 346–61.

National Research Council (2006). *Food Marketing to Children and Youth: Threat or Opportunity?,* Washington, DC, The National Academies Press.

Neumark-Sztainer, D., French, S. A., Hannan, P. J., Story, M. and Fulkerson, J. A. (2005). School lunch and snacking patterns among high school students: associations with school food environment and policies. *Int J Behav Nutr Phys Act,* 2, 14.

Nihiser, A. J., Lee, S. M., Wechsler, H., Mckenna, M., Odom, E., *et al.* (2009). BMI measurement in schools. *Pediatrics,* 124 Suppl 1 S89–97.

Nutr. Label. Stand. Menu Items Chain Restaur. (2010). HR 3590, Sec. 4205.

Nutrition Labeling and Education Act of 1990. Pub L No. 101–535, 104 Stat 2353.

Pan, A., Malik, V. S., Hao, T., Willett, W. C., Mozaffarian, D. and Hu, F. B. (2013). Changes in water and beverage intake and long-term weight changes: results from three prospective cohort studies. *Int J Obes (Lond),* 37, 1378–85.

Pomeranz, J. L. (2010). Television food marketing to children revisited: the Federal Trade Commission has the constitutional and statutory authority to regulate. *J Law Med Ethics,* 38, 98–116.

Pomeranz, J. L. (2012). The wheels on the bus go 'buy buy buy': school bus advertising laws. *Am J Public Health,* 102 1638–43.

Powell, L. M., Schermbeck, R. M., Szczypka, G., Chaloupka, F. J. and Braunschweig, C. L. (2011). Trends in the nutritional content of television food advertisements seen by children in the United States: analyses by age, food categories, and companies. *Arch Pediatr Adolesc Med,* 165, 1078–86.

Probart, C., McDonnell, E., Hartman, T., Weirich, J. E. and Bailey-Davis, L. (2006). Factors associated with the offering and sale of competitive foods and school lunch participation. *J Am Diet Assoc,* 106 242–7.

Rivard, C., Smith, D., Mccann, S. E. and Hyland, A. (2012). Taxing sugar-sweetened beverages: a survey of knowledge, attitudes and behaviours. *Public Health Nutr,* 15, 1355–61.

Roberto, C. A., Baik, J., Harris, J. L. and Brownell, K. D. (2010a). Influence of licensed characters on children's taste and snack preferences. *Pediatrics,* 126 88–93.

Roberto, C. A., Larsen, P. D., Agnew, H., Baik, J. and Brownell, K. D. (2010b). Evaluating the impact of menu labeling on food choices and intake. *Am J Public Health,* 100, 312–8.

Rolls, B. J. (2003). The supersizing of America: portion size and the obesity epidemic. *Nutr Today,* 38 42–53.

Rolls, B. J., Morris, E. L. and Roe, L. S. (2002). Portion size of food affects energy intake in normal-weight and overweight men and women. *Am J Clin Nutr,* 76 1207–13.

Rolls, B. J., Roe, L. S., Kral, T. V., Meengs, J. S. and Wall, D. E. (2004a). Increasing the portion size of a packaged snack increases energy intake in men and women. *Appetite,* 42, 63–9.

Rolls, B. J., Roe, L. S. and Meengs, J. S. (2007). The effect of large portion sizes on energy intake is sustained for 11 days. *Obesity (Silver Spring),* 15, 1535–43.

Rolls, B. J., Roe, L. S., Meengs, J. S. and Wall, D. E. (2004b). Increasing the portion size of a sandwich increases energy intake. *J Am Diet Assoc,* 104 367–72.

Sallis, J. F., Cervero, R. B., Ascher, W., Henderson, K. A., Kraft, M. K., and Kerr, J. (2006). An ecological approach to creating more physically active communities. *Ann Rev Pub Health,* 27, 297–322.

Samuelson, W. and Zeckhauser, R. (1988). Status quo bias in decision making. *Journal of Risk and Uncertainty,* 7, 7–59.

Schwartz, J., Riis, J., Elbel, B., and Ariely, D. (2012). Inviting consumers to downsize fast-food portions significantly reduces calorie consumption. *Health Affairs* 31, 399–407.

Story, M., Nanney, M. S. and Schwartz, M. B. (2009). Schools and obesity prevention: creating school environments and policies to promote healthy eating and physical activity. *Milbank Q,* 87, 71–100.

Strom, S. (2012). 'Fat Tax' in Denmark is repealed after criticism. *The New York Times.* Available from: http://www.nytimes.com/2012/11/13/business/global/fat-tax-in-denmark-is-repealed-after-criticism.html. Accessed January 2014.

Surapaneni, P., Vinales, K. L., Najib, M. Q. and Chaliki, H. P. (2011). Valvular heart disease with the use of fenfluramine-phentermine. *Tex Heart Inst J,* 38, 581–3.

Sutherland, L. A., Kaley, L. A. and Fischer, L. (2010). Guiding stars: the effect of a nutrition navigation program on consumer purchases at the supermarket. *Am J Clin Nutr,* 91, S1090–94.

Thompson, J. W. and Card-Higginson, P. (2009). Arkansas' experience: statewide surveillance and parental information on the child obesity epidemic. *Pediatrics,* 124 (Suppl 1), S73–82.

Trust for America's Health (2009). *F as in FAT: How Obesity Policies are Failing in America.* Robert Wood Johnson Foundation.

Tsai, A. G. and Wadden, T. A. (2005). Systematic review: an evaluation of major commercial weight loss programs in the United States. *Ann Intern Med,* 142, 56–66.

United Kingdom Department of Education (2013). *School Food Standards.* Retrieved from: http://www.education.gov.uk/schools/adminandfinance/schooladmin/a0012940/school-food-standards.

Vogel, L. (2011). The skinny on BMI report cards. *CMAJ,* 183, E787–8.

Vyth, E. L., Steenhuis, I. H., Roodenburg, A. J., Brug, J. and Seidell, J. C. (2010). Front-of-pack nutrition label stimulates healthier product development: a quantitative analysis. *Int J Behav Nutr Phys Act,* 7, 65.

Watson, E. (2011). GMA: There is no middle round on kids marketing proposals. *Food Navigator* Retrieved from: http://www.foodnavigator-usa.com/Markets/GMA-There-is-no-middle-ground-on-kids-marketing-proposals.

Wisotzky, M., Albuquerque, M., Pechacek, T.F., and Park, B.Z. (2004). The National Tobacco Control Program: focusing on policy to broaden impact. *Public Health Reports,* 119, 303–10.

Young, L. R. and Nestle, M. (2002). The contribution of expanding portion sizes to the US obesity epidemic. *Am J Public Health,* 92, 246–9.

Fiscal strategies to influence diet and weight management

A. M. Thow
University of Sydney, Sydney, NSW, Australia

20.1 Introduction

Fiscal policy intervention is highlighted in the Political Declaration of the United Nations High-Level Meeting on Non-Communicable Diseases (NCDs) as an important part of a comprehensive and effective approach to improve diets, reduce obesity and prevent NCDs (United Nations General Assembly, 2011). Similarly, the 2013 World Health Organization Global Action Plan for NCDs specifically identifies taxes and subsidies as a policy option for improving diets and preventing chronic disease (WHO, 2013). As part of a multi-sectoral approach, taxes and subsidies can create incentives for healthier food production and consumption, and thus form part of upstream interventions to improve diets, and prevent obesity and NCDs.

Current interest in implementing universal health coverage also means that interventions to prevent chronic NCDs are becoming more important. This was recently highlighted during the 2009 preparations for US health reform, in which soft drink taxation was proposed as an option to both reduce calorie consumption (and obesity) and raise money for public health care (Congressional Budget Office, 2008). While individuals' food preferences should be respected, the costs to the public generated by NCDs are significant; NCDs are very expensive to treat, and are not curable. Thus, NCD prevention presents an opportunity to ease the public health care burden.

The critical issues for public health policy makers regarding the use of fiscal strategies to influence diet and body weight are (1) the effect of such intervention on consumption (and flow on impacts on body weight and disease risk), (2) the best targets of such intervention, and (3) whether such intervention can be effectively implemented. This chapter summarises recent evidence for the effectiveness of fiscal interventions, considers appropriate tools and targets, and discusses experiences of intervention.

20.2 Evidence to support fiscal strategies as an intervention

The premise for taxation of unhealthy foods and/or subsidisation of healthy foods is the well-established role of price as a driver of food choice (French, 2003; Eyles

Managing and Preventing Obesity. http//dx.doi.org/10.1533/9781782420996.5.289

et al., 2012). Taxes and subsidies can create fiscal incentives for consumers to consume less (or more) of targeted foods, and thus improve overall diets.

Recent data show that certain categories of healthy and less healthy food are price elastic (price elasticity is a measure of the effect of changes in price on demand for a good) and thus indicate that fiscal intervention can be effective in reducing or increasing consumption of specific foods to improve diets (Powell *et al.*, 2013). This is largely due to the ability of consumers to substitute between foods; fiscal interventions can thus contribute to healthier food choices by encouraging substitution of healthier products for less healthy products. For example, substituting whole grain bread for low-fibre breads (Nordström and Thunström, 2009), or switching from sugar-sweetened beverages to water or unsweetened tea (Dharmasena and Capps, 2012).

This section first describes the cross-disciplinary evidence base for fiscal intervention, and then summarises effects for three different outcome measures.

20.2.1   Understanding the evidence base

Measuring responses to fiscal intervention presents a challenge. To date, there have been four different broad approaches to assessing fiscal intervention: Randomised Controlled Trials (RCTs), modelling studies based on previously collected expenditure or consumption data, longitudinal analyses of intervention, and studies of stated preference (Thow *et al.*, 2014).

Traditional public health research methods – of which the 'gold standard' is RCTs that involve prospective observation of consumer responses to interventions – can provide valuable information regarding the response of consumers in controlled settings. However, these take site-specific measures and thus are limited in their capacity to understand whole of consumption changes in diets that might result from a fiscal intervention. For example, an RCT in New Zealand assessed healthy food subsidies in a grocery store context and provided a high quality assessment of consumer responses to the intervention (Ni Mhurchu *et al.*, 2010). However, we are unable to tell from this study whether consumers made compensatory purchases elsewhere, such as those who might previously have purchased their fruit and vegetables at a different venue but shifted their purchasing because of the discount.

Modelling studies offer a way to use household expenditure and dietary data to estimate the effect of a fiscal intervention. The most robust modelling studies are able to assess, based on household purchasing and consumption data, how a household might respond to a tax or subsidy and the effect that this would have on nutrient consumption (and in some cases measures of body weight). These studies are limited by the fact that they rely on retrospective observations of responses to price fluctuations, rather than actual interventions. In their recent review, Eyles and colleagues (2012) found that the majority of modelled studies were of low quality, and that there was substantial variability in model structures, data inputs, and the types and magnitudes of food taxes and subsidies assessed, which made it difficult to compare outcomes across studies.

Studies using population-based and longitudinal data to assess intervention have been conducted in the USA, comparing states with and without soft drink taxes and assessing changes in population body weight. These studies are valuable because they assess real interventions over time, or between different populations. However, they are generally limited by their inability to account for confounding factors that might also affect body weight over the period studied. A recent review by Powell and colleagues (Powell *et al.*, 2013) found that these studies were also limited by the very low levels of taxation that have been implemented to date.

Studies of stated preference – sometimes called 'experimental studies' – collect data using laboratory or online scenarios, in which consumers make hypothetical purchases of goods. These scenarios are repeated with different prices applied to goods, to assess how consumers respond to hypothetical fiscal interventions. The limitation of this type of study is the unknown extent to which these scenarios reflect decision making in the real world (Epstein *et al.*, 2012). For example, some recent studies have used a unique 3-D web-based supermarket designed to resemble a national supermarket, with photographs of genuine products used to compose product images (Waterlander *et al.*, 2012). Participants are allocated a budget based on household composition and asked to conduct a typical shop for one week. However, participants do not receive any of the products they select and thus this hypothetical situation may not be representative of actual decision-making (Epstein *et al.*, 2012).

20.2.2 Effects on consumption

The key outcome measures of fiscal intervention relevant for public health are *consumption* (which is the direct effect that mediates subsequent health effects), *body weight* (based on changes to calorie consumption), and *chronic disease risk* (based on changes to nutrient consumption and also through body weight changes). Another relevant outcome is any *socio-economic differentials* in both economic and health effects; in particular, whether fiscal measures are regressive (are borne disproportionately by the less well-off) and whether health outcomes accrue differentially.

The direct effect of fiscal intervention is on diet. The evidence base to date indicates that taxes and subsidies can effectively improve the healthfulness of diets by decreasing consumption of less healthy foods and increasing consumption of healthier foods, respectively (An, 2012; Eyles *et al.*, 2012; Epstein *et al.*, 2012; Powell *et al.*, 2013, Thow *et al.*, 2014).

Subsidies on healthy foods (fruits, vegetables and healthy foods defined by nutrient profiling criteria) are effective in increasing consumption of the target foods (An, 2012). One RCT, conducted in supermarkets in New Zealand, found that a subsidy of 12.5% increased healthy food purchase by around 10%, with little to no effect on unhealthy nutrient consumption (Ni Mhurchu *et al.*, 2010). However, other studies suggest that subsidies can increase overall calorie consumption – either through increased consumption of healthier foods (i.e. an increase in total volume of food consumed), or through the spending of saved monies on less healthy products (Lacroix *et al.*, 2010; Giesen *et al.*, 2012).

Taxes on three types of less healthy foods have been evaluated in the literature: taxes on soft drinks; nutrient-based taxes (i.e. taxes based on the amount of a target nutrient in a food, usually salt, fat or sugar); and taxes based on nutrient profiling (i.e. using a system to classify foods as healthy or less healthy, such as an existing rating system like traffic light labelling or a measure of energy/nutrient density calculated from the nutrition information panel).

Taxes on soft drinks appear to be the most effective option for inducing consumption change away from a specific food, with strong evidence from robust modelling studies (Thow *et al.*, 2014). A recent review estimated the price elasticity of demand for sugar-sweetened beverages in the USA as −1.21 (meaning that a 20% increase in price would result in a 24% decrease in consumption) (Powell *et al.*, 2013). Some limited evidence suggests that adult consumers would substitute with fruit juices, low-fat milk, coffee, and tea (Dharmasena and Capps, 2012) and that children are likely to substitute with milk, which is a nutritionally superior alternative (Fletcher *et al.*, 2010b). The best option would be a 'specific' (applied by the volume of drink) excise tax, as this would help to reduce price disparities between brands (thus reducing incentives for substitution between brands) and also be built into the shelf price that consumers see when making their purchase, unlike a sales tax (Chriqui *et al.*, 2013).

Taxes on individual nutrients usually reduce consumption of the target nutrient (although often by a fairly small amount, and in some cases with negligible effect on the diet as a whole), but can have unintended consequences on consumption of non-target nutrients (Eyles *et al.*, 2012; Thow *et al.*, 2010). For example, a tax on saturated fat might significantly increase salt consumption (Mytton *et al.*, 2007). The more mixed findings found for these taxes may be due to the fact that these taxes apply to core foods, such as meat and dairy. Taxes can thus send mixed messages to consumers, who are told to consume such foods as part of a balanced diet; for the same reason, core foods are also likely to be less price elastic. However, within food categories (e.g. dairy) a fat tax can be effective in encouraging substitution between healthy and less healthy options (e.g. full fat and low fat dairy products) (Khan *et al.*, 2012; Miao *et al.*, 2011).

Taxes and subsidies based on nutrient profiling overcome some of the limitations of nutrient-based taxes and subsidies by taking into account both calories and nutrient density. They are thus less likely to apply to core foods. Temple and colleagues' (2011) prospective intervention study in the USA showed that a 25% tax on 'red' labelled foods (using traffic light nutrient profiling) significantly reduced consumption of unhealthy foods among obese participants (by 40%) and reduced consumption among non-obese participants by 10%. In Sweden, the most effective implementation of a nutrient profiling tax was in combination with a subsidy: a fibre subsidy and tax on unhealthy grain products resulted in a significant improvement in diets (Nordström and Thunström, 2009).

20.2.3   Effects on body weight

The potential effects of fiscal interventions on body weight are mediated through their effectiveness in reducing calorie consumption. While taxes on less healthy foods and beverages have been mainly found to reduce calorie intake, their effect on obesity is not clear. A study in the USA found that taxes on sugar sweetened beverages and fast food (pizza) of 10% could generate a significant reduction in body weight at a population level (Duffey *et al.*, 2010). Modelling studies have also found a fairly consistent relationship between reduced calorie consumption due to taxation and reductions in population body weight. However, these studies use a variety of conversion factors to estimate the effect of reduced calorie consumption on body weight. Five studies that used dynamic conversion factors (generally considered to be the most accurate) all found that the calorie reductions they predicted would reduce population body weight (Allais *et al.*, 2010; Kotakorpi *et al.*, 2011; Lin *et al.*, 2011; Sacks *et al.*, 2011; Wang *et al.*, 2012).

In contrast, four studies of existing state soft drink taxes in the US showed little difference in obesity prevalence among states with small taxes (around 5%) and states without (Powell *et al.*, 2009; Sturm *et al.*, 2010; Fletcher *et al.*, 2010a, 2010b). However, Sturm and colleagues (Sturm *et al.*, 2010) pointed out that extrapolating their finding of a small marginal effect (−0.013 BMI units) to a larger tax of 18% would produce a 20% reduction in BMI gain, which is a greater effect than any other intervention has demonstrated to date.

It is possible that subsidies for healthy food might increase population body weight through increasing calorie consumption (Epstein *et al.*, 2010; Lacroix *et al.*, 2010). However, overall, studies from the USA indicate that lower fruit and vegetable prices will reduce body weight at a population level (Powell *et al.*, 2013).

It is important to note that a limited focus on calories and body weight might mask other beneficial effects. If a soft drink tax of 5% results in children reducing consumption of soft drinks and increasing their consumption of milk (Fletcher *et al.*, 2010b), this intervention would have no effect on body weight, but would have other nutritional benefits.

20.2.4 Effects on chronic disease outcomes

Effects of fiscal intervention on diet-related NCDs (cardiovascular disease, diabetes, hypertension and stroke) are mediated both through reduced body weight as an independent risk factor for chronic disease, as well as reducing consumption of specific nutrients; namely fat, saturated fat, sugar and salt. It is also possible that people with health problems may demonstrate a greater response to taxation for public health purposes, and thus derive more substantial health benefits, but there has been limited research into these population-specific effects (Epstein *et al.*, 2012).

Fiscal intervention that considers the healthfulness of the food as a whole (rather than just nutrients) and effects on total diet is more likely to have a beneficial effect on chronic disease outcomes. The evidence to date indicates that subsidies paired with taxes in the range of 10–20% (for example: sugar tax with fruit, vegetable and fish subsidy; healthy grain subsidy with fat or sugar tax on unhealthy grain products; fat tax with fruit and vegetable subsidy; unhealthy food tax with fruit and vegetable subsidy) have been found to reduce total calories and disease risk (Tiffin and Arnoult, 2011; Nnoaham *et al.*, 2009; Nordström and Thunström, 2009; Kotakorpi *et al.*, 2011). Two studies on sugary soft drink taxes of 10–20% found that such an intervention could reduce risk factors for diabetes and other chronic diseases (Wang *et al.*, 2012; Duffey *et al.*, 2010).

In contrast, taxes on single nutrients may increase disease risk due to the effects of substitution on other unhealthy nutrients (Eyles *et al.*, 2012). For example, one UK study found that a 17.5% tax on sources of saturated fat could reduce consumption of fatty foods but also had unintended consequences on other nutrient consumption leading to increased disease risk, mainly through increased salt and decreased fruit and vegetable consumption (Mytton *et al.*, 2007).

20.3   Evidence for differential effects of fiscal strategies

Taxation of food is by nature regressive, because food is an essential commodity. This is of concern because of the potentially disproportionate (negative) effect on low-income groups (Cecchini *et al.*, 2010). Similarly, some studies have indicated that subsidies of healthy food may disproportionately benefit the well-off rather than assisting low-income households (Lacroix *et al.*, 2010; Nordström and Thunström, 2011; Dallongeville *et al.*, 2011). However, there is some indication that the health benefits of taxation may also accrue disproportionately to the poor, and thus offset this financial disadvantage to some extent (Eyles *et al.*, 2012).

Designing fiscal interventions to be less regressive might also be possible. Taxes on non-core foods and beverages are likely to be less regressive, because consumers have more capacity to reduce consumption. For example, a study in the USA found that high income consumers would pay more of a tax on soft drinks because they would be less likely to change their behaviour (Finkelstein *et al.*, 2010). Pairing taxes with subsidies would be another way to mitigate the regressive effect of taxation alone. For example, a study in Sweden on taxes and subsidies to reduce the price of healthy grain products compared to unhealthy grain products found that lower-income consumers changed their consumption to a greater degree than high-income consumers and thus benefited more from the fiscal measures (Nordström and Thunström, 2011).

20.4   Evidence for cost-effectiveness of fiscal interventions

The Organization for Economic Cooperation and Development assessed the cost effectiveness of fiscal measures affecting the prices of fruit and vegetables and foods high in fat (Cecchini *et al.*, 2010). They based their estimates on fiscal interventions that would result in a population reduction in fat consumption of $-0 \cdot 4\%$ to $-0 \cdot 6\%$ of total energy intake, and increase in fibre consumption of $3 \cdot 6$–$10 \cdot 4 \text{g/day}$, and included administrative costs in their assessment. The study found that fiscal intervention was one of the most cost-effective in terms of cumulative effectiveness, and that it was cost saving in all countries (Brazil, China, England, India, Mexico, Russia and South Africa). Disability Adjusted Life Years saved per million population over 20 years ranged from 139 in India to 1696 in Russia (the result for India was substantially lower than in other countries, because of a lower consumption of foods high in fat).

20.5 Evidence for interplay with other interventions

Price is one factor influencing food choices, and has a complex interaction with other factors. It is therefore important for fiscal interventions to be considered as part of a package, not a sole solution. In particular, education may be important in helping people to substitute appropriately; both choosing healthier alternatives to taxed foods and not increasing calorie consumption in response to subsidies (An, 2012; Epstein *et al.*, 2012). Based on their recent review, Epstein and colleagues (2012) note that some shoppers may not notice price changes without environmental prompts, and that there is a need to investigate best way of informing consumers of taxation for health.

Fiscal interventions may also reinforce efforts to educate consumers and public awareness that a product has been taxed because it is unhealthy may discourage purchases. Lacanilao and colleagues (Lacanilao *et al.*, 2011) observed this effect in Canada when warning labels were placed on products that were taxed (up to 50%) because of their high fat content. Similarly, the combination of subsidies and nutrition education may have a larger effect than subsidies alone (An, 2012).

20.6 Existing strategies and policies in place

Denmark implemented the first 'fat tax' in October 2011, just after the United Nations High-Level meeting on NCDs (Smed, 2012). This tax applied to foods with a content of saturated fat over 2.3 g/100 g, and was subsequently removed (December 2012) after intensive public lobbying by the food industry. Problems included an increase in across the border shopping, which was reported to be an attempt by consumers to avoid the tax, as well as the loss of jobs in the food industry (Snowdon, 2013).

Fifty-seven per cent of Danish households reported shopping for beer or soft drinks outside of Denmark, in neighbouring Germany – but this is an increase of only 10 percentage points from four years earlier, when 47 per cent of Danish households reported shopping over the border (Snowdon, 2013). Different types of retailers appeared to handle the tax in different ways, with discount stores such as Aldi increasing the price of butter and other foods with a high content of saturated fat to a greater extent than the associated tax increment, while more upmarket supermarkets increased prices by less than the tax increment (Jensen and Smed, 2012).

During the first three months that the tax was in place, population fat consumption decreased by 10–20%, and there was an early indication that consumers shifted from shopping at high-price supermarkets towards low-price discount stores, where the prices of butter and margarine were actually increased by more than the rate of tax (Jensen and Smed, 2012). Public health observers noted strong industry opposition, largely related to the inherent tension between economic growth predicated on increased consumption and public health interventions to reduce consumption (Nestle, 2013).

In the Pacific Islands, taxes on soft drinks were more successfully sustained in the three countries where there were overt partnerships with health – industry did not publically oppose the taxes in these three countries, and in one case supported the taxes (Thow *et al.*, 2011b). However, this was clearly not the case in Denmark, where even with a strong health justification the tax did not gain widespread public support and was vigorously opposed by the food industry. Support for the tax by the public fell from 60% to 30% during the year that the tax was in place (Snowdon, 2013).

Two contextual issues may be important in understanding these different responses. First, the burden of disease from diet-related NCDs constitutes a high proportion of total morbidity in mortality in Denmark, as it does in Pacific Island Countries, but overall life expectancy in Denmark is one of the highest in the world (Jensen and Smed, 2012). In contrast, Pacific Island populations suffer a very high total burden of disease due to diet-related diseases. Second, soft drink taxes target only one relatively small sector of the food industry, and thus have quite contained economic impacts on industry. In contrast, the saturated fat tax implemented in Denmark affected the meat, dairy and processed foods industries. As a result, the economic impact was widespread and generated a significant lobby group.

There are limited other case studies of fiscal policies as public health nutrition intervention. However, there has recently been significant government interest in soft drink taxation as an intervention; for example, taxes implemented in Hungary and Mexico. Chriqui and colleagues (2013) have documented existing public health taxes on non-alcoholic beverages in 16 countries at the national level, 7 states within the USA and 2 US cities. These taxes vary widely in their underlying rationale, rate and mechanism. Most were not implemented for public health reasons; many are small and may thus have limited effect on diets and health. The authors note that there may be potential for earmarking taxation revenue for obesity and NCD prevention.

20.7 Politics and practicalities of taxing unhealthy food

The case studies above highlight that issues of implementation are very important to consider; both the practical administrative dimensions of working within complex existing taxation systems, and also the political implications of fiscal interventions for the food industry and consumers.

Fiscal policy interventions are likely to also have upstream effects on the food supply, through the incentives that they also create for food producers and manufacturers. One of the potential benefits of 'specific' taxes and subsidies (e.g. applying a tax per gram of added sweetener in soft drinks) is that they create incentives for reformulation. However, there has been almost no research to date regarding the response of industry to fiscal measures.

Most studies are limited in their assessment of industry response, and assume that the tax is passed fully to the consumer. One study that has examined industry responses suggests that strategic pricing of firms is very important in determining the effect of taxes or subsidies on price (Bonnet and Réquillart, 2012). Only two studies have investigated industry response to an actual tax, both being case studies of the effect of removing a tax (implicit subsidies) on soft drinks (Bonnet and Réquillart, 2012; Bahl *et al.*, 2003). One study found overshifting, where the discount passed to consumers was greater than the tax removed (Bonnet and Réquillart, 2012) and the other (earlier) study found undershifting, where the discount passed to consumers was less than the tax removed (Bahl *et al.*, 2003). Epstein and colleagues (2012) review of experimental studies indicated that for retailers in a variety of settings, price discounts did not appear to negatively affect total revenue due to increased sales of targeted items. Further research into the response of industry to health-related taxes and subsidies would help understand their effects on food prices and purchase.

Case studies of soft drink taxation in the Pacific Islands suggest that active collaboration with finance in developing policies may help to improve the feasibility and thus implementation of fiscal interventions (Thow *et al.*, 2011b). Policy coherence between finance and health will require considered action by public health policy makers and practitioners because of the very strong global tax reform agenda (Thow *et al.*, 2011a).

20.8   Conclusion

Key factors to consider in fiscal intervention for diet and weight management are effectiveness, design and implementation. The options for fiscal intervention most likely to improve diets and reduce body weight are soft drink taxes and healthy food subsidies, as well as combinations of taxes and subsidies; these strategies have been found to be highly effective. These options for intervention are also the least administratively burdensome, with generally simple definitions of the target foods (e.g. where subsidies are applied to fruit and vegetables). In contrast, targeted nutrient taxes are more likely to require burdensome administrative requirements, as they apply to a wide range of different foods at a number of different tax rates. Although nutrient profile taxes are also administratively complex, tax administration could be streamlined if applied using a systematic (compulsory) nutrient profiling system.

Further research on the response of industry to taxes and subsidies, and evaluation of fiscal interventions applied in the 'real world' will help to give a better understanding of both the effectiveness of such intervention and the practical considerations that could improve implementation.

References

Allais, O., Bertail, P. and Nichele, V. (2010). The effects of a fat tax on French households' purchases: a nutritional approach. *American Journal of Agricultural Economics*, 92, 228–245.

An, R. (2012). Effectiveness of subsidies in promoting healthy food purchases and consumption: a review of field experiments. *Public Health Nutrition*, FirstView, 1–14.

Bahl, R., Bird, R. and Walker, M. B. (2003). The uneasy case against discriminatory excise taxation: soft drink taxes in Ireland. *Public Finance Review*, 31, 510–533.

Bonnet, C. and Réquillart, V. (2012). 'Sugar policy reform, tax policy and price transmission in the soft drink industry'. Transparency of Food Pricing, Seventh Framework Programme, Working Paper 4, pp. 1–30.

Cecchini, M., Sassi, F., Lauer, J. A., Lee, Y. Y., Guajardo-Barron, V. and Chisholm, D. (2010). Tackling of unhealthy diets, physical inactivity, and obesity: health effects and cost-effectiveness. *The Lancet*, 376, 1775–1784.

Chriqui, J. F., Chaloupka, F. J., Powell, L. M. and Eidson, S. S. (2013). A typology of beverage taxation: multiple approaches for obesity prevention and obesity prevention-related revenue generation. *Journal of Public Health Policy*, advance online publication 23 May 2013, doi: 10.1057/jphp.2013.17.

Congressional Budget Office (2008). *Budget Options Volume 1: Health Care*. Washington DC: Congress of the United States.

Dallongeville, J., Dauchet, L., De Mouzon, O., Requillart, V. and Soler, L.-G. (2011). Increasing fruit and vegetable consumption: a cost-effectiveness analysis of public policies. *European Journal of Public Health*, 21, 69–73.

Dharmasena, S. and Capps, O., Jr. (2012). Intended and unintended consequences of a proposed national tax on sugar-sweetened beverages to combat the U.S. obesity problem. *Health Econ*, 21(6), 669–94.

Duffey, K. J., Gordon-Larsen, P., Shikany, J. M., Guilkey, D., Jacobs, D. R., Jr and Popkin, B. M. (2010). Food price and diet and health outcomes: 20 years of the CARDIA study. *Archives of Internal Medicine*, 170, 420–426.

Epstein, L. H., Dearing, K. K., Roba, L. G. and Finkelstein, E. (2010). The influence of taxes and subsidies on energy purchased in an experimental purchasing study. *Psychological Science (Sage Publications Inc.)*, 21, 406–414.

Epstein, L. H., Jankowiak, N., Nederkoorn, C., Raynor, H. A., French, S. A. and Finkelstein, E. (2012). Experimental research on the relation between food price changes and food-purchasing patterns: a targeted review. *The American Journal of Clinical Nutrition*.

Eyles, H., Ni Mhurchu, C., Nghiem, N. and Blakely, T. (2012). Food pricing strategies, population diets, and non-communicable disease: a systematic review of simulation studies. *PLoS Med*, 9(12), e1001353.

Finkelstein, E. A., Zhen, C., Nonnemaker, J. and Todd, J. E. (2010). Impact of targeted beverage taxes on higher- and lower-income households. *Archives of Internal Medicine*, 170, 2028–34.

Fletcher, J. M., Frisvold, D. and Tefft, N. (2010a). Can soft drink taxes reduce population weight? *Contemp Econ Policy*, 28, 23–35.

Fletcher, J. M., Frisvold, D. E. and Tefft, N. (2010b). The effects of soft drink taxes on child and adolescent consumption and weight outcomes. *Journal of Public Economics*, 94, 967–974.

French, S. A. (2003). Pricing effects on food choices. *Journal of Nutrition*, 133, 841S–853S.

Giesen, J. C. A. H., Havermans, R. C., Nederkoorn, C. and Jansen, A. (2012). Impulsivity in the supermarket. Responses to calorie taxes and subsidies in healthy weight undergraduates. *Appetite*, 58, 6–10.

Jensen, J. D. and Smed, S. (2012). *The Danish Tax on Saturated Fat: short Run Effects on Consumption and Consumer Prices of Fats*. Copenhagen: Institute of Food and Resource Economics, University of Copenhagen.

Khan, R., Misra, K. and Singh, V. (2012). 'Will a Fat Tax Work': Working Paper, London.

Kotakorpi, K., Härkänen, T., Pietinen, P., Reinivuo, H., Suoniemi, I. and Pirttila, J. (2011). *The Welfare Effects of Health-based Food Tax Policy*. Tampere Economic Working Papers Net Series.

Lacanilao, R. D., Cash, S. B. and Adamowicz, W. L. (2011). Heterogeneous consumer responses to snack food taxes and warning labels. *Journal of Consumer Affairs*, 45, 108–122.

Lacroix, A., Muller, L. and Ruffieux, B. (2010). To what extent would the poorest consumers nutritionally and socially benefit from a global food tax and subsidy reform? A framed field experiment based on daily food intake. Grenoble: Grenoble Applied Economics Laboratory (GAEL).

Lin, B. H., Smith, T. A., Lee, J. Y. and Hall, K. D. (2011). Measuring weight outcomes for obesity intervention strategies: the case of a sugar-sweetened beverage tax. *Economics and Human Biology*, 9, 329–41.

Miao, Z., Beghin, J. and Jensen, H. H. (2011). 'Accounting for Product Substitution in the Analysis of Food Taxes Targeting Obesity'. Econ Papers no. 103320. Annual Meeting, 24–26 July 2011, Pittsburgh, Pennsylvania.

Mytton, O., Gray, A., Rayner, M. and Rutter, H. (2007). Could targeted food taxes improve health? *Journal of Epidemiology and Community Health*, 61, 689–694.

Nestle, M. (2013). The Danish fat tax: reflections on its demise. *Food Politics* [Online]. Available: http://www.foodpolitics.com/2012/11/the-danish-fat-tax-reflections-on-its-demise/ [accessed 01 July 2013].

Ni Mhurchu, C., Blakely, T., Jiang, Y., Eyles, H. C. and Rodgers, A. (2010). Effects of price discounts and tailored nutrition education on supermarket purchases: a randomized controlled trial. *The American Journal of Clinical Nutrition*, 91, 736–747.

Nnoaham, K. E., Sacks, G., Rayner, M., Mytton, O. and Gray, A. (2009). Modelling income group differences in the health and economic impacts of targeted food taxes and subsidies. *International Journal of Epidemiology*, 38, 1324–1333.

Nordström, J. and Thunström, L. (2011). Can targeted food taxes and subsidies improve the diet? Distributional effects among income groups. *Food Policy*, 36, 259–271.

Nordström, J. and Thunström, L. (2009). The impact of tax reforms designed to encourage healthier grain consumption. *Journal of Health Economics*, 28, 622–634.

Powell, L. M., Chriqui, J. and Chaloupka, F. J. (2009). Associations between state-level soda taxes and adolescent body mass index. *J Adolesc Health*, 45, 16.

Powell, L. M., Chriqui, J. F., Khan, T., Wada, R. and Chaloupka, F. J. (2013). Assessing the potential effectiveness of food and beverage taxes and subsidies for improving public health: a systematic review of prices, demand and body weight outcomes. *Obesity Reviews*, 14, 110–128.

Sacks, G., Veerman, J. L., Moodie, M. and Swinburn, B. (2011). 'Traffic-light' nutrition labelling and 'junk-food' tax: a modelled comparison of cost-effectiveness for obesity prevention. *International Journal of Obesity*, 35, 1001–1009.

Smed, S. (2012). Financial penalties on foods: the fat tax in Denmark. *Nutrition Bulletin*, 37, 142–147.

Snowdon, C. (2013). *The Proof of the Pudding: Denmark's Fat Tax Fiasco*. Sussex: Institute of Economic Affairs.

Sturm, R., Powell, L. M., Chriqui, J. F. and Chaloupka, F. J. (2010). Soda taxes, soft drink consumption, and children's body mass index. *Health Affairs*, 29, 1052–1058.

Temple, J. L., Johnson, K. M., Archer, K., Lacarte, A., Yi, C. and Epstein, L. H. (2011). Influence of simplified nutrition labeling and taxation on laboratory energy intake in adults. *Appetite*, 57, 184–192.

Thow, A. M., Downs, S. and Jan, S. (2014). The effectiveness of food taxes and subsidies to improve diets: Understanding the recent evidence. *Nutrition Reviews*, 72, 9, 551–565.

Thow, A. M., Heywood, P., Leeder, S. and Burns, L. (2011a). The global context for public health nutrition taxation. *Public Health Nutrition*, 14, 176–186.

Thow, A. M., Jan, S., Leeder, S. and Swinburn, B. (2010). The impact of fiscal policy interventions for diets, obesity and chronic disease: a systematic review. *Bulletin of the World Health Organization*, 88, 609–614.

Thow, A. M., Quested, C., Juventin, L., Kun, R., Khan, A. N. and Swinburn, B. (2011b). Taxing soft drinks in the Pacific: Implementation lessons for improving health. *Health Promotion International*, 26, 55–64.

Tiffin, R. and Arnoult, M. (2011). The public health impacts of a fat tax. *Eur J Clin Nutr*, 65, 427–33.

United Nations General Assembly (2011). *Political Declaration of the High-level Meeting of the General Assembly on the Prevention and Control of Non-communicable Diseases.* New York: United Nations.

Wang, Y. C., Coxson, P., Shen, Y.-M., Goldman, L. and Bibbins-Domingo, K. (2012). A penny-per-ounce tax on sugar-sweetened beverages would cut health and cost burdens of diabetes. *Health Affairs*, 31, 199–207.

Waterlander, W., Steenhuis, I., De Boer, M., Schuit, A. and Seidell, J. (2012). Introducing taxes, subsidies or both: the effects of various food pricing strategies in a web-based supermarket randomized trial. *Preventive Medicine*, Feb 23. [Epub ahead of print].

WHO (2013). Follow-up to the Political Declaration of the High-level Meeting of the General Assembly on the Prevention and Control of Non-communicable Diseases. Sixty-Sixth World Health Assembly WHA66.10 Agenda item 13.1, 13.2, 27 May 2013. Annex: Global Action Plan for the Prevention and Control of Noncommunicable Diseases 2013–2020. Geneva: World Health Organization.

Consumer responses to government dietary guidelines in the management and prevention of obesity

S. Boylan
University of Sydney, Sydney, NSW, Australia

21.1   Introduction

Dietary guidelines were introduced to encourage healthy food choice and hence reduce the rates of overweight and obesity. Despite the considerable amount of effort which has gone into developing and supporting dietary guidelines, rates of overweight and obesity continue to escalate. In fact, some argue that dietary guidelines may do more harm than good (Woolf and Nestle, 2008). Others argue that it is up to the individual to decide for themselves whether or not they should follow the guidelines (Woolf and Nestle, 2008). Arguments aside, dietary guidelines have been implemented in several countries to inform policy makers and to promote consumer behaviour change. This chapter's focus is on the consumer and will therefore attempt to answer a number of questions: how effective are dietary guidelines in (1) preventing obesity, (2) promoting healthier food choices, (3) promoting dietary behaviour change? First, a brief history of dietary guidelines will be presented.

21.2   History of dietary guidelines

21.2.1   United States

W. O. Atwater, who is seen as the instigator of the official United States (US) dietary guidance, published dietary standards in 1894 (Gifford, 2002). Almost one-hundred years later in 1980, the first Dietary Guidelines for Americans (DGA) were issued (United States Department of Agriculture and United States Department of Health and Human Services, 1980) and according to the law, the DGA must be published every five years (National Nutrition Monitoring and Related Research Act, 1990). The seven DGAs issued to date have become more detailed and prescriptive over time, with only slight changes made since the first edition. However, in 2010, in acknowledging that the 'environment and the individual choices made within it have contributed to dramatic increases in the rate of overweight and obesity', the

Managing and Preventing Obesity. http//dx.doi.org/10.1533/9781782420996.5.301

United States Department of Agriculture (USDA) and the U.S. Department of Health and Human Services (HHS) went beyond delivering education to the individual (United States Department of Agriculture and United States Department of Health and Human Services, 2010). They called for a 'co-ordinated system-wide approach ... an approach that engages all sectors of society, including individuals and families, educators, communities and organizations, health professionals, small and large businesses, and policymakers' (United States Department of Agriculture and United States Department of Health and Human Services, 2010).

21.2.2   Australia and New Zealand

On the other side of the globe, dietary guidelines in Australia have continued to focus on the individual. Australia has been publishing food guides since the 1940s, however the first dietary guidelines for Australian's did not come to fruition until 1979, with revisions made in 1992, 1999, 2003 and 2013. While the most recent guidelines offer few surprises compared to previous editions, they have taken a step forward with a greater focus on foods and food groups as opposed to nutrient-focused guidance. Across the Tasman Sea, several population-specific guidelines have been developed since New Zealand's first dietary guidelines for Healthy Adults in 1985 (Keller and Lang, 2008). Unlike their Antipodean neighbours however, the most recent New Zealand dietary guidelines for children and young people consider the influence of the social, cultural and economic environments (Ministry of Health, 2012).

21.2.3   Europe

The World Health Organisation (WHO) assessment of food-based dietary guidelines (FBDG) among the Member States of the WHO European Region (World Health Organization, 2003), found 25 countries with national, government-endorsed FBDG. There were similarities among regions with the majority of countries reported recommending a balanced diet and the use of a food pyramid or food plate to help visualise a healthy diet. However there were also important discrepancies found between sub-regions and from country to country; for example, a total fruit and vegetable intake recommendation without differentiating between the two, ranged from 3–5 portions/day to 5–9 portions/day. This however may be simply a reflection of the differing national culture and eating habits which exists from country to country. The WHO review identified shortcomings of some of the FBDGs and concluded that further effort is required in the EU region in the development of dietary guidelines (World Health Organization, 2003).

The widespread implementation of dietary guidelines in many countries indicates that there is a perception that they may be effective in promoting healthier food choices. Indeed persuasive communications are deemed helpful in engaging individuals with healthier behaviours (O'Keefe, 1990). However, given that obesity rates are now at epidemic proportions, just how effective are the dietary guidelines in preventing obesity? The next section attempts to answer this very question.

21.3 Effectiveness of dietary guidelines in preventing obesity

Unfortunately the limited research on the impact of dietary guidelines on body weight does not make it easy to answer this question (Anding *et al.*, 2001; Carels *et al.*, 2008; Duffy *et al.*, 2012). Many researchers have developed measures of 'diet quality' (e.g. Healthy Eating Indices) as a proxy of adhering to dietary guidelines (Guenther *et al.*, 2013). Those who have assessed the relationship between 'diet quality' and body weight have found an association between lower diet quality and overweight and obesity (Guo *et al.*, 2004; Gao *et al.*, 2008; Tande *et al.*, 2010). Regarding dietary guidelines *per se*, the lack of evidence regarding an impact on body weight does not necessarily mean that they do not have a role to play in obesity prevention. As with any problem-solving, in order to answer this question, it is important to first understand the exact nature of the problem itself. The complex genesis of obesity with multiple determinants from a variety of behaviours and environmental influences highlights the limitations of dietary guidelines in addressing obesity. No better illustration of the complexity of the obesity challenge is the Foresight obesity system map with over 300 solid or dashed lines indicating positive and negative influences of various domains (Vandenbroeck *et al.*, 2007).

Despite such a large and complex problem involving many environmental dimensions, there is still an important role for dietary guidance. When dealing with complexities such as obesity, it is important to remember that the individual lies at the core and remains crucial to addressing this difficult societal problem. This is particularly relevant in understanding the role of dietary guidelines in obesity prevention as they are ultimately a strategy targeted at the individual in the hope of promoting healthier food choices. So just how effective are the dietary guidelines in promoting healthier food choices?

21.4 Effectiveness of dietary guidelines in promoting healthier food choices

Most of the research conducted to date on this question has utilised nutrition surveys to examine adherence to dietary guidelines. If we were to go by these findings alone, the effectiveness of dietary guidelines gives little rise for celebration (Baghurst *et al.*, 1990; Ball *et al.*, 2004; Diethelm *et al.*, 2012; Ta *et al.*, 2012). However we cannot answer this question by solely examining the results of nutrition surveys. The relationship between health communication and behaviour change, particularly dietary change, is extremely complex and therefore examining the outcome alone (as many researchers do) may not give us the required answer. While the results of nutrition surveys provide some insight, they certainly will not offer any understanding of what works and what needs improvement. In order to disentangle the complexity, we need to take a closer look at the individual and ask how effective are the dietary guidelines in promoting behaviour change?

21.5   Effectiveness of dietary guidelines in promoting dietary behaviour change

The objectives of health communications are to raise awareness, increase knowledge, shape attitudes and thus influence behaviour change (Levine *et al.*, 2012). While it would be certainly helpful to examine the impact of these factors on behaviour change, there are a host of other covariates which may influence behaviour and may be worthy of further examination. To better understand how dietary guidelines may influence behaviour change, we should turn to theories of behaviour change – theories explain behaviour and suggest ways to achieve behaviour change. It has been stated that 'nutrition education is more likely to be effective when it focuses on behaviour ... and systematically links relevant theory, research and practice' (Contento, 2008). The next section will examine how theory and research have been applied in developing dietary guidelines.

21.5.1   The theory

There are numerous behaviour change models relevant to the impact of dietary guidelines including the Theory of Reasoned Action (TRA), Theory of Planned Behaviour (TPB), Health Belief Model (HBM), Social Cognitive Theory (SCT), and the Trans-Theoretical Model (TTM). All of these theories consider the individual, however some groups have criticised the focus on individuals. Dietary intake is an individual behaviour therefore it seems apt that theories focusing on the individual are considered. Saying this, individual behaviour can be strongly influenced at multiple levels, e.g. individual, organisational and societal (Viswanath, 2008).

It is becoming increasingly recognised that health behaviour and guiding concepts for influencing it are far too complex to be explained by a single theory (Brewer and Rimer, 2008), therefore more recent models now combine theories to help understand a specific problem in a particular context. The Integrated Behavioural Model, which has drawn upon the TRA, TPB and other influential theories, considers environmental constraints and 'other factors' (Montano and Kasprzyk, 2008). The Integrative Model of Behavioural Prediction details a range of background variables, e.g. demographics, and recognises that environmental constraints may affect the intention to perform a behaviour (Fishbein, 2008). These theories are examples of but a few which can not only help us understand health behaviour, but they also allow for a more careful measure of how interventions can change behaviour.

21.5.2   The research

One of the most utilised models which has examined dietary behaviour change is the TPB. This theory has been used to examine fat intake (Paisley and Sparks, 1998; de Bruijn *et al.*, 2008), health-related eating behaviours (Ajzen and Timko, 1986), healthy eating (Conner *et al.*, 2002) and fruit and vegetable intake (Lien *et al.*, 2002; Bogers *et al.*, 2004; Kellar and Abraham, 2005). Although the predictive utility of the TPB model has been well established, there are few studies which have examined the cognitions in the model, e.g. attitudes, beliefs and intentions, to assess whether changes in the predictors do in fact lead to behaviour change. Researchers have called for studies which explore theory specific cognition changes and their mediation of behaviour change outcomes (Michie and Abraham, 2004). Despite the wide use of TPB by researchers examining dietary behaviour change, research on the effectiveness of dietary guidelines remains largely atheoretical.

The field may not have moved forward for a number of reasons. Time is of the essence. In order to examine whether behaviour change has not only occurred, but has been maintained, needs time – a resource which most research projects lack as most are funded for less than five years (Levine *et al.*, 2012). Some have cautioned the limitation of theory testing because of its heavy dependence on correlational designs and the lack of studies which compare more than one theory (Glanz *et al.*, 2008b). Researchers may not understand how to measure and examine constructs of health behaviour theories or choose variables from different theories (Glanz *et al.*, 2008b). Glanz suggests that one of the biggest hurdles to overcome however is learning to 'tailor' the theory or model to a particular issue and population (Glanz, 2008a). This is an important step as different guidelines may be needed for different populations. Integrating theories into a comprehensive planning framework can guide research in examining an issue, population needs, resources available and the effectiveness of the program as it progresses (Glanz, 2008a). A good example of this is the application of the Socio-Ecological Model for evaluating health communication campaigns (Levine *et al.*, 2012). The Social-Ecological Model has been applied by many experts in public health, including a reference to the model in the DGA 2010 to illustrate how all elements of society – individual factors, environmental settings, sectors of influence and social and cultural norms and values – combine to shape an individual's food and physical activity (United States Department of Agriculture and United States Department of Health and Human Services, 2010).

In addition to theory application, Levine's framework highlights the need to consider the various classes of research (Levine *et al.*, 2012). While outcome research is fundamental, we must not overlook the importance of formative research and process evaluation – both of which may also apply theory. Formative research conducted during guideline development can help understand the factors which influence behaviour change including beliefs, knowledge and attitude. Consumer attitude to dietary guidelines was the focus of a recent systematic review which found that consumers want simple, clear, realistic, tailored, flexible and positive content (Boylan *et al.*, 2012). The involvement of consumers as stakeholders in health research, policy and practice, including development of dietary guidelines, has been promoted nationally and internationally (Brown *et al.*, 2013). Involving consumers is seen as not only a way to improve the quality of decisions, but also a great way to build consumer trust. As consumers are the end user of dietary guidelines, all members of the community may participate including lay consumers and more vulnerable populations (Brown *et al.*, 2013). However it has been advised that the role of consumers must be made transparent to all parties prior to any involvement to aid evaluation of consumer impact.

While there has been some formative research during the development of dietary guidelines, process evaluation has received less attention. This type of research focuses on the implementation of a program and examines the extent to which program activities are being conducted as planned. Process evaluation is extremely insightful for several reasons as it can: shed light on what elements are promising, need changing or removal from a program; examine shorter-term or more intermediate outcomes, such as *changes* in attitudes, beliefs etc. (these ultimately contribute to long-term outcomes); and examine the impact of external factors such as policy changes.

21.5.2.1 *How researchers can better examine the effectiveness of dietary guidelines*

It is clear that more thorough application and testing of health behaviour theories is required to fully understand the effectiveness of dietary guidelines. It has been recommended that application of a wider diversity of models and theories to health communication is needed, including theories of communication and language (Levine *et al.*, 2012). In order to advance what is known about health communication and to progress further, it is necessary to apply theories in the form of a theoretical framework (Angeles *et al.*, 2014). As discussed earlier, frameworks can help navigate various theories and act as a guide to implement, analyse and evaluate research. We should continue conducting formative research in developing dietary guidelines and seriously begin to consider the value of process evaluation. As well as the useful insight which this type of evaluation can provide, it may also help address the time barrier in researching the impact of dietary guidelines. Applying a model such as the Integrative Model of Behaviour Prediction may be useful in evaluating the implementation of dietary guidelines as it may offer some insight into changes at both an individual and environmental level.

21.5.3   *The practice*

It is encouraging that guideline developers are increasingly considering the individual as a key part of the process. It is also encouraging that developers are beginning to recognise environmental influences in their use of theoretical models. While there are promising moves, it is clear that there is still some way to go before we can effectively start putting research into practice. It is vital that we better understand what works and what does not work so that guideline developer's efforts are not in vain and dietary guidelines have more hope of promoting healthier food choices.

21.6   Conclusion

The relationship between dietary guidelines and behaviour change is by no means simple. In exploring this relationship, this chapter focused on the individual's role. There are of course other powerful factors at play including the built, socio-cultural and political environments – factors worthy of chapters themselves. Strategic priorities concerned with these environments' influence on dietary guideline effectiveness have been discussed elsewhere (Nitzke and Freeland-Graves, 2007; Rowe *et al.*, 2011; Watts *et al.*, 2011). These discussions highlight the importance of aligning food industry marketing messages more closely with healthy dietary practices, tailoring dietary advice to the needs of vulnerable populations, and creating a food environment which enables healthier food choices (Woolf and Nestle, 2008). However there is also a call to apply behaviour science to the development of dietary guidelines (Rowe *et al.*, 2011). It is hoped that this chapter helps point developers in the right direction and demonstrates that in ignoring the role of the individual in system function, there is little hope of creating successful change (Bar-Yam, 2005).

References

Ajzen, I. and Timko, C. (1986) 'Correspondence between health attitudes and behavior', *Basic Appl Soc Psych*, 7, 259–276.

Anding, J. D., Suminski, R. R. and Boss, L. (2001) 'Dietary intake, body mass index, exercise, and alcohol: are college women following the dietary guidelines for Americans?', *J Am Coll Health*, 49, 167–171.

Angeles, R. N., Dolovich, L., Kaczorowski, J. and Thabane, L. (2014) 'Developing a theoretical framework for complex community-based interventions', *Health Promot Pract*, 15, 100–108.

Baghurst, K. I., Record, S. J., Baghurst, P. A., Syrette, J. A., Crawford, D. and Worsley, A. (1990) 'Sociodemographic determinants in Australia of the intake of food and nutrients implicated in cancer aetiology', *Med J Aust*, 153, 444–452.

Ball, K., Mishra, G. D., Thane, C. W. and Hodge, A. (2004) 'How well do Australian women comply with dietary guidelines?', *Public Health Nutr*, 7, 443–452.

Bar-Yam, Y. (2005) *Making Things Work: Solving Complex Problems in a Complex World*, Cambridge, MA, NECSI – Knowledge Press.

Bogers, R. P., Brug, J., van Assema, P. and Dagnelie, P. C. (2004) 'Explaining fruit and vegetable consumption: the theory of planned behaviour and misconception of personal intake levels', *Appetite*, 42, 157–166.

Boylan, S., Louie, J. C. Y. and Gill, T. P. (2012) 'Consumer response to healthy eating, physical activity and weight-related recommendations: a systematic review', *Obes Rev*, 13, 606–617.

Brewer, N. T. and Rimer, B. K. (2008), 'Perspectives on health behaviour theories that focus on individuals', in: Glanz, K., Rimer, B. K. and Viswanath, K. (eds) *Health Behaviour and Health Education: Theory, Research, and Practice*, San Francisco, Jossey-Bass, pp. 149–165.

Brown, K. A., Hermoso, M., Timotijevic, L., Barnett, J., Lillegaard, I. T. L., *et al.* (2013) 'Consumer involvement in dietary guideline development: opinions from European stakeholders', *Public Health Nutr*, 16, 769–776.

Carels, R. A., Young, K. M., Coit, C., Clayton, A. M., Spencer, A., *et al.* (2008) 'Can following the caloric restriction recommendations from the dietary guidelines for americans help individuals lose weight?', *Ann Behav Med*, 35, S43–S43, 328–335.

Conner, M., Norman, P. and Bell, R. (2002) 'The theory of planned behavior and healthy eating', *Health Psychol*, 21, 194–201.

Contento, I. R. (2008) 'Nutrition education: linking research, theory, and practice', *Asia Pac J Clin Nutr*, 17 (Suppl 1), 176–179.

de Bruijn, G. J., Kroeze, W., Oenema, A. and Brug, J. (2008) 'Saturated fat consumption and the Theory of Planned Behaviour: exploring additive and interactive effects of habit strength', *Appetite*, 51, 318–323.

Diethelm, K., Jankovic, N., Moreno, L. A., Huybrechts, I., De Henauw, S., *et al.* (2012) 'Food intake of European adolescents in the light of different food-based dietary guidelines: results of the HELENA (Healthy Lifestyle in Europe by Nutrition in Adolescence) Study', *Public Health Nutr*, 15, 386–398.

Duffy, P., Yamazaki, F. and Zizza, C. A. (2012) Can the dietary guidelines for Americans 2010 help trip America's waistline? *Choices: the magazine of food, farm and resouce issues.* Agricultural & Applied Economics Association, 1st Quarter 27(1).

Fishbein, M. (2008) 'A reasoned action approach to health promotion', *Med Decis Making*, 28, 834–844.

Gao, S. K., Beresford, S. A., Frank, L. L., Schreiner, P. J., Burke, G. L. and Fitzpatrick, A. L. (2008) 'Modifications to the Healthy Eating Index and its ability to predict obesity: the Multi-Ethnic Study of Atherosclerosis', *Am J Clin Nutr*, 88, 64–69.

Gifford, K. D. (2002) 'Dietary fats, eating guides, and public policy: history, critique, and recommendations', *American Journal of Medicine*, 113 (Suppl 9B), S89–S106.

Glanz, K. (2008a), 'Using theory in research and practice', in: Glanz, K., Rimer, B. K. and Viswanath, K. (eds) *Health Behaviour and Health Education: Theory, Research and Practice*, San Francisco, Jossey-Bass, pp. 405–406.

Glanz, K., Rimer, B.K., and Viswanath, K. (2008b), 'Theory, research and practice in health behaviour and health education', in: Glanz, K., Rimer, B. K. and Viswanath, K. (eds) *Health Behaviour and Health Education: Theory, Research and Practice*, San Francisco, Jossey-Bass, pp. 23–40.

Guenther, P. M., Casavale, K. O., Reedy, J., Kirkpatrick, S. I., Hiza, H. A., *et al.* (2013) 'Update of the Healthy Eating Index: HEI-2010', *J Acad Nutr Diet*, 113, 569–580.

Guo, X., Warden, B. A., Paeratakul, S. and Bray, G. A. (2004) 'Healthy Eating Index and obesity', *Eur J Clin Nutr*, 58, 1580–1586.

Kellar, I. and Abraham, C. (2005) 'Randomized controlled trial of a brief research-based intervention promoting fruit and vegetable consumption', *Brit J Health Psych*, 10, 543–558.

Keller, I. and Lang, T. (2008) 'Food-based dietary guidelines and implementation: lessons from four countries: Chile, Germany, New Zealand and South Africa', *Public Health Nutr*, 11, 867–874.

Levine, E., Abbatangelo-Gray, J., Mobley, A. R., McLaughlin, G. R. and Herzog, J. (2012) 'Evaluating MyPlate: an expanded framework using traditional and nontraditional metrics for assessing health communication campaigns', *J Nutr Educ Behav*, 44, S2–S12.

Lien, N., Lytle, L. A. and Komro, K. A. (2002) 'Applying theory of planned behavior to fruit and vegetable consumption of young adolescents', *Am J Health Promot*, 16, 189–197.

Michie, S. and Abraham, C. (2004) 'Interventions to change health behaviours: evidence-based or evidence-inspired?', *Psychol Health*, 19, 29–49.

Ministry of Health (2012) *Food and Nutrition Guidelines for Healthy Children and Young People (Aged 2–18 Years) A Background Paper*, Wellington, Ministry of Health.

Montano, D. E. and Kasprzyk, D. (2008), 'Theory of Reasoned Action, Theory of Planned Behaviour, and the Integrated Behaviour Model', in: Glanz, K., Rimer, B. K. and

Viswanath, K. (eds) *Health Behaviour and Health Education: Theory, Research, and Practice*, San Francisco, Jossey-Bass, pp. 67–96.

National Nutrition Monitoring and Related Research Act (1990). Public Law 101–445, Title III, 7 U.S.C5301 et seq.

Nitzke, S. and Freeland-Graves, J. (2007) 'Position of the American Dietetic Association: total diet approach to communicating food and nutrition information', *J Am Diet Assoc*, 107, 1224–1232.

O'Keefe, D. J. (1990) *Persuasion: Theory and Research*, Newbury Park, CA, Sage.

Paisley, C. M. and Sparks, P. (1998) 'Expectations of reducing fat intake: the role of perceived need within the theory of planned behaviour', *Psychol Health*, 13, 341–353.

Rowe, S., Alexander, N., Almeida, N., Black, R., Burns, R., *et al.* (2011) 'Food science challenge: translating the dietary guidelines for Americans to bring about real behavior change', *J Food Sci*, 76, R29–37.

Ta, M. L., VanEenwyk, J. and Bensley, L. (2012) 'Limited percentages of adults in Washington State meet the Dietary Guidelines for Americans recommended intakes of fruits and vegetables', *J Acad Nutr Diet*, 112, 699–704.

Tande, D. L., Magel, R. and Strand, B. N. (2010) 'Healthy Eating Index and abdominal obesity', *Public Health Nutr*, 13, 208–14.

United States Department of Agriculture and United States Department of Health and Human Services (1980) *Nutrition and Your Health: Dietary Guidelines for Americans*, Washington D.C.

United States Department of Agriculture and United States Department of Health and Human Services (2010) *Dietary Guidelines for Americans, 2010*, Washington D.C.

Vandenbroeck I. P., Gossens J. and Clemens, M. (2007) *Foresight Tackling Obesities: Future Choices – Building the Obesity System Map*. UK, Department of Innovation Universities and Skills.

Viswanath, K. (2008), 'Perspectives on models of interpersonal health behaviour', in: Glanz, K., Rimer, B. K. and Viswanath, K. (eds) *Health Behaviour and Health Education: Theory, Research, and Practice*, San Francisco, Jossey-Bass, pp. 271–281.

Watts, M. L., Hager, M. H., Toner, C. D. and Weber, J. A. (2011) 'The art of translating nutritional science into dietary guidance: history and evolution of the Dietary Guidelines for Americans', *Nutr Rev*, 69, 404–412.

Woolf, S. H. and Nestle, M. (2008) 'Do dietary guidelines explain the obesity epidemic?', *Am J Prev Med*, 34, 263–265.

World Health Organization (2003) *Food based dietary guidelines in the WHO European Region*, Copenhagen.

The impact of marketing of 'junk' foods on children's diet and weight

B. Kelly[1], L. King[2]
[1]University of Wollongong, Wollongong, NSW, Australia;
[2]University of Sydney, Sydney, NSW, Australia

22.1 Introduction

Contemporary Western(ised) society is typified by pervasive and aggressive brand promotion, through all communication platforms. Food promotion in particular is a dominant area of marketing, particularly the marketing by large multinational food companies that manufacturer less healthy foods and beverages (Cairns *et al.*, 2013). The ubiquitous marketing of these unhealthy foods contributes to creating a negative food culture that undermines international and national nutrition recommendations and guidelines for disease prevention. Specifically, frequent exposure to persuasive promotions for unhealthy foods serves to normalise these food products as part of everyday life, create positive brand images, and ultimately encourage (over) consumption of these foods (Hoek and Gendall, 2006).

The *Diet, Nutrition and the Prevention of Chronic Diseases* report published by the Food and Agriculture Organization and the World Health Organization (WHO) in 2003 concluded that the heavy marketing of fast food outlets and energy dense, micronutrient poor foods and beverages ('junk foods') is a probable causal factor in overweight and obesity, and is a target for future interventions (World Health Organization, 2003). Since this time, limiting children's exposure to unhealthy food marketing has been on the international public health agenda.

Over the past decade there have been at least seven major systematic reviews of the scientific evidence relating to the impact of food marketing on children (Dalmeny *et al.*, 2003; Hastings *et al.*, 2003, 2006; Escelante de Cruz, 2004; Livingstone, 2006; McGinnis *et al.*, 2006; Cairns *et al.*, 2009). The most recent systematic review, commissioned by the World Health Organization in 2008, identified that food marketing has a modest impact on nutrition knowledge, food preferences and consumption patterns, and that these effects operate at both the brand and food category level (Cairns *et al.*, 2009). In other words, not only does food marketing contribute to brand switching within a food category, but also leads to switching between less marketed foods to more highly marketed food types. These findings are concerning as the most commonly promoted foods have been identified as sugar-sweetened breakfast

Managing and Preventing Obesity. http//dx.doi.org/10.1533/9781782420996.5.311

cereals, savoury snacks, fast food restaurants, confectionery and soft drinks (Cairns *et al.*, 2009).

This chapter provides a detailed overview of the scope and impact of food marketing on children, including:

1. the extent of children's exposure to unhealthy food promotions, as evidenced by studies measuring the prevalence of promotions through a range of media;
2. policy responses to unhealthy food promotion, including at the international level and exemplars of good practice by national and provincial governments, and policy actions by the food and advertising industries; and
3. evidence linking food promotions to food consumption and nutrition and weight outcomes.

In the latter section, we provide a conceptual framework of cause and effect to indicate how immediate impacts of exposure to promotions (e.g. brand awareness and recall) can be linked to subsequent, downstream behavioural and health-related outcomes.

22.2   Extent of children's exposure to food and beverage marketing

Research studies have repeatedly demonstrated that children are exposed to high levels of unhealthy food and beverage marketing across a range of media, including on commercial television (Adams *et al.*, 2009; Kelly *et al.*, 2010; Boyland *et al.*, 2011; Powell *et al.*, 2011), on product packaging (Harris *et al.*, 2010), in children's magazines (Kelly and Chapman, 2007; Jones *et al.*, 2012), on popular children's websites (Kelly *et al.*, 2008a; Lingas *et al.*, 2009), in outdoor advertisements near schools and other child-serving institutions (Kelly *et al.*, 2008b; Hillier *et al.*, 2009), and through sponsorship arrangements with children's sport (Maher *et al.*, 2006; Kelly *et al.*, 2011) and schools (Molnar *et al.*, 2008).

For example, in an international study comparing patterns of television advertising across 11 countries in 2009, including from Australasia, North and South America and Eastern and Western Europe, almost 68,500 advertisements were identified in 2,449 hours of television recordings, and food was the most frequently promoted product type (18% of all ads). Two-thirds of food advertisements were for unhealthy products, although this increased to almost 90% in some countries, including Germany, the USA and Canada (Kelly *et al.*, 2010). Another study showed that, of all outdoor food advertising within a 500 m radius around 40 randomly sampled primary schools in Sydney, Australia, 80% were for unhealthy foods and beverages (Kelly *et al.*, 2008b). In the USA, an analysis of the 30 most popular children's websites identified advertisements for 93 unique food products, most of which were foods that would not be permitted to be sold in school canteens (Lingas *et al.*, 2009).

Marketers use increasingly integrated approaches in marketing campaigns, whereby multiple media channels are used to promote commercial messages (Cairns *et al.*, 2013). This integrated approach ensures that children are repeatedly exposed to promotions throughout all facets of daily life: in the home, at school, during recreational activities and through peer-to-peer interactions. The use of multiple platforms increases the credibility of commercial messages, where these are viewed as independent sources of information (Voorveld *et al.*, 2011). While relatively unstudied, marketers are progressively using new media, including through Web 2.0 platforms, which refers to the use of consumer-generated content, such as on social networking sites like Facebook and YouTube (Freeman and Chapman, 2007).

Furthermore, evidence highlights the common use of persuasive techniques specifically designed to appeal to and attract children (Boyland *et al.*, 2012). In analyses of techniques used on websites of 130 food companies known to have the greatest expenditure on all marketing promotions in the USA, almost half of the sites had a designated children's section and most of these children's sections contained 'advergaming' (branded online games) and other interactive components (Henry and Story, 2009). Only one in ten sites with a children's section were for products that met nutrition criteria for healthy products. In an Australian study assessing the use of promotional characters, including cartoons and celebrities on food packaging across three large supermarkets, more than 350 unique products displaying promotional characters were identified, of which three-quarters were classified as unhealthy (Hebden *et al.*, 2011). Almost all promotional characters were company-owned cartoon characters, considered to be of primary appeal to children.

22.3   International policy to reduce the impact of unhealthy food and beverage marketing to children

Limiting children's exposure to the promotion of unhealthy foods and beverages has been increasingly recognised as a target for childhood obesity prevention policy. In 2010, the World Health Organization released a set of recommendations on the marketing of these products to children, which aim to guide countries in developing new and/or strengthening existing policies in this area (World Health Organization, 2010). Specifically, these recommendations establish that the aim of such policies should be to reduce the impact of marketing of unhealthy foods and beverages on children, whereby 'impact' refers to the extent of children's exposure to this marketing and the persuasive power of promotions. Governments were identified as the key stakeholders in the development of food marketing policy, including policy implementation, monitoring and evaluation (World Health Organization, 2010).

In contrast, most policy development in this area has been undertaken by the food and advertising industries, through the development of self-regulatory approaches (Hawkes, 2007). These codes of practice typically claim to ensure 'socially responsible marketing' of foods and beverages, rather than to explicitly reduce children's exposure to this marketing (Yale Rudd Center for Food Policy and Obesity, 2013). This is an important distinction, as policy evaluations use different measures and make different conclusions depending on policy objectives. For example, the Australian food retail industry code stipulates that food advertisements must provide healthy lifestyle messages (Australian Food and Grocery Council, 2009). Indicators of policy implementation success could therefore relate to the presence of messages related to physical activity or balanced diets in unhealthy food advertisements, rather than assessing changes to children's exposure to unhealthy food promotions. Independent studies that have assessed changes to children's marketing exposure following the introduction of industry codes of practice have identified that these policies have had no impact on children's exposure to unhealthy food advertising on television, including studies from Australia (King *et al.*, 2010; Hebden *et al.*, 2011), Canada (Kent *et al.*, 2012), and the USA (Kunkel *et al.*, 2009).

There are notable instances where national and provincial governments have taken a strong stance against unhealthy food marketing to children and introduced statutory regulation to limit children's exposure, including in Norway, South Korea, the UK, and in Quebec, Canada. Evaluations of these regulations have demonstrated positive changes in the food marketing environment for children. For example, the South Korean government introduced the *Special Act on Safety Management of Children's Dietary Life* in 2010, which restricts advertisements for unhealthy 'children's foods' from being advertised on television between 17:00 and 19:00 daily and during children's programs broadcast outside of these times (Korean Ministry of Food and Drug Safety; Kim *et al.*, 2013). Subsequently, gross ratings points (GRPs) for unhealthy food advertisements, which represent the size of the audience exposed to an advertisement within a given time period, have decreased by 82% during restricted broadcast times and by 50% at other times since the introduction of the regulations (Kim *et al.*, 2013).

In the UK, the government introduced a ban on the scheduling of advertisements for foods and beverages high in fat, sugar and/or salt during programs with a disproportionately high child audience (when the viewing audience over represents the population distribution of children by at least 20%). Following the full implementation of this regulation in 2009, young children were estimated to see 52% fewer unhealthy food advertisements compared to 2004, and were exposed to 84% fewer food advertisements featuring licensed characters, 56% fewer advertisements with branded characters and 41% fewer advertisements with promotions (Office of Communication, 2010).

22.4   Food marketing effects on food consumption and nutrition and weight outcomes

22.4.1   *Children as a vulnerable audience*

Information from psychological research indicates that children are highly vulnerable to marketing. Younger children are thought to consider commercial information to be mostly true and unbiased (Wackman DB and Wartella E, 1977), and do not recognise the *selling* intent of marketing (to promote a product based on its features and qualities) until at least seven or eight years (Kunkel *et al.*, 2004). It is not until later still that children recognise the *persuasive* intent of marketing that advertisers use appealing and compelling techniques to increase interest in a product (Carter *et al.*,

2011). Even adolescents, however, are thought to be more vulnerable to marketing effects than adults, due to the neurological changes that occur during this development period and their relative inexperience in processing and navigating commercial messages (Pechmann *et al.*, 2005). At this time, adolescents are susceptible to social pressures and peer influences (Pechmann *et al.*, 2005), which are exploited by the marketing industry, such as through peer-to-peer marketing on social networking websites. Brands are also symbolised in marketing communications targeting adolescents to represent desired image attributes, such as 'coolness' and sexuality (Pechmann *et al.*, 2005).

22.4.2   Challenges for researchers in determining the impact of marketing on children

Due to the pervasive nature of food marketing in most societies, research to identify a causal association between food marketing exposure and nutrition and weight outcomes, such as could be elucidated through randomised controlled trials, is difficult. This is because most children are exposed to large volumes of promotions, thereby impeding the identification of a control group for comparison. The considerable extent of this 'baseline' marketing exposure also means that any experimental trials that variably expose children to episodes of marketing, with the intent to determine the effect of this exposure on food behaviours, are swamped by previous exposures. Therefore, exposures to test advertisements are diminutive compared to children's lifetime exposures to marketing, and responses to test advertisements are likely to be smaller than would be the case with cumulative exposure over time.

22.4.3   Schema of effects of food marketing exposures

Despite these considerable difficulties in undertaking research to define the effects of food marketing on children, there is available evidence to indicate the logical sequence of marketing effects: where promotions impact on children's brand awareness and recall, brand preference, brand purchase, consumption patterns, and consequently nutrition and weight outcomes (see Table 22.1). Research can test associations between marketing exposures and outcomes along this hierarchy of effects, with proximate outcomes of exposure, including changes to brand recall and attitudes, being simpler to test and confirm than distal effects on nutrition status and body weight. This sequence is influenced by the extent of exposures, with repetition of exposure serving to reinforce commercial messages and strengthen the sequence of attitudes and behaviours. The delivery of messages through multiple media also ensures repeated and continued exposure, and consolidates brand awareness. Preferences for products can then be actualised, particularly where there is exposure to point-of-purchase prompts, such as outdoor advertising near shops and promotions at the point-of-sale or on food packages.

Table 22.1 **Schema of cumulative effects of integrated cross-media marketing**

Marketing exposure	Unconscious awareness/ immediate brand recall	Awareness/ prolonged brand recall	Brand preferences	Intent to try/ purchase request	Purchase
Initial exposure (e.g. TV)					
Repeated exposures (e.g. TV)					
Persuasive elements (cartoons)					
Additional exposures through other media (e.g. sport sponsorship, Internet)					
Outdoor ads near shops					
Point of purchase/ packaging promotions					
Peer influences					

The following sections describe methods that have been used to assess the impact of food marketing exposures along this hierarchy of effects, and provide a summary of findings from available research.

22.4.3.1 Food marketing and brand awareness and recall

The first step in the logic chain linking children's food marketing exposure to nutrition and weight outcomes relates to the effect of exposure on awareness of promoted brands and marketing campaigns. Recall of brands and campaigns can be assessed either directly, by questioning children about marketing campaigns that they have seen; or indirectly, using association tasks to match brands to food types or related attributes. These types of studies have identified that children have high recall of food promotions, including being able to associate brand logos with food types (Arredondo *et al.*, 2009; Ueda *et al.*, 2012), and matching brands to sponsored sporting events and teams (Pettigrew *et al.*, 2013). In general, brand awareness is related to the amount of advertising that a child is exposed to and increases with age (Fan and Li, 2010).

22.4.3.2 Food marketing and food preferences

The development of brand awareness subsequently influences food preferences by increasing children's familiarity with brands and reducing food neophobia, or the trial of new foods (Dias and Agante, 2011), and through the normalisation of these products. The effect of food marketing on brand preferences can be identified in studies that ask children about perceived attributes or qualities of promoted products or of perceived consumers of products. For example, children can be asked to rate brands along dimensions such as 'fun-boring' or 'exciting-unexciting'. Desire for promoted products can also be demonstrated in experimental trials which measure reported preference for a food product after short-term episodic exposure to a food promotion, as compared to children who are not exposed to the food promotion. Such experimental trials have found that children who are exposed to unhealthy food promotions, that may be embedded in online games or television programs, are more likely to subsequently report preferring related unhealthy foods than children who are exposed to healthy food or non-food promotions (Dias and Agante, 2011; Redondo, 2012).

Further, there is a growing body of evidence to indicate that children prefer food products that are associated with promotional characters, such as when these are shown on their packaging. In these studies, children are often presented with foods with or without a branded character on the packaging and asked to rate their preference for these foods. The presence of characters has been shown to significantly increase children's liking of the foods (Roberto *et al.*, 2010; Lapierre *et al.*, 2011).

22.4.3.3 Food marketing and food purchases and requests

A range of methods have been used to assess the impact of food marketing on product purchases. One outstanding study compared household expenditure data for fast food between French- and English-speaking households in Quebec, Canada and between English-speaking households in Ontario (Dhar and Baylis, 2011). A ban has been in place on advertising to children in Quebec since 1980, although this only applies to channels originating from this province. Channels that are broadcast into Quebec from neighbouring provinces and countries are English-language channels. This study found that French-speaking households with children in Quebec were significantly less likely to purchase fast food compared to similar households in Ontario. Comparatively, there were no differences in purchases of fast food between English-speaking households in these two provinces. Therefore, fast food purchases were lower for households with children in Quebec, who were not exposed to other sources of television advertising. This study design overcomes limitations of controlled, laboratory-based experiments, which may not represent real-world behaviours.

Other studies have surveyed parents about the extent that children request advertised food products; and observed parent and child interactions within supermarkets to identify the frequency that parents accede to these requests. Most parents generally agree that food advertising leads children to pester them for food products (Ogba and Johnson, 2010; Yu, 2012), and parents agree to buy up to half of all products requested by children when grocery shopping (Atkin, 1978).

22.4.3.4 Food marketing and food consumption

Most studies in this domain have included experimental trials to assess the impact of exposure to unhealthy food promotions (versus non-food or healthy food promotions) on immediate changes to food consumption, either while watching television with embedded advertisements or immediately afterwards. Factors that may influence the amount of food consumed by children, other than exposure to the food promotions, include children's pre-test hunger, preference for the test food, time of day of the testing and importantly, prior accumulated exposure to advertising.

One early innovative study that sought to overcome limitations of the short-term nature of many experimental trials was conducted at a two-week summer camp, whereby children were exposed to controlled advertising and snack choices (Goris *et al.*, 2010). In this study, children who were exposure to almost five minutes per day of television advertisements for confectionery chose significantly less fruit as a snack over the two weeks compared to children who saw advertisements for fruit, public service announcements to limit sugar intake, or no advertisements.

Other studies have used correlational techniques to determine cross-sectional associations between children's exposure to television advertisements for fast food and sugary drinks and their consumption of these products. In one US study, dietary intake and anthropometric data from a national cohort of children was compared to industry data on children's exposure to television advertisements over three years (Andreyeva *et al.*, 2011). Higher intakes of soft drink and fast food were observed with increased exposure to advertisements for these products: for every additional 100 soft drink advertisements viewed over three years, consumption of soft drinks increased by 9.4%; and for the same magnitude of increase in exposure to fast food advertisements, consumption of fast food increased by 1.1%. Advertisements for these product types also had a corresponding effect on the consumption of other unhealthy foods and drinks not shown in these advertisements. This suggests that advertisements for unhealthy food/drinks may have dualistic effects on increasing consumption of other unhealthy products.

Responses to food marketing may differ between children of different weight status. In an experimental trial from the USA, overweight children were found to consume 40 kcal more when food was presented in branded packages compared to when this was presented in unbranded packages (Forman *et al.*, 2009). Conversely, non-overweight children consumed 45 kcal less in the branded condition. Similarly, in a UK study, obese children were found to consume 471 kcal more from snack foods after they were exposed to unhealthy food advertisements, compared to when they were exposed to non-food advertisements within a two week period (Halford *et al.*, 2008). This compared with an increase of 306 kcal in the overweight and 250 kcal in the normal-weight children.

22.4.3.5 Food marketing and nutrition and weight outcomes

The final component of the hierarchy of effects of food marketing is the impact of marketing exposures on nutrition and weight outcomes. Few longitudinal studies are available that follow children over time to determine the impact of higher and lower marketing exposures on nutrition and weight outcomes prospectively. As discussed in section 22.4.2, such studies are difficult as there is little variation in marketing exposures between children within the same culture, with most children exposed to large volumes of food promotions. However, some studies have compared differences in exposure to commercial television and compared this to weight status over a five year period (Zimmerman and Bell, 2010). Based on parent report of television viewing, each hour of commercial television that younger children (aged <7 years) watched per day in 1997 was associated with a 0.1 increase in BMI z-scores in 2002. There was no association between children's exposure to non-commercial television and weight status at follow up, indicating that in-program advertisements were contributing to weight outcomes rather than the act of watching television itself.

Mathematical modelling studies have sought to determine the magnitude of obesity that can be attributed to exposure to unhealthy food marketing. One such study compared data from a US national dietary survey to children's television viewing habits (Veerman *et al.*, 2009). In this study, an increase in television food advertising exposure by 25 minutes per week was estimated to cause a child to consume one additional snack per week (1.4% energy increase). The researchers estimated that a 4.5% reduction in energy intake would occur if television food advertising exposure reduced from 80.5 min/week to nothing. However, the estimation of marketing effects on energy intake was based on just one study conducted in 1983.

A later study made estimates of advertising impact on energy intake based on expert opinion rather than measured data. The study used an estimate of energy intake attributable to television food advertising exposure, derived from experts in a Delphi survey, and applied this estimate to obesity prevalence data from multiple countries with higher and lower advertising exposures (Goris *et al.*, 2010). The contribution of television food advertising exposure to energy intake was highest in countries with the greatest obesity prevalence and the highest rates of advertising, for which 40% of obese children were predicted to have not been obese in the absence of food advertising exposure (Goris *et al.*, 2010).

22.5 Future trends

It is acknowledged that patterns of food marketing across different media are changing, largely through the advent of new media, such as social media, that provide unique opportunities to engage consumers. The traditional mode of television viewing is being superseded (by younger generations at least) with new methods of viewing content, and importantly of skipping blocks of advertisements. This poses new challenges for monitoring exposure to this marketing and for regulating marketing practices, whilst providing opportunities for highly personalised and seductive messages to vulnerable children and adolescents.

The World Health Organization's recommendations and implementation actions have arguably raised the profile and awareness of this problem, particularly amongst emerging economies, and have the potential to provide sound guidance for governments to take action. Research is also accumulating, both in documenting the extent of food marketing across different countries, so as to guide policy responses, and in refining our understanding of the effects of this marketing.

Nevertheless, internationally the negative impacts of food marketing on children's nutrition and health is likely to continue into the foreseeable future. Fundamental change is required to transform cultural norms, whereby the promotion of 'junk' food to children is no longer seen as acceptable. Such change will require widespread population awareness of the issue, political impetus for action and a food industry that is committed to being socially responsible.

There has been no overall abatement in the extent or persuasive nature of food advertising (with some notable exceptions). This is largely the case because industry self-regulatory approaches have become the major policy response, despite the accumulating evidence that industry policies have been designed to minimise any changes to marketing practices and have had minimal impact on reducing children's exposure to unhealthy food marketing. The development of these self-regulatory approaches has, however, allowed industry to claim that it is committed to responsible marketing to children and stalled any government intervention in many countries.

22.6   Sources of further information and advice

This chapter provides a structured overview of research related to the extent of food marketing to children, the types of effects that marketing has on children's nutrition and health, and some indications of the effectiveness of policy responses. The chapter also indicates some of the methodological approaches and issues related to generating evidence in this area. The reference list provides a good starting point for readers interested in exploring some of these issues further. For future developments in this field readers could refer to the following sources:

- World Health Organization, 2013. Publications related to marketing of food and non-alcoholic beverages to children. Available at: http://www.who.int/dietphysicalactivity/publications/marketing/en/index.html
- Rudd Center for Food Policy and Obesity, 2013. Pledges on food marketing to children Worldwide. Available at: http://www.yaleruddcenter.org/marketingpledges/
- Rudd Center for Food Policy and Obesity, 2013. Food marketing to youth. Available at: http://yaleruddcenter.org/what_we_do.aspx?id=4
- International Association for the Study of Obesity (IASO). Marketing to children. Available at: http://www.iaso.org/policy/marketing-children/

References

Adams A, Hennessy-Priest K, Ingimarsdóttir S, Sheeshka J, Østbye T and White, M (2009). Changes in food advertisements during 'prime-time' television from 1991 to 2006 in the UK and Canada. *British Journal of Nutrition*, 102, 584–93.

Andreyeva T, Kelly IR. and Harris JL (2011). Exposure to food advertising on television: associations with children's fast food and soft drink consumption and obesity. *Economics & Human Biology*, 9, 221–33.

Arredondo E, Castaneda D, Elder J, Slymen D and Dozier D (2009). Brand name logo recognition of fast food and healthy food among children. *Journal of Community Health*, 34, 73–8.

Atkin CK (1978). Observation of parent–child interaction in supermarket decision-making. *Journal of Marketing*, 42, 41–5.

Australian Food and Grocery Council (2009). *The Responsible Children's Marketing Initiative* [Online]. Available: http://www.afgc.org.au/industry-codes/advertising-kids.html [Accessed 14 June 2013].

Boyland EJ, Harrold JA, Kirkham TC and Halford JC (2011). The extent of food advertising to children on UK television in 2008. *Int J Pediatr Obes*, 6, 455–461.

Boyland EJ, Harrold JA, Kirkham, TC and Halford, JCG. (2012). Persuasive techniques used in television advertisements to market foods to UK children. *Appetite*, 58, 658–64.

Cairns G, Angus K and Hastings G (2009). The extent nature and effects of food promotion to children: a review of the evidence to December 2008. Prepared for the World Health Organization. United Kingdom: Institute for Social Marketing, University of Stirling

Cairns G, Angus K, Hastings G and Caraher M (2013). Systematic reviews of the evidence on the nature, extent and effects of food marketing to children. A retrospective summary. *Appetite*, 62, 209–15.

Carter OBJ, Patterson LJ, Donovan RJ, Ewing MT and Roberts CM (2011). Children's understanding of the selling versus persuasive intent of junk food advertising: implications for regulation. *Social Science & Medicine*, 72, 962–8.

Dalmeny K, Hanna E and Lobstein T (2003). Broadcasting bad health: why food advertising needs to be controlled. International Association of Consumer Food Organisations.

Dhar T and Baylis K (2011). Fast-food consumption and the ban on advertising targeting children: the Quebec experience. *Journal of Marketing Research*, 48, 799–813.

Dias M and Agante L (2011). Can advergames boost children's healthier eating habits? A comparison between healthy and non-healthy food. *Journal of Consumer Behaviour*, 10, 152–60.

Escelante de Cruz A (2004). The junk food generation. A multi-country survey of the influence of television advertisements on children *Consumers International*

Fan Y and Li Y (2010). Children's buying behaviour in China. *Marketing Intelligence & Planning*, 28, 170–87.

Forman J, Halford JCG, Summe H, MacDougall M and Keller KL (2009). Food branding influences ad libitum intake differently in children depending on weight status. Results of a pilot study. *Appetite*, 53, 76–83.

Freeman B and Chapman S (2007). Is 'YouTube' telling or selling you something? Tobacco content on the YouTube video-sharing website *Tobacco Control*, 16, 207–10.

Goris JM, Petersen S, Stamatakis E and Veerman JL (2010). Television food advertising and the prevalence of childhood overweight and obesity: a multicountry comparison. *Public Health Nutrition*, 13, 1003–12.

Halford JC, Boyland EJ, Hughes GM, Stacey, L, McKean S and Dovey TM (2008). Beyond-brand effect of television food advertisements on food choice in children: the effects of weight status. *Public Health Nutrition*, 11, 897–904.

Harris JL, Schwartz MB and Brownell KD (2010). Marketing foods to children and adolescents: licensed characters and other promotions on packaged foods in the supermarket. *Public Health Nutr*, 13, 409–17.

Hastings G, McDermott L, Angus K, Stead M and Thomson S (2006). *The Extent, Nature and Effects of Food Promotion to Children: a Review of the Evidence.* Technical Paper prepared for the World Health Organization. *In:* Organization, W. H. (ed.). Geneva

Hastings G, Stead M, McDermott L, Forsyth A, MacKintosh AM, *et al.* (2003). *Review of Research on the Effects of Food Promotion to Children.* Food Standard Agency.

Hawkes C (2007). Regulating and litigating in the public interest: regulating food marketing to young people worldwide: trends and policy drivers. *Am J Public Health*, 97, 1962–73.

Hebden L, King L, Kelly B, Chapman K and Innes-Hughes C (2011). A menagerie of promotional characters: promoting food to children through food packaging. *J Nutr Educ Behav*, 43, 349–55.

Hebden LA, King L, Grunseit A, Kelly B and Chapman K (2011). Advertising of fast food to children on Australian television: the impact of industry self-regulation. *Med J Aust*, 195, 20–4.

Henry AE and Story M (2009). Food and beverage brands that market to children and adolescents on the Internet: a content analysis of branded web sites. *Journal of Nutrition Education and Behavior*, 41, 353–9.

Hillier A, Cole BL, Smith TE, Yancey AK, Williams JD, Grier SA and McCarthy WJ (2009). Clustering of unhealthy outdoor advertisements around child-serving institutions: a comparison of three cities. *Health Place*, 15, 935–45.

Hoek J and Gendall P (2006). Advertising and obesity: a behavioral perspective. *Journal of Health Communication*, 11, 409–23.

Jones SC, Gregory P and Kervin L (2012). Branded food references in children's magazines: 'advertisements' are the tip of the iceberg. *Pediatr Obes*, 7, 220–9.

Kelly B, Baur LA, Bauman AE, King L, Chapman K and Smith BJ (2011). Food and drink sponsorship of children's sport in Australia: who pays? *Health Promot Int*, 26, 188–95.

Kelly B, Bochynska K, Kornman K and Chapman K (2008a). Internet food marketing on popular children's websites and food product websites in Australia. *Public Health Nutrition*, 11, 1180–7.

Kelly B and Chapman K (2007). The extent and nature of food marketing in children's magazines. *Health Promotion International*, 22, 284–91.

Kelly B, Cretikos M, Rogers K and King L (2008b). The commercial food landscape: outdoor food advertising around primary schools in Australia. *Australian and New Zealand Journal of Public Health* 32, 522–8.

Kelly B, Halford JC, Boyland EJ, Chapman K, Bautista-Castano I, *et al.* (2010). Television food advertising to children: a global perspective. *Am J Public Health*, 100, 1730–6.

Kent MP, Dubois L and Wanless A (2012). A nutritional comparison of foods and beverages marketed to children in two advertising policy environments. *Obesity*, 20, 1892–37.

Kim S, Lee Y, Yoon J, Chung SJ, Lee SK and Kim H (2013). Restriction of television food advertising in South Korea: impact on advertising of food companies. *Health Promot Int*, 28, 17–25.

King L, Hebden L, Grunseit A, Kelly B, Chapman K and Venugopal K (2010). Industry self regulation of television food advertising: Responsible or responsive? *International Journal of Pediatric Obesity*.

Korean Ministry of Food and Drug Safety. *The Special Act on the Safety Management of Children's Dietary Life* [Online]. Seoul: Food Safety Bureau. Available: http://www.kfda.go.kr/eng/index.do?nMenuCode=66 [Accessed 17 April 2013].

Kunkel D, McKinley C and Wright P (2009). The impact of industry self-regulation on the nutritional quality of foods advertised on television to children. *In:* Now, C. (ed.). University of Arizona.

Kunkel D, Wilcox B, Cantor J, Palmer E, Linn S and Dowrick P (2004). *Report of the APA Taskforce on Advertising to Children*. Section: Psychological issues in the increasing commercialization of childhood. Washington, DC: American Psychological Association.

Lapierre MA, Vaala SE and Linebarger DL (2011). Influence of licensed spokescharacters and health cues on children's ratings of cereal taste. *Archives of Pediatrics & Adolescent Medicine*, 165, 229–34.

Lingas EO, Dorfman L and Bukofzer E (2009). Nutrition content of food and beverage products on Web sites popular with children. *Am J Public Health*, 99 (Suppl 3), S587–92.

Livingstone S (2006). *New Research on Advertising Foods to Children: an Updated Review of the Literature*. Published as Annex 9 to Ofcom Television Advertising of Food and Drink Products to Children consultation. London: Office of Communications (Ofcom).

Maher A, Wilson N, Signal L and Thomson G (2006). Patterns of sports sponsorship by gambling, alcohol and food companies: an Internet survey. *BMC Public Health*, 6, 95.

McGinnis MJ, Gootman JA and Kraak VI (2006). *Food Marketing to Children and Youth: threat or Opportunity?* [Online]. Food and Nutrition Board, Board on Children, Youth and Families, Institute of Medicine of the National Academies. Available: http://books.nap.edu/catalog/11514.html [Accessed 6 January 2012].

Molnar A, Garcia DR, Boninger F and Merrill B (2008). Marketing of foods of minimal nutritional value to children in schools. *Prev Med*, 47, 504–7.

Office of Communication (2010). *HFSS Advertising Restrictions – Final Review* [Online]. London: Ofcom. Available: http://stakeholders.ofcom.org.uk/market-data-research/other/tv-research/hfss-final-review/ [Accessed 18 June 2013].

Ogba I and Johnson R (2010). How packaging affects the product preferences of children and the buyer behaviour of their parents in the food industry. *Young Consumers*, 11, 77–89.

Pechmann C, Levine L, Loughlin S and Leslie F (2005). Impulsive and self-conscious: adolescents' vulnerability to advertising and promotion. *Journal of Public Policy and Marketing*, 24, 202–21.

Pettigrew S, Rosenberg M, Ferguson R, Houghton S and Wood L (2013). Game on: do children absorb sports sponsorship messages? *Public Health Nutrition*, doi:10.1017/S1368980012005435.

Powell LM, Schermbeck RM, Szczypka G, Chaloupka FJ and Braunschweig CL (2011). Trends in the nutritional content of television food advertisements seen by children in the United States: analyses by age, food categories, and companies. *Arch Pediatr Adolesc Med*, 165, 1078–86.

Redondo I (2012). The effectiveness of casual advergames on adolescents' brand attitudes. *European Journal of Marketing*, 46, 1671–88.

Roberto CA, Baik J, Harris JL and Brownell KD (2010). Influence of licensed characters on children's taste and snack preferences. *Pediatrics*, 126, 88–93.

Ueda P, Tong L, Viedma C, Chandy SJ, Marrone G, *et al.* (2012). Food marketing towards children: brand logo recognition, food-related behavior and BMI among 3–13–year-olds in a south Indian town. *PLoS One*, 7, e47000.

Veerman JL, Van Beeck EF, Barendregt JJ and Mackenbach JP (2009). By how much would limiting TV food advertising reduce childhood obesity? *The European Journal of Public Health*, 19, 365–9.

Voorveld HAM, Neijens PC and Smit EG (2011). Opening the black box: understanding cross-media effects. *Journal of Marketing Communications*, 17, 69–85.

Wackman DB and Wartella E (1977). A review of cognitive development theory and research and the implication for research on children's responses to television. *Communications Reserach*, 4, 203–24.

World Health Organization (2003). *Diet, Nutrition and the Prevention of Chronic Diseases.* Geneva: World Health Organization.

World Health Organization (2010). *Set of Recommendations on the Marketing of Foods and Non-alcoholic Beverages to Children.* Geneva: WHO Press.

Yale Rudd Center for Food Policy and Obesity (2013). *Pledges on Food Marketing to Children Worldwide* [Online]. New Haven: Yale Rudd Center Available: http://www.yaleruddcenter. org/marketingpledges/ [Accessed 14 June 2013].

Yu J (2012). Mothers' perceptions of the negative impact on TV food ads on children's food choices. *Appetite*, 59, 372–6.

Zimmerman FJ and Bell JF (2010). Associations of television content type and obesity in children. *American Journal of Public Health*, 100, 334–40.

Front-of-pack and point-of-purchase labelling schemes designed for obesity prevention

M. Rayner
University of Oxford, Oxford, UK

23.1 Introduction

In this chapter I will first provide some definitions of point-of-purchase labelling and front-of-pack food labelling and then describe some different types of food labelling that have been designed to help people make healthier food choices. I will then describe some trends in such labelling. Next I will a propose a simple conceptual framework for the way food labelling might affect health, and then I will go on to provide a brief survey of the evidence for its effects on food purchasing behaviour and health (including obesity). Finally I will describe some trends in national and international policy on food labelling. Some themes of this chapter are that (i) there is inadequate research into the effects of food labelling on health and (ii) food labelling is a hotly contested issue and decisions about it are made principally on the basis of values rather than on logic or evidence.

23.2 Definitions and scope

The terms 'front-of-pack labelling' and 'point-of-purchase labelling' mean different things to different people and so the International Network for Food and Obesity/Non-Communicable Disease Research, Monitoring and Action Support (INFORMAS) has sought to develop an agreed taxonomy for food labelling components and a set of definitions for those different components based, wherever possible, on those of the Codex Alimentarius Commission (Codex) (1). Codex is the body established by the Food and Agriculture Organization of the United Nations and the World Organization, 50 years ago, to set international standards for foods including food labelling.

Codex defines food labelling as: 'Any written, printed or graphic matter that is present on the label, accompanies the food, or is displayed near the food, including that for the purpose of promoting its sale or disposal' (2). All food labelling may therefore be described as 'point-of-purchase'.

Managing and Preventing Obesity. http//dx.doi.org/10.1533/9781782420996.5.325

Food labelling is potentially an important, source of useful information for consumers. It is also a source of marketing claims, by food producers which have the potential to mislead consumers in their food choices by, for example, highlighting the positive attributes of a product while ignoring other, less desirable characteristics.

Food labelling is increasingly found in a variety of different venues including food retail outlets, quick service/fast food and other types of restaurants, school and workplace cafeterias, etc. Increasingly electronic media are used to display food labelling information and claims. The setting sets constraints on the type of food labelling that can be used. There is, for example, less space to present food labelling on menu boards in fast food restaurants than on most food packets.

Food labels have information and/or make claims about foods including their price, taste, methods of production, etc. Some food labelling components are more pertinent to health than others. The components that are most directly relevant to health include dates by which foods should be eaten (for reasons connected with food safety), cooking instructions (for similar reasons), ingredient lists, nutrition information (including nutrient declarations in the form of back-of-pack tables or lists and more interpretive front-of-pack schemes) and claims about the 'healthiness' of the food (nutrition and health claims). But other labelling components may also be indirectly important including labelling about methods of production, etc.

Nutrition information – 'a description intended to inform the consumer of nutritional properties of a food' according to Codex (3) – is the food labelling component most obviously connected with the management of overweight and obesity. Nutrition information is increasingly found front of pack but in other places close to the point of purchase of both packaged and unpackaged foods.

A number of different front-of-pack schemes for nutrition information – called 'supplementary nutrition information' by Codex – have been devised ranging from those which merely reproduce information found in back or side-of-pack nutrient declarations to more interpretative schemes employing a variety of methods to guide the consumer towards more healthier choices. Note these schemes have generally been designed to promote healthier eating in general rather than calorie reduction. INFORMAS, following the US Institute of Medicine (4), subdivides such schemes into 'nutrient specific systems' and 'summary indicator systems'.

Nutrient specific systems – illustrated by the %Guideline Daily Amount (GDA) nutrition information system recommended by the trade association – Food Drink Europe (5) and other similar bodies and the more interpretative traffic-light labelling system recommended by the UK Government (6) – display the level of different nutrients separately. In the case of the traffic-light labelling, three colours are used to indicate the levels of fat, saturated fat, total sugar, or salt. Green indicates a low level, amber medium and red high.

Summary indicator systems – illustrated by the star rating system under consideration by the Australian Government (7) – combine a number of nutrient levels into a single score or classification and then display these in a variety of ways. In the case of the star rating system the levels of energy, saturated fat, total sugar, sodium, protein, fibre and fruit, vegetable and nuts are combined into a score and foods are awarded a number of stars depending on that score: five stars indicating the healthiest products and half a star the least healthy products.

If supplementary nutrition information systems are to go beyond merely reproducing information found in the nutrient declaration then they need nutrient criteria for their use. For example %GDA systems need the GDAs to be specified and whether the percentages are to be given per 100 g or per serving; star rating systems need the thresholds for awarding one, two, three (etc.) stars to be specified. The nutritional criteria, underlying supplementary nutrition information systems, have come to be known as 'nutrient profile models' and the science of 'nutrient profiling' as: 'The science of classifying or ranking foods according to their nutritional composition for reasons related to preventing disease and promoting health' (8).

As well as a proliferation of supplementary nutrition information systems there has, over recent years, been an increase in the use of various symbolic or iconic nutrition and health claims on food packets. These types of front-of-pack labelling are sometimes seen as an alternative to supplementary nutrition information: particularly by the food industry. They too are often underpinned by nutrient profile models.

Nutrition claims are claims about the composition of foods (nutrients and other health-related ingredients either separately or in combination). Worded nutrition claims include claims as 'low in fat' and 'high in fibre'. An example of a symbolic nutrition claim would be the symbol used in the UK (9) to indicate that the food can constitute one of the Government's recommended target of '5-a-day' for fruit and vegetable intake, i.e. a serving of the food contains a portion of fruit or vegetable.

Health claims are claims about the relationship between consumption of the food or a constituent and health. Worded claims range from general claims such 'good for you' to more specific claims as 'good for your heart'. Examples of symbolic health claims include the 'Tick scheme' developed by the Australian Heart Foundation (10), the Nordic Keyhole scheme originally developed by the Swedish National Food Administration (11) and the health logo scheme developed by the Choices International Foundation (12). Such symbolic health claims differ from supplementary nutrition information in that they can only be found on foods with a healthy nutrient profile. Supplementary nutrition information is designed for all foods – both healthy and unhealthy – and is therefore potentially much more useful to consumers. Some examples of supplementary nutrition information, and symbolic health and nutrition claims are shown in Figure 23.1.

The nutrition information to be found in catering outlets is generally more limited than that found on packets, e.g. nutrient-specific information systems are generally concerned with fewer nutrients – sometimes just calories. There are a few instances where summary indicator systems or symbolic health claims have been used by caterers.

23.3   Current status of front-of-pack and point-of-purchase labelling schemes

Current international and national policy on supplementary nutrition information (and on symbolic nutrition and health claims) is in flux with little consensus as to which forms are most useful to consumers. Government, non-governmental consumer and

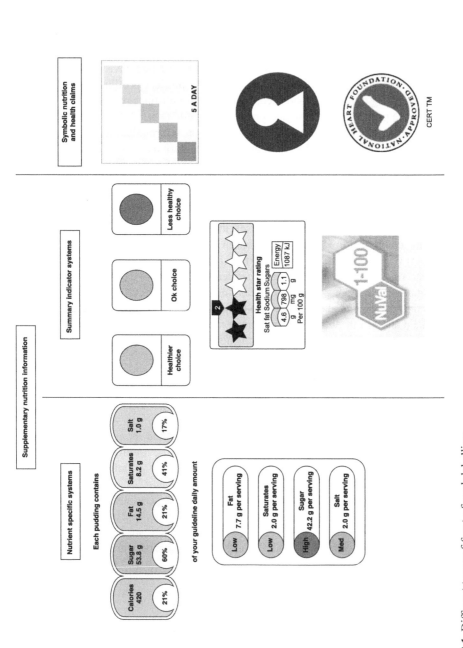

Figure 23.1 Different types of front-of-pack labelling.

Nutrient specific systems: top: %GDA system; bottom: traffic–light labelling of nutrients.

Summary indicator systems: top: traffic-light labelling of foods; middle: Australian star rating system; bottom: US NuVal system.

Symbolic nutrition and health claims: top: UK Government 5-a-day logo; middle: Nordic Keyhole; bottom: Australian Hearth Foundations Tick logo.

public health organisations and commercial organisations all have different preferred schemes. In general it can be said that consumer and public health organisations favour schemes that are more interpretative than industry bodies do. In addition consumer and public health organisations favour labelling schemes that signal less healthy foods as well as healthier foods.

Codex has yet to produce any guidance on supplementary nutrition information or symbolic nutrition and health claims (13) and there is little international or national legislation which governs their use. An exception is the recent European Union Food Information regulation which sets boundaries on what food producers may provide by way of supplementary nutrition information (14).

A good recent survey of initiatives to promote different forms of supplementary nutrition information is provided by the European Food Information Council (15). However this, and similar surveys of labelling policy, e.g. that of the World Cancer Research Fund (16), tell us more about intent than actuality.

There is little information about the actual prevalence of food labelling components in their various forms. A recent review of food labelling prevalence studies found 23 studies but methods varied considerably making comparisons between the results of surveys difficult (1). Nevertheless some general observations are possible. First, supplementary nutrition information is increasing in its prevalence in many parts of the world – particularly nutrient-specific systems. Secondly, nutrition claims are much more common than health claims. Thirdly, the prevalence of some symbolic nutrition and health claims is also growing in some countries: in particular the Nordic Keyhole symbol and possibly the Choices International symbol. For example the Nordic Keyhole symbol – originally developed in Sweden – has spread to Norway and Denmark. It is claimed that by 2012 there were over a 1500 food products in Danish stores that bear the symbol (17).

Supplementary nutrition information in catering establishments is also on the increase, in particular in the US where some states have passed laws making it compulsory in certain circumstances. The format of this supplementary nutrition information is normally very simple with merely kcal or kJ per serving being declared.

23.4   Impact of front-of-pack and point-of-purchase labelling schemes and interventions involving such schemes

The impact of food labelling on consumer health is highly contentious and there is a lack of good quality research to help resolve various important questions such as which form of supplementary nutrition information is most useful to consumers (18–20).

It is clear that for food labelling to have an impact on health it needs to do so through a complex chain – or more precisely a web of physiological, cognitive and behavioural processes – a simplified version of this web is shown in Figure 23.2. These processes include those that take place in the eye and the neural pathways

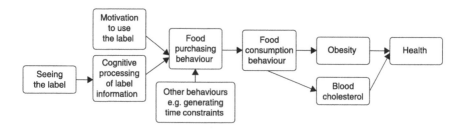

Figure 23.2 A simple conceptual model for the relationship between food labelling and health.

that connect the eye to the visual cortex and other parts of the brain; cognitive functions such as the processing of numerical and verbal information, motivational states in relation to label use, food purchasing behaviour with its many constraints: time, money, etc.; physiological processes resulting from an excess or deficit in energy and/ or particular nutrients and leading to poor or good health.

It is easy to see why food labelling research can quickly get bogged down in confusing detail. More usefully it is generally agreed that consumers say that they use food labels and will use food labelling if asked to do so in laboratory settings but that this does not translate into much actual use in real life. Whether label use leads to healthier food choices is also disputed. It is possible that some types of labelling – such as poorly substantiated health claims – might even lead to behaviour which increases the risk of diet-related diseases (21).

It is also agreed that, compared with other factors influencing food purchasing behaviour (such as familiarity with products or their prices), food labelling is likely to have relatively small effects. This makes detecting and quantifying its effects difficult. It should, however, be remembered that even if the effects on individuals are small, food labelling is so ubiquitous that the effect on a population wide basis could be large.

It is often contended that food labelling information has a bigger effect on food producer behaviour than on consumer behaviour (22). For example, it is anecdotally reported that food producers in the UK reformulated their foods when starting to use traffic-light labelling to reduce the number of red 'lights' on packets and this effect on the food supply has exceeded any effect of the scheme on consumer purchasing decisions.

Studies of the effects of existing food labelling on purchasing behaviour may have only detected small effects but it is also agreed that different, more informative formats for food labelling and increased label use might improve health-related food purchasing behaviour. So various researchers have sought to devise and test the effectiveness of interventions to enhance food label use (23–25). Some of these interventions have included redesigning formats but most have merely have involved seeking to enhance the use of food labelling through educational means. Many of these interventions have been combined with other elements. Such intervention studies have had mixed results. Interventions based on education alone have had the smallest effects (24).

23.5   Future trends in front-of-pack and point-of-purchase labelling schemes

It is difficult predict future developments in food labelling, including research into food labelling. It seems possible that since the 'obesity epidemic' shows few signs of abatement governments might turn to ever more drastic measures to tackle the problem, including measures involving food labelling. Increasingly, governments are exploring (and in some cases introducing) legislation in relation to supplementary nutrition information (16). And indeed quite a few countries round the world are exploring health warnings for unhealthy foods (a particular, if extreme, type of supplementary nutrition information). Thailand, Indonesia, Peru and Chile have all recently passed legislation to require health warnings on certain foods (15). The requirement for such health warnings seem to be based on similar requirements for health warnings for other health-damaging products such as tobacco and alcohol. It remains to be seen whether health warnings are effective.

It is also seems clear that food labelling information is increasingly likely to be conveyed through electronic means as well as on food packaging. Recently, for example, 'apps' have been developed which provide, in effect, supplementary nutrition information via a mobile phone (26).

23.6   Sources of further information and advice

There is an increasing number of reviews covering different aspects of the research into supplementary nutrition information and symbolic health and nutrition claims. Some of these reviews are systematic and therefore to be preferred over unsystematic reviews. Two commonly cited systematic reviews are those by Cowburn and Stockley published in 2005 (18) and a review, with methods based on those of Cowburn and Stockley, by Grunert and Wills published in 2007 (19). Since these reviews are now somewhat out of date a more recent systematic review such as that by Heike and Taylor (20) is useful. A forthcoming Cochrane review – for which the protocol has already been published (27) – may provide interesting reading. A common problem shared by these reviews is a lack of an agreed terminology for different labelling components – a problem that the INFORMAS paper on labelling (1) attempts to address.

References

(1) Rayner, M., Wood, A., Mhurchu, C. N., Swinburn, B., Vandevijvere, S., *et al.* (2013). Monitoring the health-related labelling of foods and non-alcoholic beverages in retail settings. *Obesity Reviews*, 14(S1), 70–81. doi:10.1111/obr.12077

(2) Codex Alimentarius Commission. Codex General Standard for the Labelling of Prepackaged Foods (CODEX STAN 1–1985). 2010. Rome, amended 1991, 1999, 2001, 2003, 2005, 2008 and 2010.

(3) Codex Alimentarius Commission. Guidelines on Nutrition Labelling (CAC/GL 2–1985). 2012. Rome, adopted 1985, revised 1993 and 2011, amended 2003, 2006, 2009, 2010, 2012, annex adopted 2011.

(4) Institute of Medicine Committee on Examination of Front-of-Package Nutrition Rating Systems and Symbols (2011). Phase II, Front-of-Package Nutrition Rating Systems and Symbols. IOM, Washington, D.C.

(5) CIAA (Confederation of the Food and Drink Industries in the EU) GDAs – The Facts. Your Choice. http://gda.fooddrinkeurope.eu/asp2/guideline-daily-amounts.asp (Accessed March 31, 2014).

(6) Department of health (UK) and others. Guide to Creating a Front of Pack (FoP) Nutrition Label for Pre-packed Products Sold Through Retail Outlets. http://multimedia.food.gov. uk/multimedia/pdfs/pdf-ni/fop-guidance.pdf. (Accessed March 31, 2014).

(7) Choice (Australia) Health Star Rating Comparison of Popular Food Products Finds Few Stars.   http://www.choice.com.au/media-and-news/consumer-news/news/is-this-what-krafty-companies-dont-want%20you-to-know.aspx. (Accessed March 31, 2014).

(8) World Health Organization. Guiding Principles and Framework Manual for the Development or Adaptation of Nutrient Profile Models. WHO, Geneva, in press.

(9) Department of Health (UK). *5 a Day Logo and Portion Indicator*. http://webarchive. nationalarchives.gov.uk/+/www.dh.gov.uk/en/Publichealth/Healthimprovement/ FiveADay/FiveADaygeneralinformation/DH_4001493 (Accessed March 31, 2014).

(10) Heart Foundation (Australia). *Heart Foundation Tick*. http://www.heartfoundation.org. au/healthy-eating/heart-foundation-tick/Pages/default.aspx (Accessed March 31, 2014).

(11) The National Food Agency (Sweden). *The Keyhole Symbol*. http://www.slv.se/en-gb/ Group1/Food-labelling/Keyhole-symbol/ (Accessed March 31, 2014).

(12) The Choices Programme. *Making the Choice the Easy Choice*. http://www.choices-programme.org/ (Accessed March 31, 2014).

(13) World Health Organization (WHO) *Joint FAO/WHO Workshop on Front-of-Pack Nutrition Labelling*. http://www.who.int/nutrition/events/2013_FAO_WHO_workshop_ frontofpack_nutritionlabelling/en (Accessed March 31, 2014).

(14) Regulation (EU) No 1169/2011 of the European Parliament and of the Council of 25 October 2011 on the provision of food information to consumers, amending Regulations (EC) No 1924/2006 and (EC) No 1925/2006 of the European Parliament and of the Council.

(15) European Food Information Council (2014) *Global Update on Nutrition Labelling*, EUFIC, Brussels.

(16) World Cancer Research Fund International. *WCRF International Food Policy Framework for Healthy Diets: NOURISHING*. http://www.wcrf.org/policy_public_affairs/nourish-ing_framework/ (Accessed March 31, 2014).

(17) Norden. *The Nordic Keyhole – Healthy Choices made Easy*. http://www.noeglehullet. dk/NR/rdonlyres/11A129E1–E6E4–4D41–9024–23F4F929DAA8/0/Island_SE_NO_ DK010612.pdf (Accessed March 31, 2014).

(18) Cowburn G and Stockley L (2005) Consumer understanding and use of nutrition labelling: a systematic review. *Public Health Nutrition* 8(1): 21–8.

(19) Grunert KG and Wills JM (2007) A review of European research on consumer response to nutrition information on food labels. *J Public Health* 15: 385–399 Doi 10.1007/ s10389–007–0101–9

(20) Hieke D and Taylor CR (2012) A critical review of the literature on nutritional labeling. *Journal of Consumer Affairs*, 46: 20–156. doi: 10.1111/j.1745–6606.2011.01219.x

(21) Chandon P and Wansink B (2007). The biasing health halos of fast-food restaurant health claims: lower calorie estimates and higher side-dish consumption intention. *J Consumer Res* 34(3): 301–314.

(22) Sacks G, Rayner M and Swinburn B (2009). Impact of front-of-pack 'traffic-light' nutrition labelling on consumer food purchases in the UK. *Health Prom Int* 24(4): 344–352.

(23) Jay M, Adams J, Herring SJ, Gillespie C, Ark T, *et al.* (2009). A randomized trial of a brief multimedia intervention to improve comprehension of food labels. *Prev Med.* 48(1): 25–31.

(24) Vijaykumar S, Lwin MO, Chao J and Au C (2013). Determinants of food label use among supermarket shoppers: a Singaporean perspective. *J Nutr Educ Behav* 45(3): 204–212.

(25) Thorndike AN, Riis J, Sonnenberg LM and Levy DE (2014). Traffic-light labels and choice architecture: promoting healthy food choices. *Amer J Prev Med* 46(2): 143–149.

(26) Bupa. *Foodswitch*. https://www.bupa.com.au/foodswitch (Accessed March 31, 2014).

(27) Crockett RA, Hollands GJ, Jebb SA and Marteau TM (2011) *Nutritional Labelling for Promoting Healthier Food Purchasing and Consumption*, Cochrane Collaboration, published online.

Index

Lightning Source UK Ltd.
Milton Keynes UK
UKOW06n0946110315

247683UK00012B/221/P